Modern Acupuncture

Learn From the Master

Volume 1

By

Dr. Chandrashekhar Pardeshi
MBBS DGO MD

Table of Contents

Section II - Acupuncture Therapy   95

Advantages, Anatomy, Nerve Supply, Master Points, Motor
Sensory Points, Internal Organs, Technique, Electro-Acupuncture,
Press-Needles/ Tacks/ Pellets/ Seeds, Bloodletting, Side Effects,
Precautions, Contraindications, Indications.

Foreword

With great pleasure and deep respect, I endorse Modern Acupuncture: Learn from the Master, authored by Dr. Chandrashekhar Pardeshi. With his distinguished background in obstetrics and gynecology, as well as his decades-long dedication to acupuncture, Dr. Pardeshi brings a rare and valuable perspective to this field.

This book culminates years of meticulous clinical practice, thoughtful reflection, and scientific inquiry. Dr. Pardeshi has distilled his vast experience into a comprehensive guide that captures the principles, techniques, and modern applications of acupuncture in a way that is both accessible and profound.

Whether you are an experienced acupuncturist seeking to enhance your practice or a student just beginning your journey, this book will be an essential companion. It offers practical techniques, clinical wisdom, and a rational approach that defines effective and compassionate care.

Dr. Pardeshi's journey—from a leading consultant in obstetrics and gynecology to a full-time acupuncturist—speaks volumes about his conviction in the therapeutic potential of acupuncture. Every chapter of this work reflects his transformative encounter with this healing art and his unwavering commitment to integrating it with modern medical thinking.

I wholeheartedly recommend Modern Acupuncture: Learn from the Master to all practitioners who wish to deepen their knowledge and elevate their clinical skills. This book is more than a reference—it is a legacy of insight, dedication, and healing. May it guide and inspire you, as it has inspired many others.

Warm regards,

Dr. Rumi Beramji
President, Maharashtra Acupuncture Council
Senior Acupuncturist, Beramji Hospital

Preface

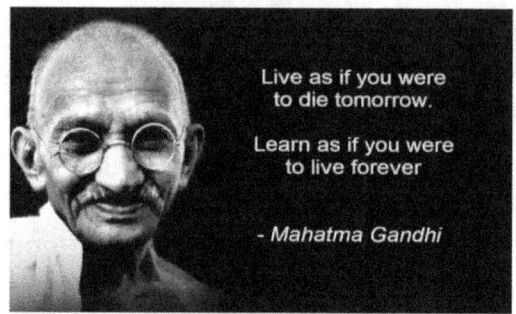

Live as if you were
to die tomorrow.

Learn as if you were
to live forever

- Mahatma Gandhi

Welcome to Modern Acupuncture – Learn from the Master, a gateway to a transformative journey through the intricate and inspiring world of acupuncture. This book is not merely a compilation of techniques; it is a deeply personal exploration of an ancient healing art, shaped by clinical experience and a lifelong pursuit of integrative knowledge.

My journey into acupuncture began with a search for relief from a chronic shoulder injury. As a practicing obstetrician and gynecologist immersed in Western medicine, I had little exposure to traditional healing methods. Yet, a single acupuncture treatment brought me unexpected and lasting relief. This experience forever changed my perception of healing and ignited a passion to understand the science behind this remarkable therapy.

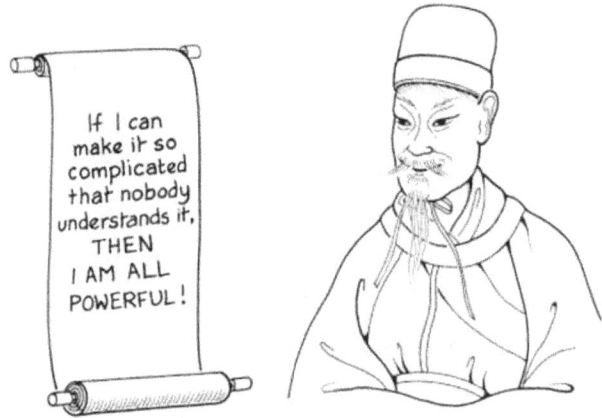

If I can make it so complicated that nobody understands it, THEN I AM ALL POWERFUL!

Acupuncture is Made Unnecessarily Complicated

Source - Felix Mann

Motivated by curiosity and conviction, I delved into over a hundred foundational texts, absorbing the philosophies of Eastern medicine while grounding my learning in the rigors of Western science. My quest took me beyond books to the Republic of China, where I engaged directly with skilled practitioners, gaining practical insights that bridged the gap between theory and application.

My tenure as Vice President of the Maharashtra Acupuncture Council allowed me to contribute to advancing acupuncture education. In that role, I developed training programs that equipped future practitioners with a strong, science-based foundation in this sophisticated discipline.

This book culminates two decades of exploration, reflection, and hands-on clinical experience. It was born out of a desire to make acupuncture more accessible, logical, and practical for both learners and professionals. I have witnessed newcomers and seasoned clinicians struggle with the abstract complexity surrounding acupuncture education. This inspired me to create a guide that is practical, clinically relevant, and grounded in scientific clarity, without losing the essence of traditional wisdom.

Modern Acupuncture – Learn from the Master presents a redefined approach to acupuncture, integrating the art's classical roots with a contemporary, neurophysiological framework. I hope this book empowers you to understand acupuncture as a treatment modality and a profound healing tool.

May these pages enrich your practice, deepen your insight, and inspire a new appreciation for the elegance and power of acupuncture in today's medical landscape.

With unwavering dedication,

Dr. Chandrashekhar Pardeshi, MBBS, DGO, MD
Obstetrician, Gynecologist, and Acupuncturist
Former Vice President, Maharashtra Acupuncture Council (India)

Acknowledgments

The creation of 'Modern Acupuncture, *Learn From the Master'* has been an enriching journey, made possible by the support, encouragement, and contributions of many individuals to whom I owe my sincere gratitude.

First and foremost, I would like to express my heartfelt thanks to my wife, Dr. Rajni Pardeshi, a fellow acupuncturist, whose unwavering support and understanding have created the space and stability I needed to dedicate myself fully to this work over the past two years.

I am profoundly grateful to the esteemed members of the medical community who generously shared their time, insights, and critical feedback, helping refine and strengthen this book:

- Dr. Rumi Beramji (MBBS) – President, Maharashtra Acupuncture Council
- Dr. Ravindra Shivde (MBBS, MD)
- Dr. Mohan Sali (MBBS, MD)
- Dr. Hiralal Samanta (MBBS, DCH)

Special thanks also go to Aarti Pardeshi and my student Venkateshwara, whose contributions enriched the content and presentation of this work.

I am indebted to the authors whose published works have been sources of inspiration and reference. Their contributions are acknowledged in the reference section and have significantly shaped the academic and practical foundation of this book. I also appreciate the creators of the online resources cited in this document.

Lastly, I invite all readers to join in this ongoing journey. I welcome your feedback if you discover any errors or have suggestions for improvement. As a token of appreciation, I would be delighted to offer you a complimentary copy of my next eBook.

With sincere gratitude,

Dr. Chandrashekhar Pardeshi, MBBS, DGO, MD
Acupuncturist, Obstetrician, and Gynecologist
Nashik, India

Introduction

Welcome to Modern Acupuncture – Learn From the Master, a structured and insightful journey into acupuncture. This two-volume work bridges traditional healing with modern medical science, offering a clear and practical guide for learners at all levels.

Volume 1: Building a Strong Foundation

This volume lays the scientific groundwork essential for effective acupuncture practice. Through a focused study of anatomy and physiology, you'll develop a deep understanding of how acupuncture influences body systems, including the nervous, musculoskeletal, endocrine, immune, digestive, respiratory, and reproductive systems.

Key areas include:

- Acupuncture points and meridians
- Scientific mechanisms of acupuncture
- Classical and modern needling techniques
- Safety and clinical effectiveness

You'll also be introduced to various systems such as:

- Traditional Chinese Medicine (TCM)
- Tung's Acupuncture
- Scalp, Abdominal, and Auricular Acupuncture
- Myofascial Trigger Points
- Bloodletting methods

A Practical Resource for All Practitioners

Whether you are beginning your acupuncture journey or refining years of practice, this book offers clinical clarity, practical insights, and integrative wisdom. It aims to empower you with tools and understanding to apply acupuncture safely and effectively in modern healthcare.

Let this volume guide you in integrating ancient wisdom with scientific reasoning as you explore acupuncture as an art and a healing science.

With dedication,
Dr. Chandrashekhar Pardeshi, MBBS, DGO, MD

Section I - Human Body

Anatomy and Physiology

1.1 An Introduction to Anatomy

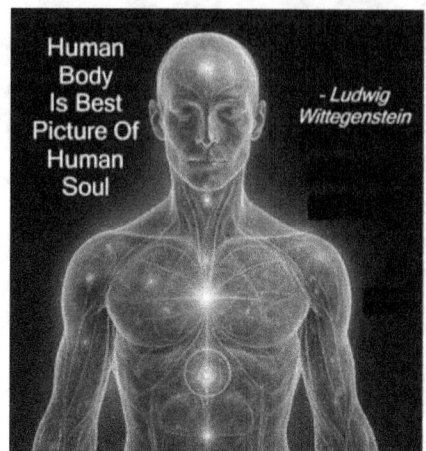

Anatomy forms the cornerstone of acupuncture practice. It offers a detailed understanding of the human body's structure, examining the size, shape, position, and interrelationships of organs, tissues, and cells. This foundational knowledge empowers acupuncturists to navigate the body's landscape with precision, confidence, and safety.

Exploring the Body's Blueprint

Anatomy is traditionally divided into two primary domains:

- **Macroscopic (Gross) Anatomy**: Focuses on structures visible to the naked eye, such as bones, muscles, and organs.
- **Microscopic Anatomy**: Involves the use of microscopes to study tissues and cells, revealing their composition, organization, and function.

Why Anatomy Matters in Acupuncture

A solid grasp of anatomy provides several critical advantages in clinical acupuncture:

- **Accurate Point Location**: Anatomical landmarks guide practitioners in precisely locating acupuncture points.
- **Safe and Effective Practice**: Understanding the positioning of nerves, vessels, and organs minimizes risk and enhances treatment outcomes.
- **Rational Clinical Decisions**: Insight into the anatomical basis of disease supports better diagnostic and therapeutic planning.

Embryology and Neurology: The Deeper Connections

Acupuncture's theoretical framework often draws from embryological development and neural pathway mapping. Understanding how tissues and nerves originate and interact deepens the practitioner's ability to apply treatment purposefully and effectively. For example, the nerve supply of the forearm and abdomen has a common foetal developmental nerve root supply. Therefore, abdominal conditions can be treated by needling the forearm and vice versa.

DNA and RNA

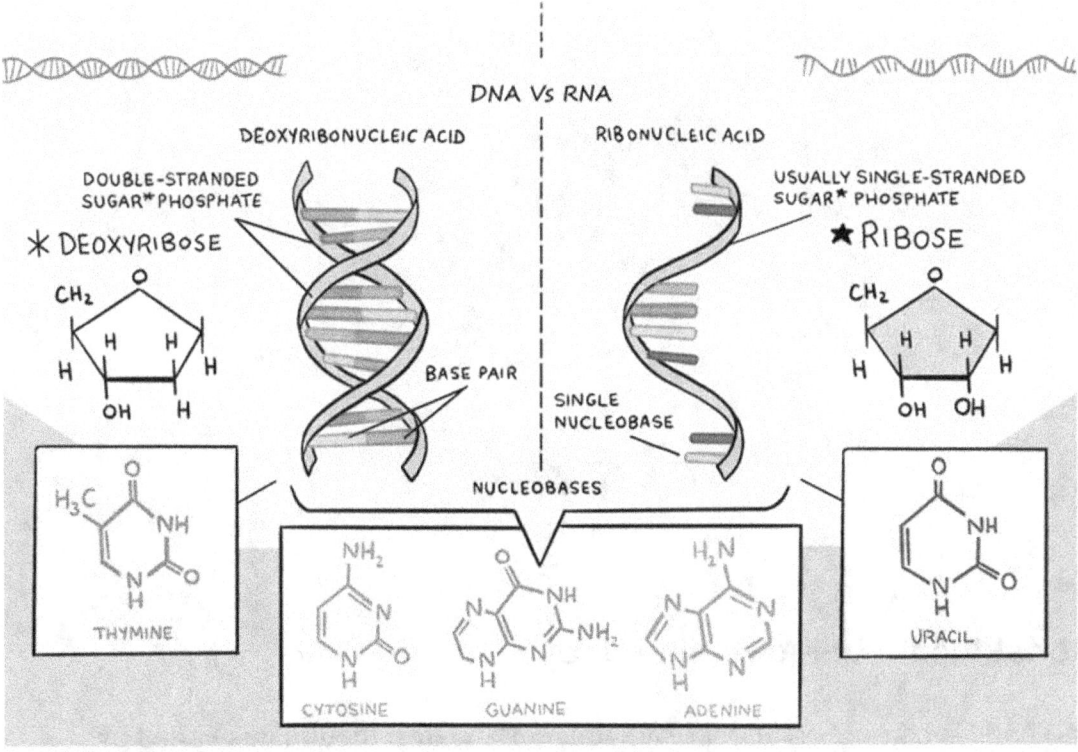

Fig. 1.1.1 RNA and DNA

- **DNA (Deoxyribonucleic Acid)** governs the nucleus's genetic expression and cellular function.
- **RNA (Ribonucleic Acid)**: Acts as a messenger, copying and translating DNA instructions into proteins vital for cell function.

Interestingly, not all cells contain DNA; mature red blood cells expel their nucleus during development.

Cells

Cells are the fundamental building blocks of life. Trillions exist in the human body, each performing unique roles. However, not all body components are composed of cells. The

extracellular matrix, composed of proteins like collagen and surrounding fluid, provides structural support.

Additionally, the body harbours trillions of non-human cells, including the gut and skin microbiota. Up to 2 kg of body weight may consist of these microorganisms in an average 70 kg human.

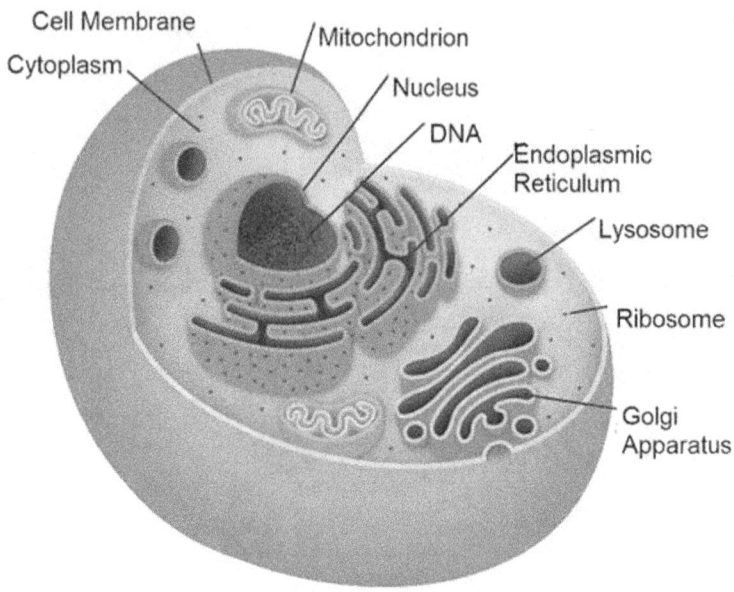

Fig. 1.1.2 Cell

Basic Constituents of the Human Body

The human body is composed of approximately **60% water**, though this varies by tissue:

- Lungs: 85%
- Kidneys & Muscles: 79%
- Heart & Brain: 73%
- Skin: 63%
- Bone: 31%

Elemental composition includes:

- **Oxygen (65%)**, **Carbon (18%)**, **Hydrogen (10%)**, **Nitrogen (3%)**, and trace elements.
  These elements form **molecules**, which build cells, the fundamental units of all tissues.

Tissues

A **tissue** is a group of specialized cells performing a shared function. The body has four primary types:

1. **Epithelial tissue** – forms body coverings and linings
2. **Connective tissue** – supports and binds other tissues
3. **Muscle tissue** enables movement
4. **Nervous tissue** – transmits electrical signals

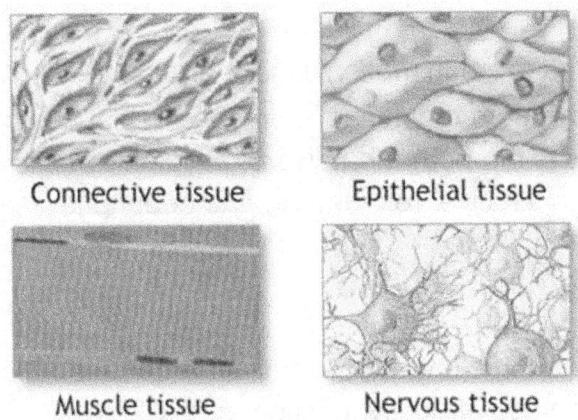

Connective tissue   Epithelial tissue

Muscle tissue   Nervous tissue

Fig. 1.1.3 Types of Tissue

Epithelial vs. Endothelial Cells:
Epithelial cells cover internal and external surfaces, while endothelial cells, a specialized subtype, line the **circulatory system**.

Organs

An **organ** is a structured assembly of tissues designed to perform specific functions, such as the heart, lungs, or liver. Most organs are housed within **body cavities**:

- **Thoracic cavity** – lungs and pleura
- **Abdominal cavity** – stomach, intestines, liver, etc.
- **Cranial cavity** – brain
- **Pelvic cavity** – reproductive and urinary organs

Although external, the skin is the body's largest organ and serves as its first line of defence.

-Dr. Pardeshi Acupuncture-

1.2   Introduction to Physiology

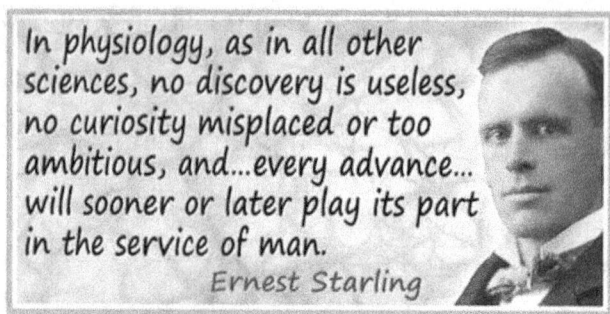

In physiology, as in all other sciences, no discovery is useless, no curiosity misplaced or too ambitious, and...every advance... will sooner or later play its part in the service of man.
Ernest Starling

Physiology is the science of life in motion. Unlike anatomy, which focuses on static structures, physiology explores the dynamic processes that sustain and regulate the human body. If anatomy is the body's hardware, physiology is its software, coordinating every function that keeps us alive, responsive, and adaptable.

Levels of Physiological Function

Physiology operates at multiple levels of biological organization, each contributing uniquely to the understanding of bodily function:

- **Cellular Physiology**: Examines the essential processes that maintain cellular viability and activity, including transport, metabolism, and communication.
- **Organ Physiology**: This field focuses on the functional roles of individual organs, such as the heart, lungs, liver, or kidneys, and how they contribute to homeostasis.
- **Systems Physiology**: Integrates the activities of multiple organs into coherent systems, such as the nervous, endocrine, and circulatory systems, that work together to sustain life.
- **Pathophysiology**: Examines how normal physiological processes are disrupted in disease, providing critical insights for diagnosis and therapeutic interventions.

Core Functions of Human Physiology

The body performs a broad spectrum of interdependent and finely regulated functions. These include:

- **Homeostasis**: The regulation of a stable internal environment, such as pH, temperature, and electrolyte balance, despite external variability.
- **Respiration**: The uptake of oxygen and expulsion of carbon dioxide, essential for cellular energy production.

- **Circulation**: The movement of blood to distribute nutrients, gases, hormones, and to remove metabolic waste.
- **Digestion and Absorption**: Food's mechanical and enzymatic breakdown into absorbable nutrients, fuelling cellular activity.

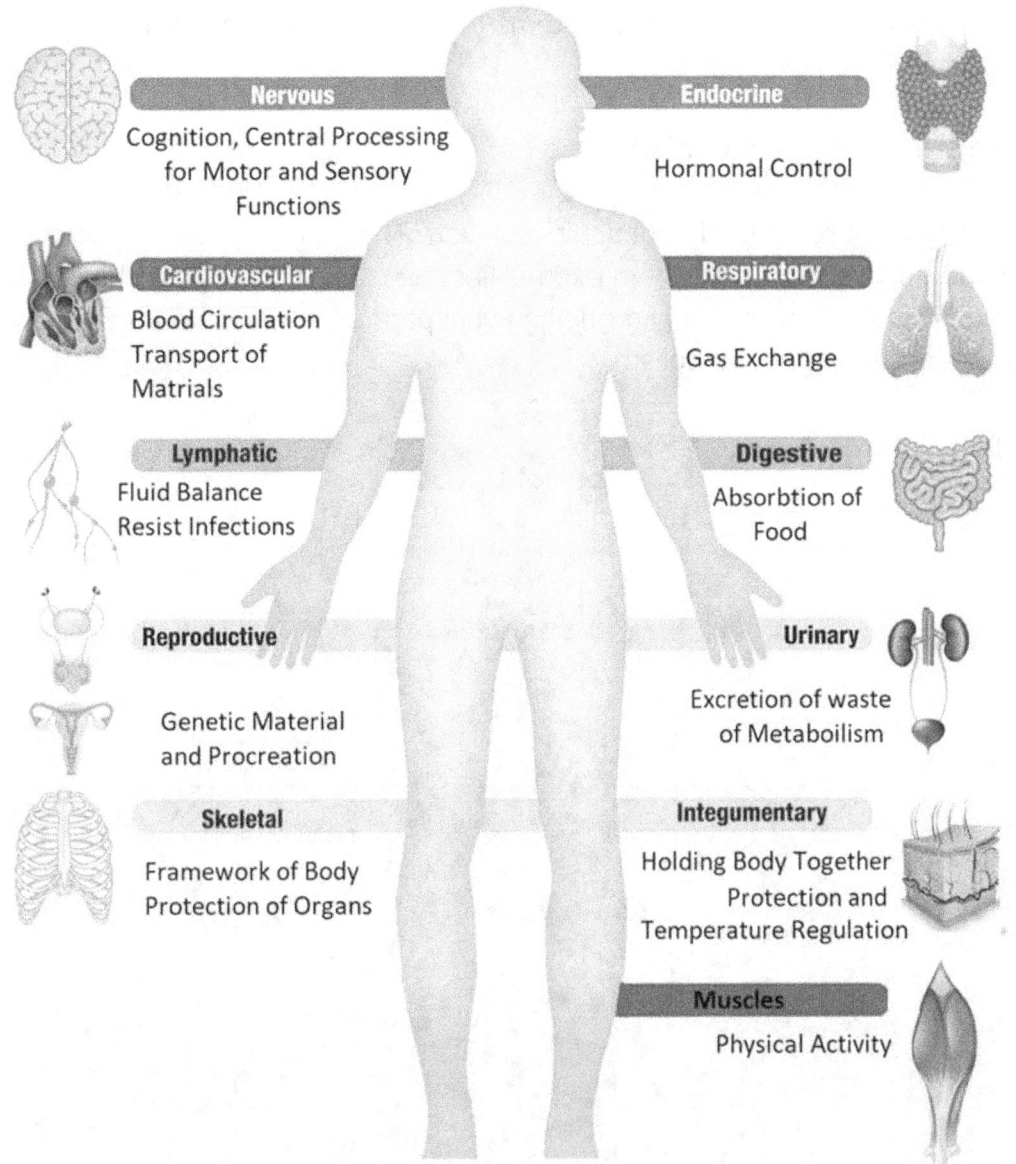

Nervous
Cognition, Central Processing for Motor and Sensory Functions

Endocrine
Hormonal Control

Cardiovascular
Blood Circulation Transport of Matrials

Respiratory
Gas Exchange

Lymphatic
Fluid Balance Resist Infections

Digestive
Absorbtion of Food

Reproductive
Genetic Material and Procreation

Urinary
Excretion of waste of Metaboilism

Skeletal
Framework of Body Protection of Organs

Integumentary
Holding Body Together Protection and Temperature Regulation

Muscles
Physical Activity

Fig.1.2 Physiological System

- **Excretion**: The removal of metabolic waste through organs such as the kidneys, lungs, and skin, preventing toxic buildup.
- **Movement**: Voluntary and involuntary muscle actions enabling locomotion, posture, and internal organ function.

- **Sensory Perception**: The reception and processing of external stimuli via specialized organs, allowing interaction with the environment.
- **Hormonal Regulation**: The control of physiological activities through hormones, which act as chemical messengers coordinating growth, metabolism, and reproduction.
- **Reproduction**: The biological systems that enable procreation and the perpetuation of the species.

The Symphony of Integration

These physiological systems do not act in isolation. They are intricately interwoven. For example, the neuroendocrine system exemplifies the close collaboration between the nervous and endocrine systems in regulating vital parameters, such as blood pressure, temperature, and energy metabolism.

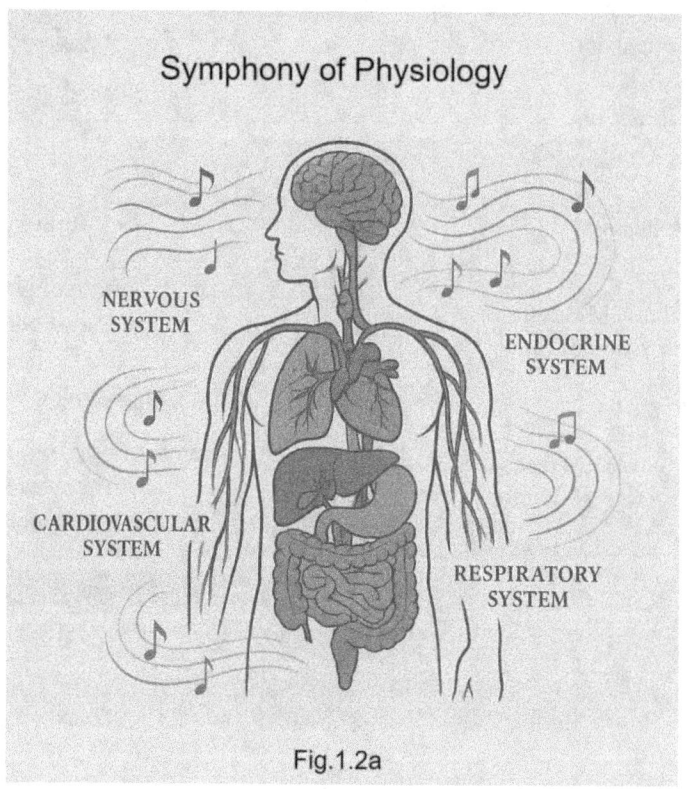

Fig.1.2a

Physiology provides a scientific foundation for understanding the mechanisms of acupuncture. By integrating knowledge of nerve pathways, hormone systems, circulation, and immune responses, modern acupuncture moves beyond tradition to offer a holistic, evidence-informed approach to healing.

-Dr. Pardeshi Acupuncture-

1.3   Nervous System

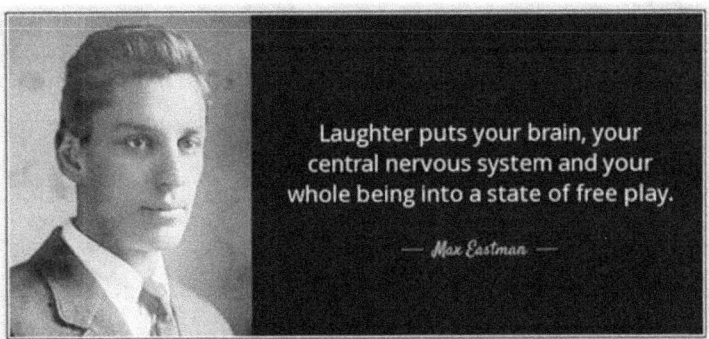

Laughter puts your brain, your central nervous system and your whole being into a state of free play.

— Max Eastman —

The nervous system is the body's sophisticated communication and control network, integral to the action of acupuncture. It collects, interprets, and responds to sensory information, enabling regulation of movement, perception, cognition, and emotion. The brain functions as the central command center, while nerves branching from the brain and spinal cord transmit signals throughout the body. Acupuncture is believed to exert its therapeutic effects by modulating this intricate network through targeted stimulation of specific points.

Divisions of the Nervous System

The nervous system is anatomically and functionally divided into the central nervous system (CNS) and the peripheral nervous system (PNS):

- **Central Nervous System (CNS)**: This system comprises the brain and spinal cord, analogous to a computer's CPU. It processes sensory data, initiates motor responses, and governs cognition, memory, and emotion.
- **Peripheral Nervous System (PNS)**: Consists of all neural structures outside the CNS, including cranial nerves, spinal nerves, and ganglia, much like the cables and connectors of a communication system. It transmits information to and from the CNS.

Functionally, the PNS is subdivided into:

- **Somatic Nervous System (SNS)** – responsible for voluntary movements and sensory processing.
- **Autonomic Nervous System (ANS)** – governs involuntary functions such as heart rate, digestion, and glandular activity.

Understanding these divisions is essential for acupuncturists, as acupuncture often modulates autonomic and somatosensory pathways to produce therapeutic effects.

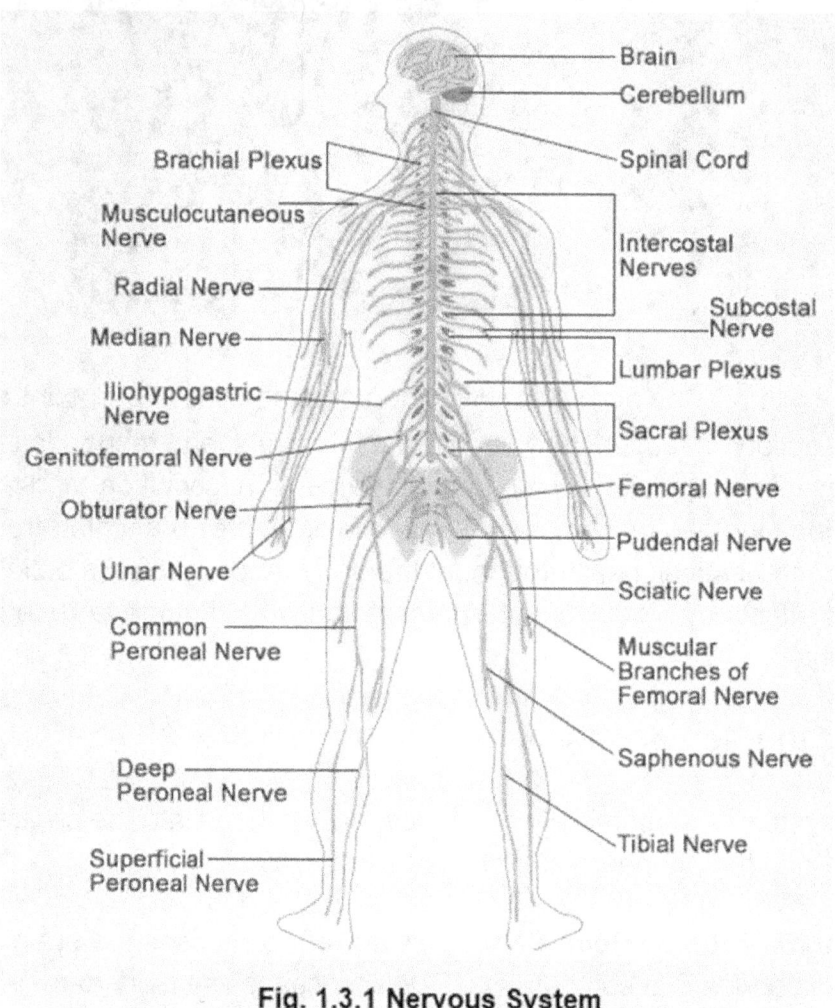

Fig. 1.3.1 Nervous System

Cellular Components of the Nervous System

Nervous tissue is primarily composed of two types of cells:

- **Neurons**: The functional units of communication. They transmit electrical impulses and are responsible for sensory perception, integration, and response.
- **Glial Cells**: Provide structural and metabolic support to neurons, maintain homeostasis, and participate in signal modulation.

The nervous system is organized into grey matter (rich in neuronal cell bodies and dendrites) and white matter (comprised mainly of axons with myelin sheaths). This structural distinction is vital for understanding signal transmission pathways.

Functions of the Central Nervous System

The CNS performs three primary functions:

1. **Sensory Function**
   Detects changes in the internal and external environment. Sensory stimuli include:
   - External: Taste (chemical), smell (chemical), touch (mechanical), vision (light), and hearing (sound).
   - Internal: Organ stretch, pain, and proprioception.
2. **Integration Function**
   Processes incoming sensory information by comparing it with past experiences and current internal states, enabling coordinated, context-specific responses.
3. **Motor and Reflex Function**
   Initiates voluntary or involuntary responses. The somatic system governs voluntary actions (e.g., moving a limb), while the autonomic system mediates involuntary responses (e.g., pupil constriction, sweating).

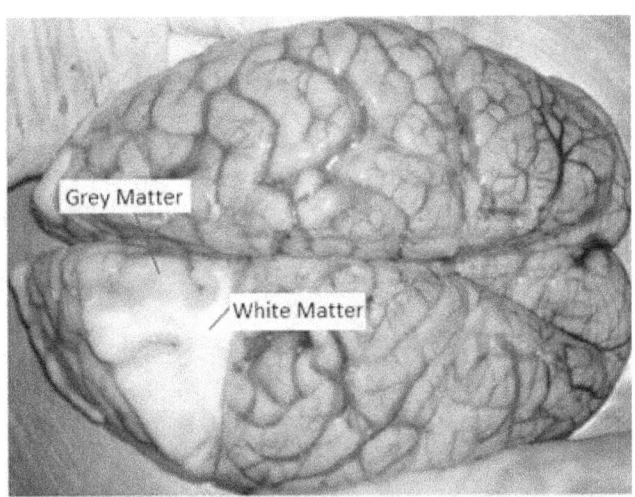

Fig. 1.3.2 Brain - Grey and White Matter

Peripheral Nervous System: Somatic and Autonomic Divisions

1. Somatic Nervous System (SNS)

This system includes spinal and cranial nerves, motor and sensory fibres, and associated ganglia. It controls:

- Voluntary motor actions: Skeletal muscle movement.
- Conscious sensory input: Touch, proprioception, and pain.

- Reflex arcs: Involuntary yet protective responses.

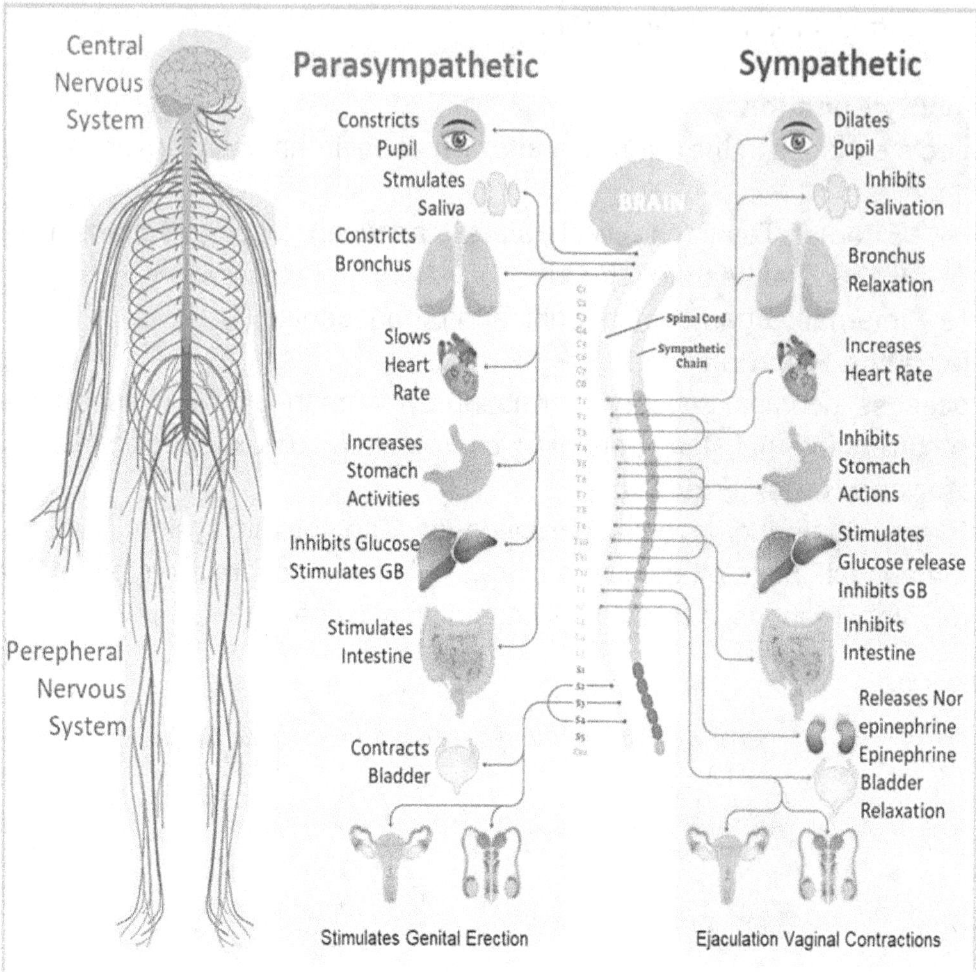

Fig. 1.3.3 Functions of Nervous System

2. Autonomic Nervous System (ANS) Fig. 1.3.3

The ANS regulates involuntary physiological processes and is divided into:

- **Sympathetic Nervous System**:
  Prepares the body for 'fight or flight.' It:
  - Increases heart rate and respiratory rate
  - Dilates pupils and airways
  - Mobilizes energy stores
  - Inhibits digestion and urination
- **Parasympathetic Nervous System**:
  Maintains and restores homeostasis during restful states ('rest and digest'). It:
  - Slows the heart rate

- o Stimulates digestion and waste elimination
- o Supports tissue repair and energy conservation

Many organs are dually innervated, with sympathetic and parasympathetic inputs modulating their activity in response to physiological demands.

Relevance to Acupuncture

Acupuncture is now increasingly understood to influence the **nervous system** through central and peripheral mechanisms. Stimulation of acupoints can:

Modulate neurotransmitter and neurohormone release, activate afferent nerve fibres, influence spinal segmental circuits and brain centres, restore autonomic balance

Modern research suggests that acupuncture-induced changes in neurochemical signalling play a crucial role in its therapeutic effects, particularly in modulating pain, regulating homeostasis, and influencing the immune response.

-Dr. Pardeshi Acupuncture-

1.4 Spine

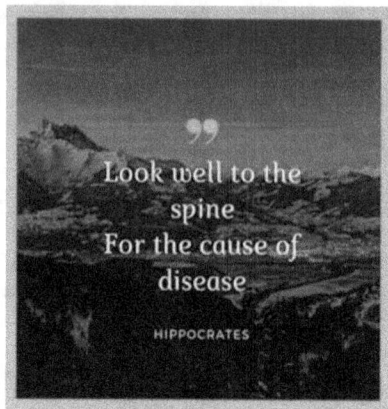

The spine, or vertebral column, is the central structural axis of the human body. It is composed of 24 individual vertebrae arranged in a vertical stack. Each vertebra is separated by an intervertebral disc, a gel-filled cushion that acts as a shock absorber, preventing friction during movement. Strong vertebral ligaments stabilize this structure, while tendons and muscles facilitate movement. The small joints between vertebrae, known as facet joints, allow controlled flexibility of the spine.

Functions of the Spine

The spine serves several vital roles:

- **Structural support** for the head and torso
- **Postural stability** for upright movement
- **Mobility and flexibility** for bending and twisting
- **Protection** of the spinal cord and spinal nerves
- **Transmission of nerve signals** to and from the brain and peripheral organs

These combined functions make the spine a biomechanical and neurophysiological marvel, central to acupuncture's action on neural pathways.

Anatomical Regions of the Spine

The spine is divided into five major regions, each with characteristic curvature and function:

- **Cervical Spine (C1–C7)**
  - 7 vertebrae
  - Anterior (lordotic) curvature

- o Supports the head and allows rotation, flexion, and extension
- **Thoracic Spine (T1–T12)**
  - o 12 vertebrae
  - o Posterior (kyphotic) curvature
  - o Anchors the rib cage and protects thoracic organs

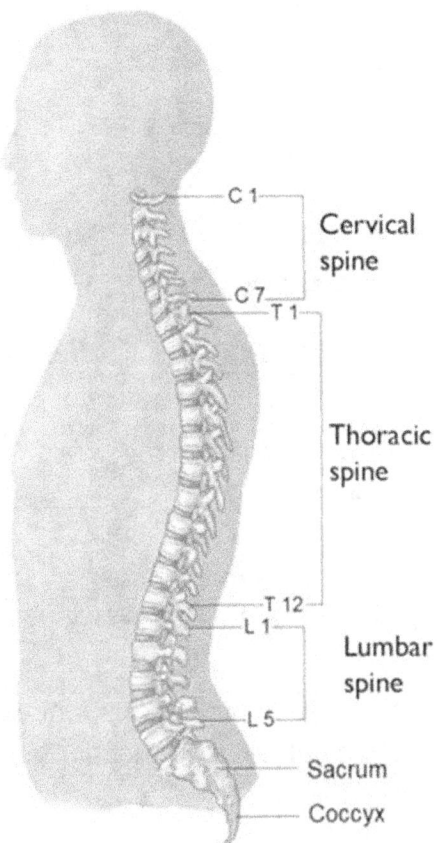

C 1

Cervical spine

C 7
T 1

Thoracic spine

T 12
L 1

Lumbar spine

L 5

Sacrum

Coccyx

Fig. 1.4.1 Curvatures of Spine

- **Lumbar Spine (L1–L5)**
  - o 5 vertebrae
  - o Anterior curvature
  - o Bears the most body weight and absorbs stress from lifting and walking
- **Sacrum**
  - o 5 fused vertebrae
  - o Connects to the pelvis and distributes spinal load
- **Coccyx (Tailbone)**
  - o 4 fused vertebrae
  - o Vestigial structure provides minor support

The natural **'S'-shaped curvature** of the spine enhances its ability to absorb mechanical stress and distribute body weight efficiently.

Structure of a Vertebra:

Each vertebra has a **vertebral body** in front and a **vertebral arch** behind, forming the **vertebral foramen**—a hollow canal for the **spinal cord**. Key structural features include:

- **Spinous Process** – Posterior bony projection; attachment site for muscles

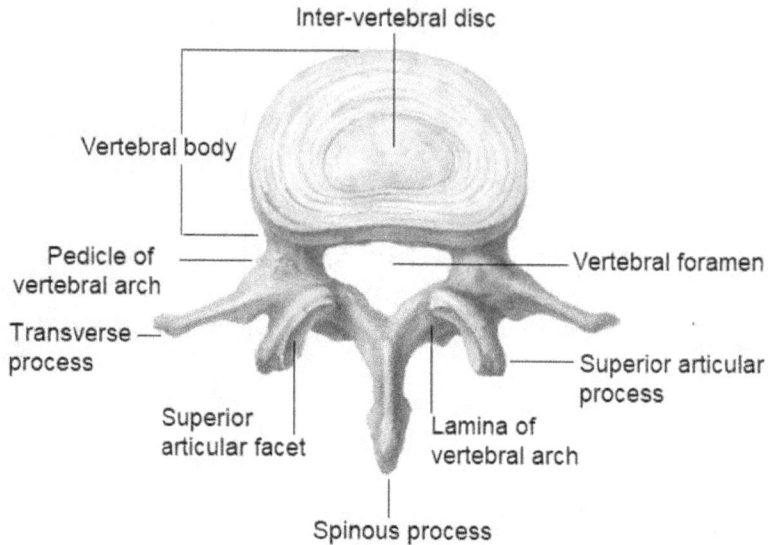

Fig. 1.4.2 Anatomy of a Vertebra

- **Transverse Processes** – Lateral projections; anchor points for spinal muscles
- **Facet Joints** – Paired synovial joints connecting adjacent vertebrae and permitting movement (see Fig. 1.4.2)

Intervertebral Discs

Each disc has two major components:

- **Annulus fibrosus**: Outer fibrous ring providing structural integrity
- **Nucleus pulposus**: Inner gelatinous core rich in water content that acts as a shock absorber

These discs play a significant role in maintaining spinal flexibility and absorb compressive forces during movement.

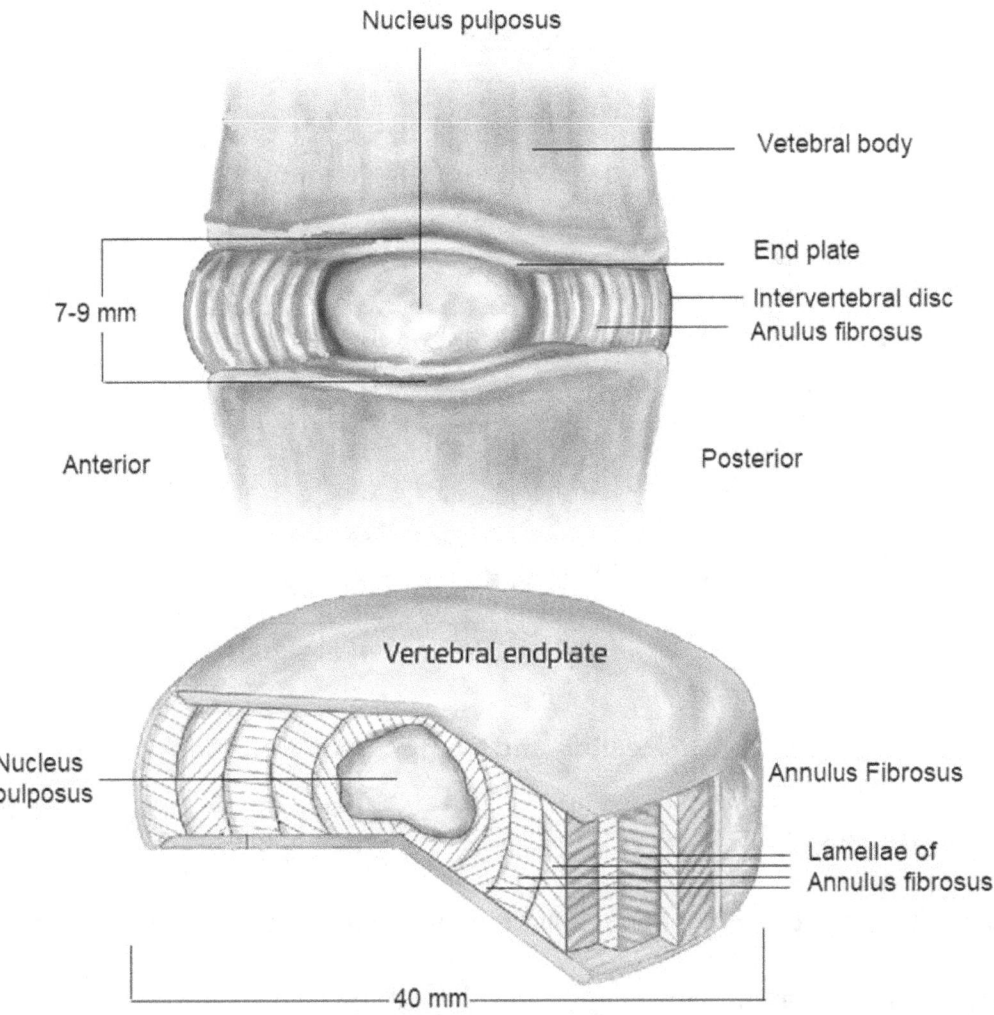

Fig. 1.4.3 Intervertebral Disc

Paraspinal Muscles

The paraspinal muscles, located on both sides of the spine, control spinal movement, posture, and balance. Though small and often overlooked, these muscles play a significant role in segmental stability. Injury or chronic stress can cause them to go into **protective spasm**, sometimes mimicking or exacerbating actual spinal pathology.

Neural Foramina and Nerve Exit

Between adjacent vertebrae lies the **neural foramen**, through which **spinal nerve roots** exit the spinal canal on both sides (see Fig. 1.4.4). These nerve roots transmit signals between the **spinal cord** and **peripheral tissues**, and can become compressed due to disc herniation or bony changes, resulting in pain, weakness, or sensory deficits.

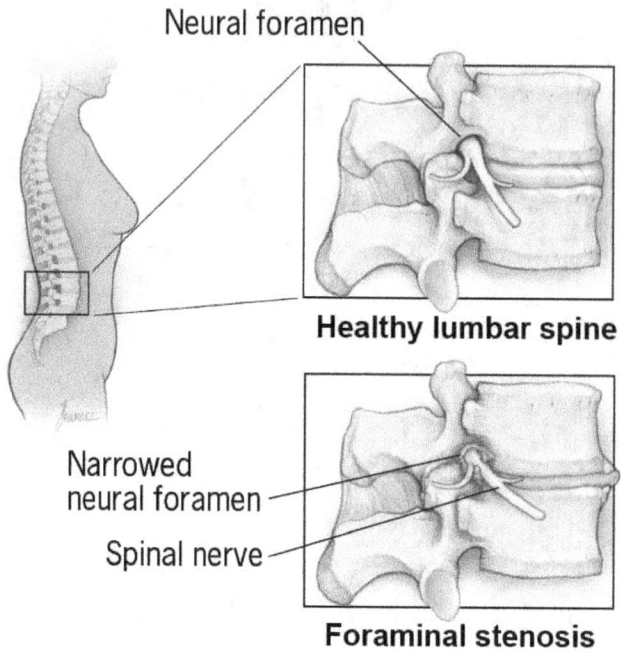

Neural foramen

Healthy lumbar spine

Narrowed
neural foramen

Spinal nerve

Foraminal stenosis

Fig. 1.4.3a Healthy and Compressed Foramen

Spinal Segments

Each **spinal segment** is a functional unit of the spine and includes:

1. Two adjacent vertebrae
2. An intervertebral disc
3. Two facet joints
4. A pair of neural foramina

This repeated structure enables uniform function and serves as a blueprint for understanding **segmental pathology** and **selecting acupuncture points**. Imaging studies like MRI often localize degenerative changes or nerve compression at specific segments.

Spinal Cord and Nerve Roots

The **spinal cord** is the primary conduit for signal transmission between the brain and the **peripheral organs**. It begins at the **brainstem** and descends through the spinal canal, terminating around the **L1–L2 vertebral level**, where it continues as a bundle of nerves called the **cauda equina**.

Each spinal cord region gives rise to paired **nerve roots**, which innervate specific body regions. The **Hua Tuo Jiaji acupuncture points**, located 0.5 cun lateral to the midline on the back, correspond closely to the exit zones of these nerve roots and provide access for segmental neuromodulation.

Sacral nerve roots, emerging from the **sacral foramina**, innervate pelvic organs and are frequently targeted in acupuncture for reproductive, urinary, and bowel disorders.

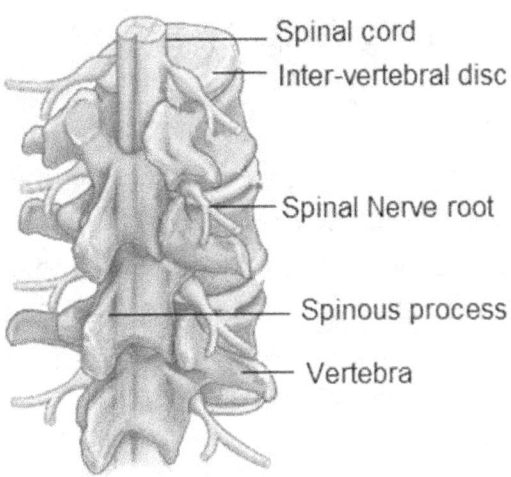

Fig. 1.4.4 Spine

Clinical Relevance to Acupuncture

The spine is a central anatomical and functional structure in acupuncture. It is a reference for locating key points on the Governing Vessel (Du Mai) and Urinary Bladder meridians. It is closely associated with the spinal cord, nerve roots, autonomic ganglia, and musculoskeletal tissues. Acupuncture along the spine has a dual influence on both segmental and systemic health.

Segmental innervation and dermatomes

Each spinal segment corresponds to a specific dermatome and myotome, as reflected in the sensory and motor functions associated with it. Acupuncture applied to paraspinal points can influence the organs and tissues innervated by that segment, making spinal points powerful tools for treating visceral disorders, referred pain, and neurological conditions.

-Dr. Pardeshi Acupuncture-

1.5 Sensory Organs

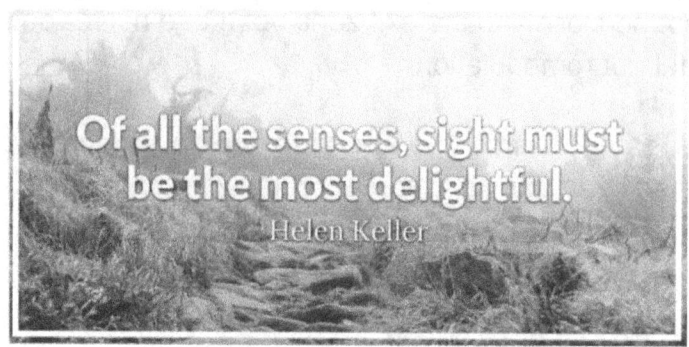

Of all the senses, sight must be the most delightful.
Helen Keller

The sensory system comprises specialized organs and neural pathways that detect and process environmental stimuli. These systems enable the perception of external and internal cues, forming the basis for cognition, behaviour, and motor responses. Sensory input is collected by specific receptors within sense organs and converted into electrical signals through a process known as transduction. These signals are then relayed to the central nervous system for interpretation. All sensory functions serve to inform, protect, or regulate physiological responses.

A. General Sense Organs

General senses include sensations such as touch, pressure, temperature, pain, and proprioception. These are mediated by widely distributed receptors in the skin, muscles, tendons, joints, and visceral organs.

- **Mechanoreceptors** detect mechanical deformation, such as pressure, stretch, and vibration.
- **Thermoreceptors** respond to temperature changes externally (skin) and internally (viscera).
- **Chemoreceptors** monitor chemical parameters like pH (H^+ ions), CO_2, and O_2 levels, stimulating taste and olfactory senses.
- **Nociceptors** are pain receptors that respond to noxious stimuli resulting from injury or inflammation.

1. Pain Sensation

Pain is a distinct protective sensory modality, separate from other senses. It is both a discriminative experience—allowing localization and intensity evaluation—and an emotional one, often associated with potential or actual tissue damage. Nociceptors detect intense stimuli, such as extreme heat, pressure, or chemical exposure, and relay this information via redundant neural pathways to ensure a rapid protective response. Individuals lacking pain sensation (congenital analgesia) are prone to unrecognized injuries, often leading to early mortality. Notably, the brain itself lacks nociceptors—hence, brain tissue injury does not elicit pain. This suggests that headaches are not caused by pain within the brain parenchyma.

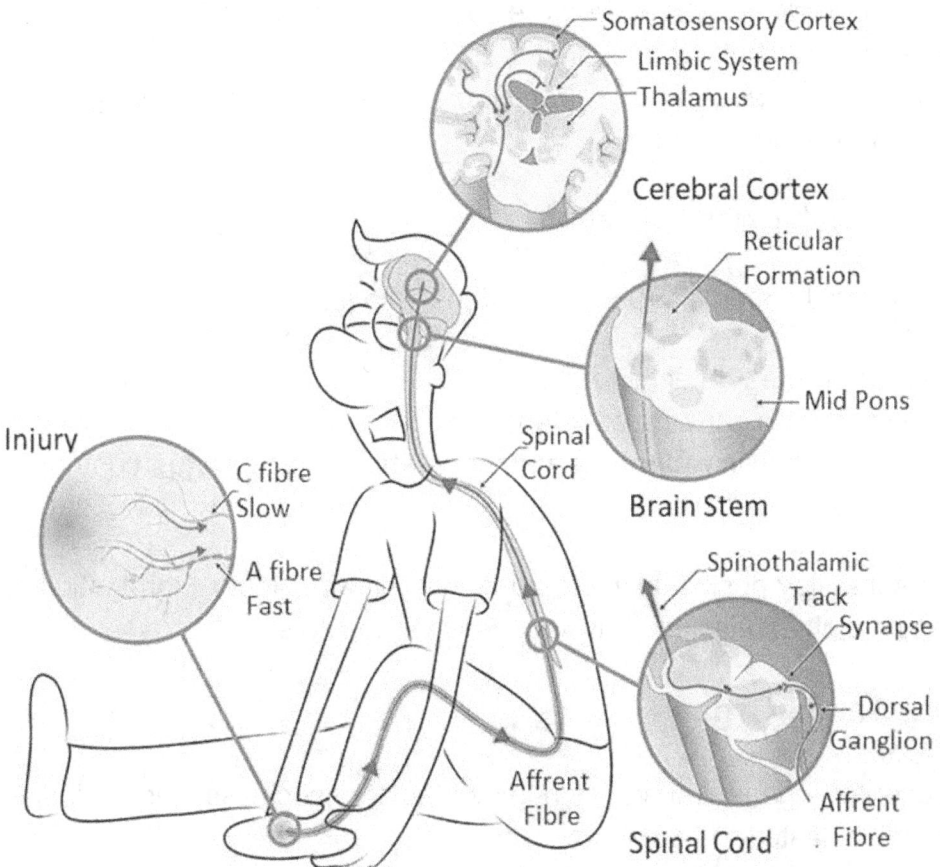

Fig. 1.5.1 Pain Pathway

Acupuncture's primary clinical domain is pain management, making acupuncturists highly specialized in the modulation of nociceptive pain.

2. Temperature Sensation

Thermoreceptors located in the skin detect changes in environmental temperature:

- **Cold receptors** are more numerous and most active around 25°C. They become inactive below 3°C, which explains the numbness associated with frostbite.
- **Heat receptors** respond above 37°C and peak at 45°C. Beyond this, nociceptors are triggered to prevent thermal injury.

The face, particularly the ears and nose, has a high density of thermal receptors, which explains its heightened sensitivity in cold environments.

3. Touch Sensation

- **Light Touch:** Mediated by Meissner's corpuscles (found in fingertips, lips, genitals), Merkel discs (at dermo-epidermal junction), and hair follicle receptors.
- **Pressure and Vibration:** Detected by Pacinian corpuscles (deep dermis), Ruffini endings, and Krause's bulbs. Pacinian corpuscles are particularly sensitive to rapid changes in pressure.

4. Proprioception (Stretch Sensation)

Proprioceptors are located in muscles, tendons, and joints:

- **Muscle spindles** detect stretch.
- **Golgi tendon organs** monitor tension.
- **Joint kinaesthetic receptors** and the **vestibular apparatus** contribute to spatial orientation and posture.

These receptors relay positional information to the brain, aiding coordination and balance, and maintain baseline muscle tone via reflex arcs.

B. Special Sense Organs

Complex receptor organs and cranial nerves mediate special senses, including vision, hearing, balance, taste, and smell.

1. Eye – Vision

The eye contains multiple structures enabling photoreception:

- **Retina:** Contains rods (black-and-white vision) and cones (color vision).
- **Lens and ciliary body: Focus light onto** the retina.
- **Iris & Pupil:** Regulate light entry.
- **Cornea & Sclera:** Maintain shape and transparency.

Optic nerve: Transmits visual data to the brain.

Common Visual Defects Relevant to Acupuncture:

- **Myopia:** Elongated eyeball or steep cornea.

- **Hyperopia:** Short eyeball or flat lens.
- **Presbyopia:** Age-related lens stiffening.
- **Nyctalopia:** Poor rod function in low light.
- **Other indications:** Diabetic retinopathy, diplopia, eyelid twitching, ocular pain.

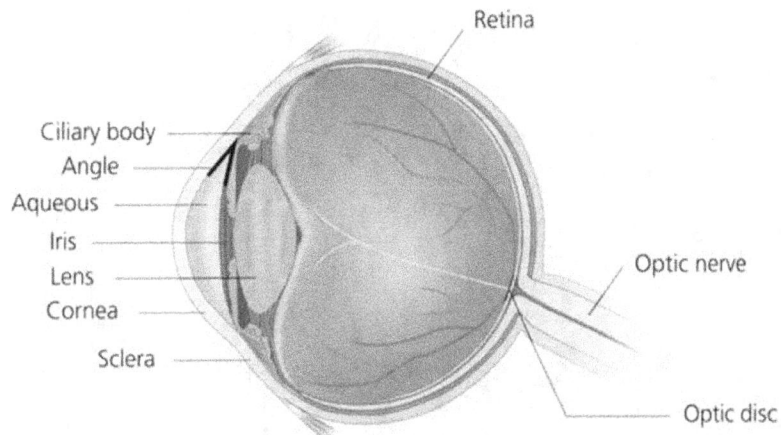

Fig. 1.5.2 Anatomy of Eye

2   Ear – Hearing

The ear consists of three parts:

- **Outer Ear:** The Pinna and canal collect sound.
- **Middle Ear:** Ossicles (malleus, incus, stapes) amplify vibrations.
- **Inner Ear:** The Cochlea transduces vibrations into nerve impulses relayed via the auditory nerve.

Hearing Process:

Sound waves → tympanic membrane → ossicles → cochlea → brain (via auditory nerve).

3. Taste (Gustation)

Taste buds are located mainly on the tongue and respond to:

- **Sweet, sour, salty, bitter, umami.**

Each taste bud contains receptor cells with microvilli, or taste hairs, that detect dissolved chemicals and send impulses via the facial, glossopharyngeal, or vagus nerves.

4. Ear – Equilibrium

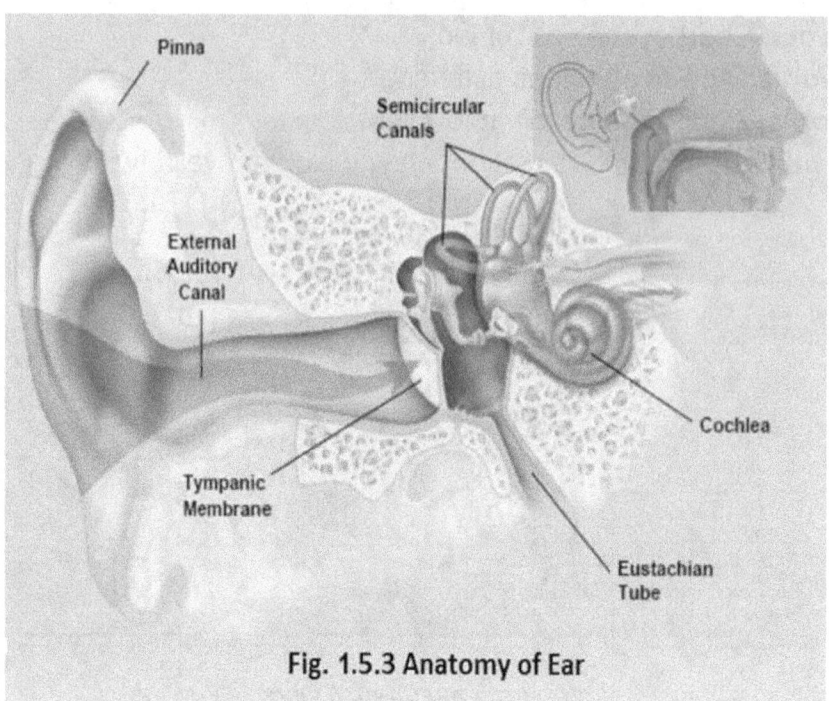

Fig. 1.5.3 Anatomy of Ear

The vestibular apparatus mediates balance:

- **Static equilibrium:** Detected by maculae in the utricle and saccule (position relative to gravity).
- **Dynamic equilibrium:** Detected by semicircular canals (angular movement).

These signals are integrated with visual input to maintain posture and spatial orientation.

5. Smell (Olfaction)

Olfactory receptors are located in the nasal epithelium. Airborne molecules dissolve in mucus and bind to receptor hairs, triggering impulses that travel to the olfactory bulb and the brain. Olfaction is closely linked to memory and complements the sense of taste.

Clinical Relevance to Acupuncture

Acupuncture has a significant therapeutic effect on sensory organs through local needling and systemic neurohormonal modulation. The five primary sensory organs—eyes, ears, nose, tongue, and skin—are closely linked to corresponding internal organs via Traditional Chinese Medicine (TCM) meridian theory and modern neurophysiology.

1. Eyes

- **Associated Organ (TCM):** Liver
- **Clinical Applications:**
  - Needling points like GB 20, BL 1, and LI 4 may improve vision, eye strain, dry eyes, glaucoma, or optic nerve dysfunction.
  - Scalp acupuncture and electroacupuncture have shown benefits in retinitis pigmentosa and macular degeneration.

2. Ears

- **Associated Organ (TCM):** Kidney
- **Clinical Applications:**
  - Points such as SI 19, GB 2, and SJ 17 are used for tinnitus, hearing loss, Meniere's disease, and otitis media.
  - Auricular acupuncture targets the entire body via somatotopic representation on the ear.

3. Nose

- **Associated Organ (TCM):** Lung
- **Clinical Applications:**
  - Points like LI 20, LI 4, and GV 23 are used for rhinitis, sinusitis, nasal congestion, and anosmia.
  - Electroacupuncture may reduce inflammation and mucosal swelling in allergic rhinitis.

4. Tongue

- **Associated Organ (TCM):** Heart
- **Clinical Applications:**
  - The tongue's appearance aids diagnosis; treatment targets speech issues, taste disorders, and mouth ulcers.
  - Points like CV 23, HT 5, and ST 4 are used in aphasia, dysarthria, and glossitis.

5. Skin (Tactile Organ)

- **Associated Organ (TCM):** Lung
- **Clinical Applications:**
  - Acupuncture treats itching, eczema, neuralgia, numbness, and neuropathy.

- Points such as LI 11, SP 6, and UB 40 are used for dermatological and cutaneous nerve conditions.
- Skin is also the interface for needling sensation, triggering local and systemic neuromodulation.

Scientific Perspective

From a modern viewpoint:

- Acupuncture stimulates afferent sensory nerves, modulating activity in the central nervous system.
- It can affect neurotransmitters (e.g., serotonin, endorphins) and autonomic balance, influencing sensory organ function.
- Functional MRI and electrophysiological studies support sensory and brain activation after acupuncture near sensory organ areas.

Summary

Acupuncture offers both local and systemic benefits for disorders of sensory organs. A practitioner's knowledge of anatomical pathways, meridian theory, and neurophysiology enhances therapeutic outcomes. Combining targeted points with proper technique can restore function, reduce symptoms, and improve quality of life in conditions affecting vision, hearing, smell, taste, and touch.

-Dr. Pardeshi Acupuncture-

1.6 Musculoskeletal System

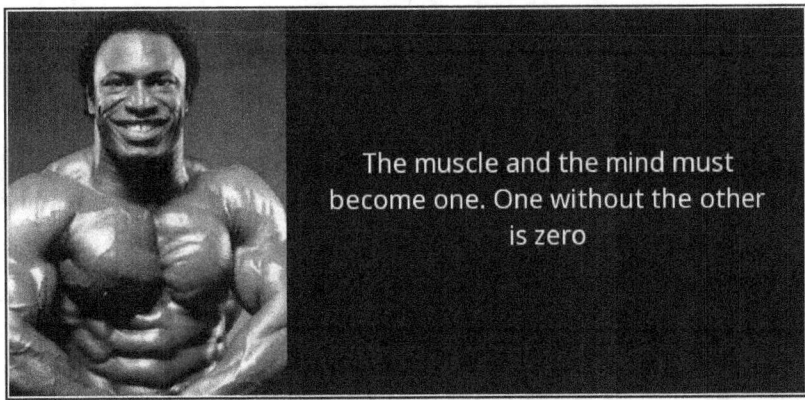

The muscle and the mind must become one. One without the other is zero

The musculoskeletal system is the body's complex framework, consisting of bones, muscles, cartilage, ligaments, and tendons. It provides our body with:

- Structure and Support: Bones form the framework, giving us shape and stability.
- Movement: Muscles contract and pull on bones, allowing for movement at joints.
- Protection: Bones shield vital organs like the brain and heart.
- Blood Cell Production: Bone marrow produces red and white blood cells within some bones.
- Mineral Storage: Bones store calcium and phosphorus, which are essential for various bodily functions.

Skeletal System:

The human skeleton comprises fused and individual bones supported by ligaments, tendons, muscles, and cartilage. It is a complex structure comprising two distinct divisions: the axial skeleton, which includes the vertebral column, and the appendicular skeleton.

Axial Skeleton:
The axial skeleton (80 bones) is formed by the vertebral column (32 - 34 bones; the number of the vertebrae differs from human to human as the lower two parts, sacral bone, and coccygeal bone, may vary in length), a part of the rib cage (12 pairs of ribs and the sternum), and the skull (22 bones and seven associated bones). The axial skeleton maintains humans' upright posture, which transmits the weight from the head, trunk, and upper extremities to the lower extremities at the hip joints. Many ligaments and erector spinae muscles support and balance the spine's bones.

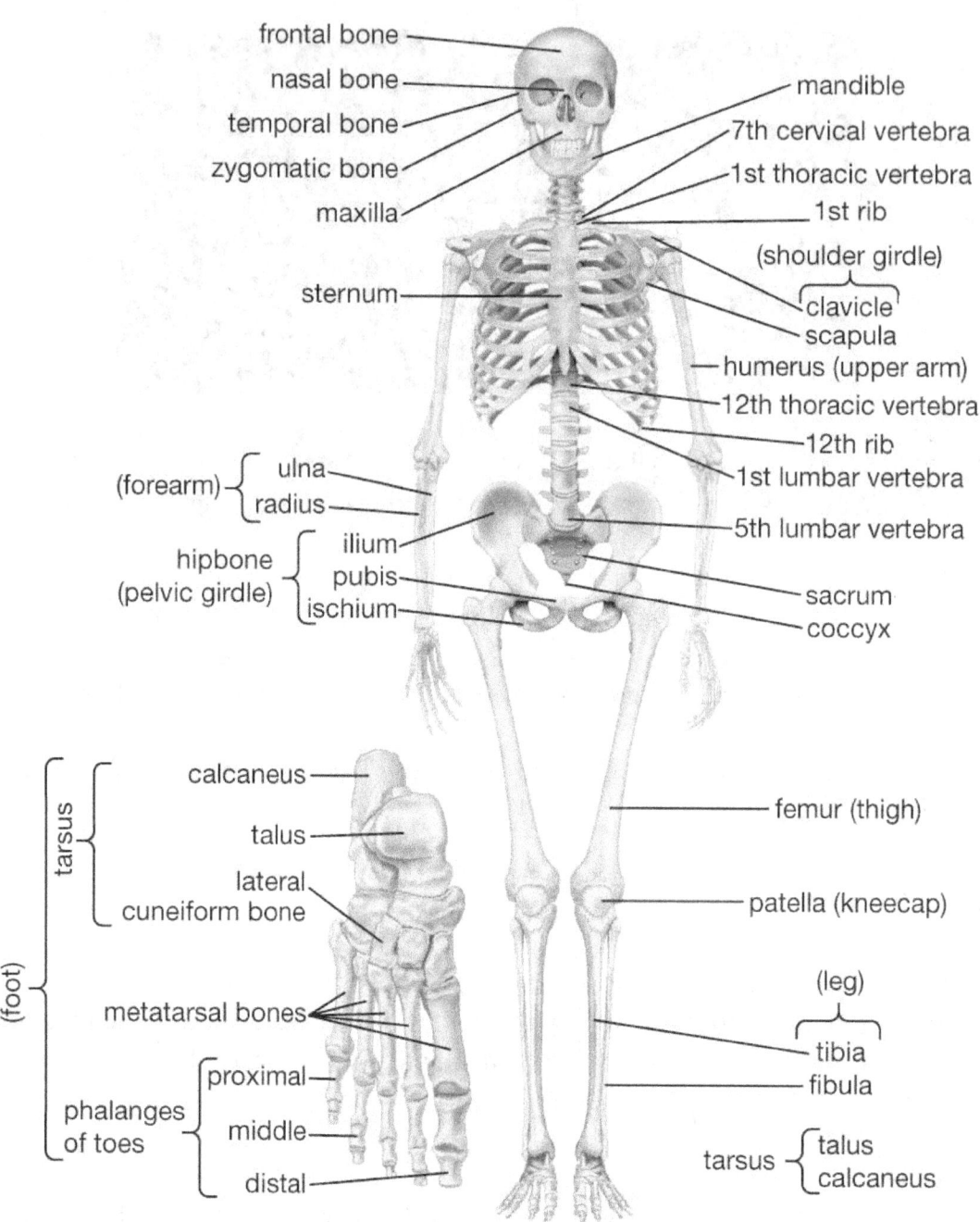

Fig 1.6.1A Human Skeleton Anterior View

Source: Encyclopedia Britanica Inc

Appendicular Skeleton:

The pectoral girdles, the upper limbs, the pelvic girdle or pelvis, and the lower limbs form the appendicular skeleton (126 bones). These structures enable locomotion and protect the vital organs of digestion, excretion, and reproduction.

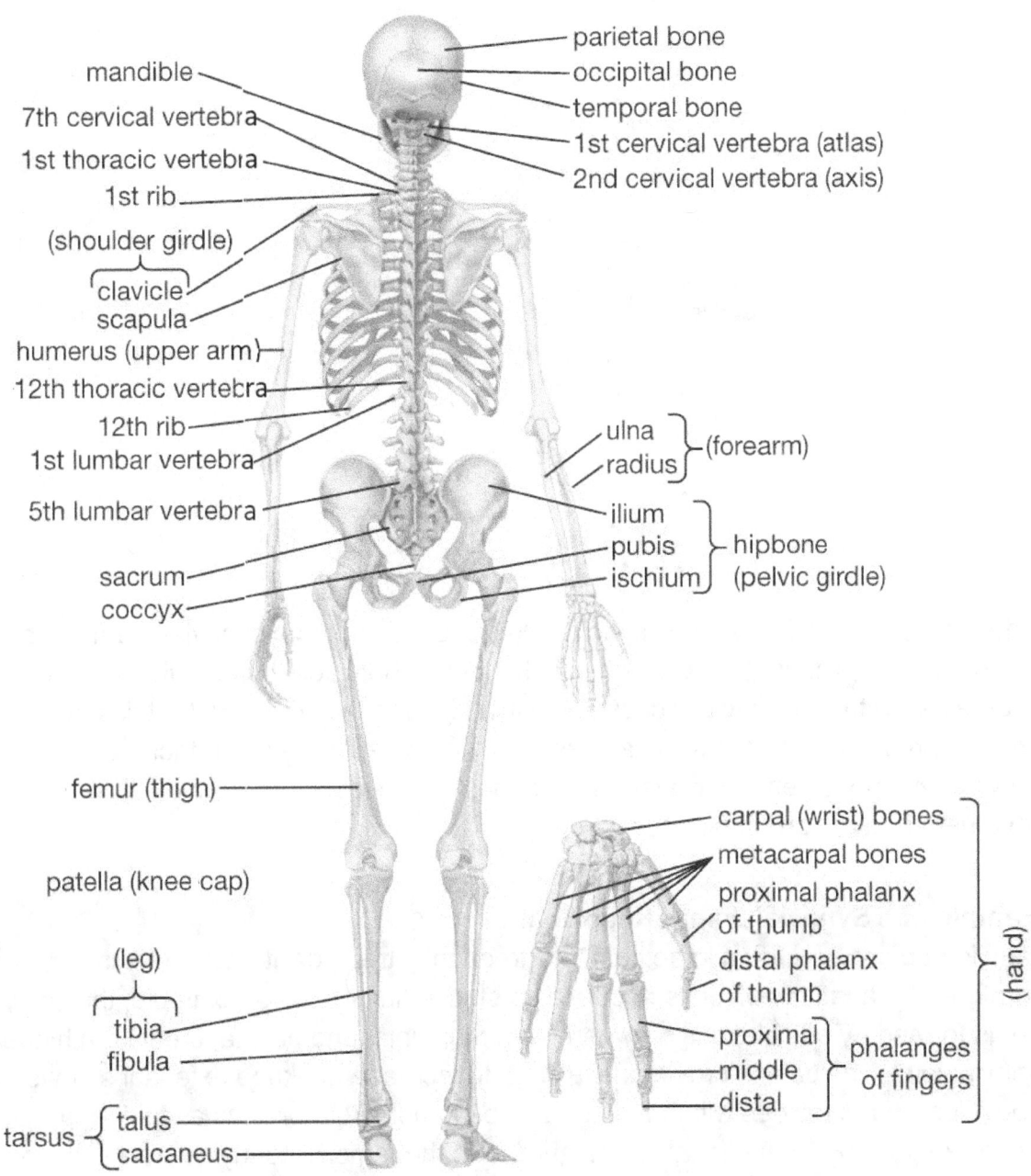

Fig. 1.6.1 P Human Skeleton Posterior View

Source: Encyclopedia Britanica

Joints:
They connect individual bones and allow them to move relative to each other, causing movement. The main types of joints are Synovial (knee), Hinge (elbow), Ball and Socket (hip), Condyloid (metacarpophalangeal), Saddle (sterno-clavicular), Pivot (wrist), Plane (metacarpal) joints.

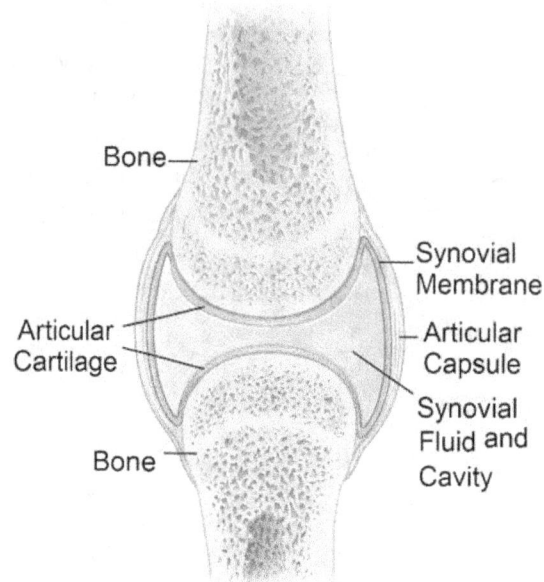

Fig. 1.6.2 Typical Synovial Joint

Synovial joints are lubricated by synovial fluid produced by the synovial membranes and are not directly joined. This fluid reduces the friction between the articular surfaces and is contained within an articular capsule, which binds the joint with its taut tissue. Amphiarthrosis or synarthrosis is a false joint, characterized by an attachment that allows some movement. However, these almost immovable joints enable little or no movement and are predominantly fibrous.

Example of a Synovial Joint - Knee Joint:
Many joint pains, including knee pain, are frequently treated with acupuncture; therefore, the anatomy of joints needs to be studied in detail. For example, the knee joint is formed by articulations between the femur, tibia, and patella, creating a hinge synovial joint. The patella provides a fulcrum to increase the knee extensor's power as it is developed and resides within the quadriceps femoris tendon. It is a stabilizing structure that reduces frictional forces applied to the femoral condyles. The knee joint is mainly created to allow flexion, extension, and a slight medial and lateral rotation. Nerve and blood supply of the knee joint: The Femoral, tibial, and common fibular nerves supply muscles and the knee joint. Genicular branches of the femoral and popliteal

arteries supply blood to the knee joint. Blood supply to the knee comes through the genicular anastomosis.

Inner surfaces of joint: The inner surface of the knee joint consists of tibiofemoral and patella-femoral articulations. The joint surfaces are enclosed within a single cavity and lined with hyaline cartilage. The patellofemoral joint allows the quadriceps femoris tendon (a primary knee extensor) to be inserted directly over the knee, thereby increasing the muscle's efficiency. It is on the anterior aspect of the distal femur that articulates with the patella. The knee joint's tibio-femoral component is the weight-bearing part and is formed by the medial and lateral condyles of the femur that articulate with the tibial condyles.

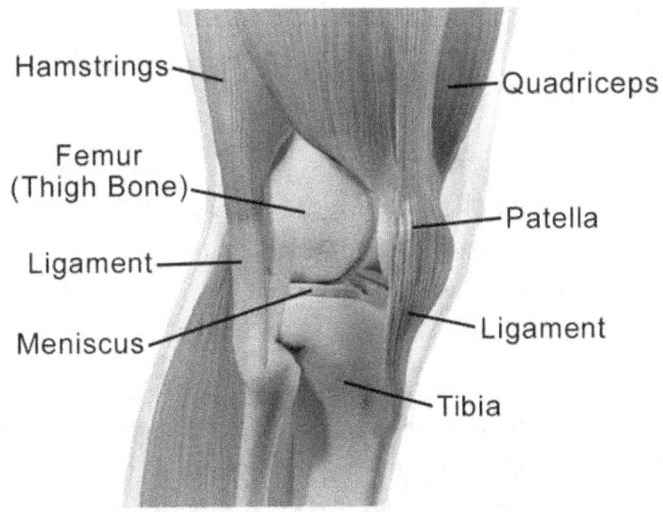

Fig. 1.6.3 Anatomy of Knee Joint

The menisci are C-shaped medial and lateral fibro-cartilaginous structures. They are attached at both ends to the intercondylar area of the tibia. The minor lateral meniscus has no extra attachments, rendering it reasonably mobile. The medial meniscus is fixed to the tibial collateral ligament, joint capsule, and intercondylar attachment. The tibial collateral ligament damage usually causes a medial meniscal tear. Menisci serve two functions: increasing surface area to dissipate forces further and acting as shock absorbers. Secondly, they add stability to the joint by deepening the articular surface of the tibia. Bursae are synovial fluid-filled sacs found between moving structures in a joint.

The Ligaments of the Knee Joint:
The patellar ligament is attached from the patella to the tibial tuberosity. It is a continuation of the tendon of the quadriceps femoris beyond the patella. Collateral ligaments are strap-like on both sides, stabilizing the knee's hinge motion and preventing extreme medial or lateral movements. A medial or tibial collateral ligament, a broad and flat ligament, attaches to the femur's medial epicondyle above and the tibia's medial condyle below. The lateral or fibular collateral ligament, thinner and rounder than

the tibial collateral, attaches to the femur's lateral epicondyle above and a depression on the lateral surface of the fibular head below. Cruciate ligaments cross each other, connecting the tibia and femur. The anterior cruciate ligament attaches the tibia at the anterior intercondylar region and blends with the medial meniscus. It goes up posteriorly and attaches to the femur in the intercondylar fossa. The primary function of the anterior cruciate ligament is to prevent an anterior dislocation of the tibia onto the femur. Likewise, the posterior cruciate ligament prevents posterior dislocation of the tibia onto the femur.

Knee movements: The quadriceps femoris muscle, inserted into the tibial tuberosity, causes knee joint extension. The Hamstrings, Gracilis, Sartorius, and Popliteus muscles are responsible for knee flexion. The biceps femoris performs lateral rotation. The Gracilis, Semitendinosus, Semimembranosus, Sartorius, and Popliteus muscles cause medial rotation.

Bursa:
A bursa is a small fluid-filled sac of white fibrous tissue lined with a synovial membrane. It provides a cushion between bones and tendons or muscles around a joint. Synovial fluid fills the bursa around almost every major joint, and a synovial membrane that extends outside the joint capsule may also form a bursa.

Ligaments:
A ligament is a small band of dense, white, fibrous elastic tissue. Ligaments connect the ends of bones to form a joint. Most ligaments limit dislocation or prevent specific movements that may cause breaks. Since they are elastic, they lengthen when under pressure. The ligament may be susceptible to breaking when this occurs, resulting in an unstable joint. Ligaments also restrict some actions, like hyperextension (knee) and hyperflexion. They also prevent specific directional movement.

Tendons
A tendon is a robust, flexible band of fibrous connective tissue that connects muscles to bones. The extracellular connective tissue between muscle fibers binds to the distal and proximal ends of tendons. The tendon binds to the periosteum of individual bones at the muscle's origin and insertion. As muscles contract, tendons transmit the forces to the relatively rigid bones, pulling on them and causing movement. Tendons can stretch substantially, functioning as springs during locomotion, saving energy.

Upper Limb
The upper limb consists of the upper arm, lower arm, and hand. The arm is located between the shoulder and elbow joints; the forearm is between the elbow and wrist, and the hand is located distal to the wrist. Each upper limb has 30 bones. The upper arm has a single humerus bone. The forearm has paired bones, the ulna (medially) and

the radius (laterally). The base of the hand has eight carpal bones, and the palm has five metacarpal bones. The fingers and thumb contain 14 phalanges.

The primary life activities depend upon the upper limb, which moves the hand around the body. The hand may reach in all directions because the shoulder girdle provides a wide range of motion exceeding a hemisphere.

Muscle System

There are three types of muscles - skeletal, smooth, and cardiac. Skeletal and cardiac muscles have striations visible under a microscope due to the particular components within their cells. Only skeletal and smooth muscles are part of the musculoskeletal system. Skeletal muscles are attached to bones and arranged in opposing groups around joints.

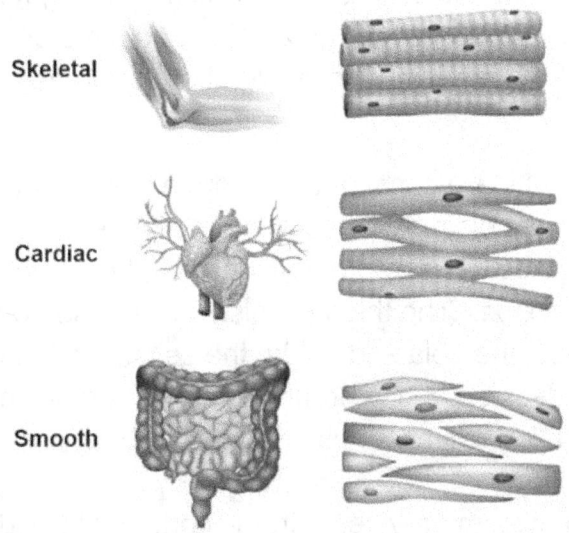

Types of Muscles

Smooth muscles control the flow of substances within the lumens of hollow organs and are not consciously controlled. For example, cardiac muscles are located in the heart and are responsible for circulating blood. Skeletal muscles get a stimulus from the central nervous system through nerves that cause the muscles to contract.

The muscles carry out many functions; in summary, they are -

Respiration: Muscles carry out lifelong respiration.
Circulation: The heart is a muscle-powered pump.
Stability: The stability of the body's motion depends on muscle force.
Posture: Muscles give the correct anatomical posture.
Mobility: Every body movement is executed by the power of the muscles.

Vision: Constant eye movements provide a clear and focused vision. Movements of the eyelids protect the eye.

Digestion and excretion: Food continues to move further through the intestine with the help of smooth muscle. Urination: Urine from the kidneys to the bladder is carried out by the muscles in the bladder.

Childbirth: Children cannot be born without the muscular movements of the uterus.

Organ Protection: Muscles protect the intestines and other organs.

Temperature regulation: Muscle action generates heat to maintain a stable body temperature.

Trunk

The trunk or torso is the human body's central part, or core, extending from the neck and limbs. It includes the thoracic segment, the abdominal segment, and the perineum. The 51 trunk bones comprise 26 vertebrae, 24 ribs, and the sternum. The 26 vertebrae comprise seven cervical, 12 thoracic, and five lumbar vertebrae, plus the sacrum.

Lower Limb

The bones of the lower limbs are considerably more extensive and more robust than comparable bones of the upper limbs. The lower limb is the principal part of locomotion and is essential at every step. The lower limb consists of the thigh (the upper leg), the leg (the lower leg), and the foot. The thigh consists of a single bone, the femur. The leg consists of two long bones: the tibia and fibula, the sesamoid bone, the patella, and the kneecap. The foot comprises 26 bones grouped into the tarsals, metatarsals, and phalanges. Thus, the lower limbs must support the body's weight while walking, running, or jumping.

In summary, the skeletal system provides a framework for the body, offering structural support to the entire body. Individuals or groups of bones provide a framework for attaching soft tissues and organs.

Protection of organs: Skeletal elements surround many soft tissues and organs, providing protection. For example, the rib cage protects the heart and lungs, the skull protects the brain, the vertebrae protect the spinal cord, and the pelvis protects the delicate reproductive organs.

Clinical Relevance of the Musculoskeletal System to Acupuncture

The musculoskeletal system, bones, joints, muscles, tendons, ligaments, and connective tissues, is one of acupuncture's most commonly treated systems. Acupuncture addresses pain, inflammation, stiffness, limited mobility, and functional disorders by stimulating neurovascular, myofascial, and segmental pathways.

Key Mechanisms of Action

1. **Neuromodulation**
   - Acupuncture activates A-delta and C-fibres, triggering segmental inhibition in the spinal cord and promoting endogenous opioid release (e.g., endorphins, enkephalins).
   - It modulates central pain processing centres, reducing chronic pain and muscle hypertonicity.
2. **Local Effects**
   - Improves microcirculation and tissue oxygenation at the needled site.
   - Reduces inflammatory cytokines in injured tissues.
   - Releases tight myofascial trigger points and reduces muscle spasms.
3. **Motor Point Activation**
   - Needling motor points or myotomal zones can restore muscle tone and strength, improve coordination, and reduce neuromuscular fatigue.
4. **Postural and Segmental Regulation**
   - Treating paraspinal points influences spinal alignment and segmental innervation, which is helpful in radiculopathy, sciatica, and facet joint dysfunction.

Clinical Applications in Musculoskeletal Disorders

Condition	Commonly Used Points	Effect
Cervical spondylosis	GB 20, GV 14, SI 3, LI 4	Relieves neck stiffness and radiating pain
Shoulder pain (Frozen shoulder)	LI 15, SJ 14, SI 9, Ashi points	Improves range of motion, reduces inflammation
Back pain (Lumbar strain, Disc)	BL 23, BL 25, GV 3, UB 40, Ashi	Relaxes muscles, reduces disc pressure
Knee osteoarthritis	ST 35, EX-LE4 (Heding), SP 9, UB 40	Improves mobility, reduces synovial swelling.
Sciatica	GB 30, UB 40, UB 57, UB 62	Relieves nerve root irritation
Tennis/Golfer's Elbow	LI 10, LI 11, SJ 5, Ashi	Reduces tendon inflammation
Plantar fasciitis	KI 1, UB 57, UB 60	Stimulates fascia healing
Post-fracture rehabilitation	Local motor points, ST 36, SP 6	Enhances healing, reduces stiffness

Modern Evidence and Integration

- Randomised controlled trials support acupuncture's efficacy in chronic low back pain, knee OA, neck pain, and fibromyalgia.
- Integrates with physical therapy, rehabilitation, orthopaedics, and sports medicine.
- Electroacupuncture enhances outcomes in resistant conditions by improving neuromuscular reactivation.

Summary

Acupuncture plays a vital role in managing musculoskeletal disorders. It offers pain relief, functional improvement, and tissue recovery without the need for drugs or invasive procedures. Its combination of neurophysiological effects, anatomical precision, and energetic balance makes it an ideal modality for both acute and chronic conditions affecting the musculoskeletal system.

-Modern Acupuncture-

1.7   Endocrine System

> MOLECULES MOVE NOT ONLY FROM THE
> BRAIN TO THE ENDOCRINE SYSTEM BUT
> ALSO FROM THE ENDOCRINE SYSTEM,
> INDEED, FROM ALL PARTS OF THE BODY TO
> THE BRAIN.
> - RICHARD BERGLAND -

The endocrine system functions as the body's internal conductor, orchestrating physiological harmony through the precise release of **hormones**—chemical messengers synthesized and secreted by specialized glands. These hormones enter the bloodstream and act on distant target organs to regulate essential processes, including growth, metabolism, reproduction, immunity, and emotional state.

Importance and Regulation:

Hormonal balance is vital for homeostasis. However, this finely tuned system is sensitive to several influencing factors:

- **Aging**: Natural decline in hormone production can affect metabolism, reproductive function, and repair mechanisms.
- **Chronic Stress**: Sustained stress elevates cortisol levels, disrupting the regular hormonal feedback loops.
- **Environmental Toxins**: Chemicals like endocrine disruptors can interfere with hormone synthesis, release, or receptor function.
- **Genetics**: Inherited conditions may predispose individuals to endocrine dysfunctions, such as thyroid disorders or diabetes.
- **Disease States**: Conditions like autoimmune diseases, tumours, or infections can impair hormone production and signalling pathways.

Understanding endocrine interactions is crucial in acupuncture, as many conditions responsive to acupuncture, such as menstrual irregularities, metabolic syndromes, and mood disorders, often involve underlying hormonal imbalances.

Major Endocrine Glands and Their Functions

Parathyroid: This gland controls the amount of calcium in the body.

Ovaries: Ovaries are present only in women. They secrete estrogen, progesterone, female sex hormones, and even testosterone.

Testes: The testes produce the male sex hormone testosterone and produce sperm.

Hypothalamus: The hypothalamus is not included in the endocrine gland but is responsible for releasing hormones from other glands and controls thirst, sleep, sex drive, body temperature, hunger, and moods.

Brain: Though not grouped as an endocrine gland, it secretes neurohormones and directly or indirectly affects many body functions.

All Organs and Tissues: They secrete specific messaging substances into the blood.

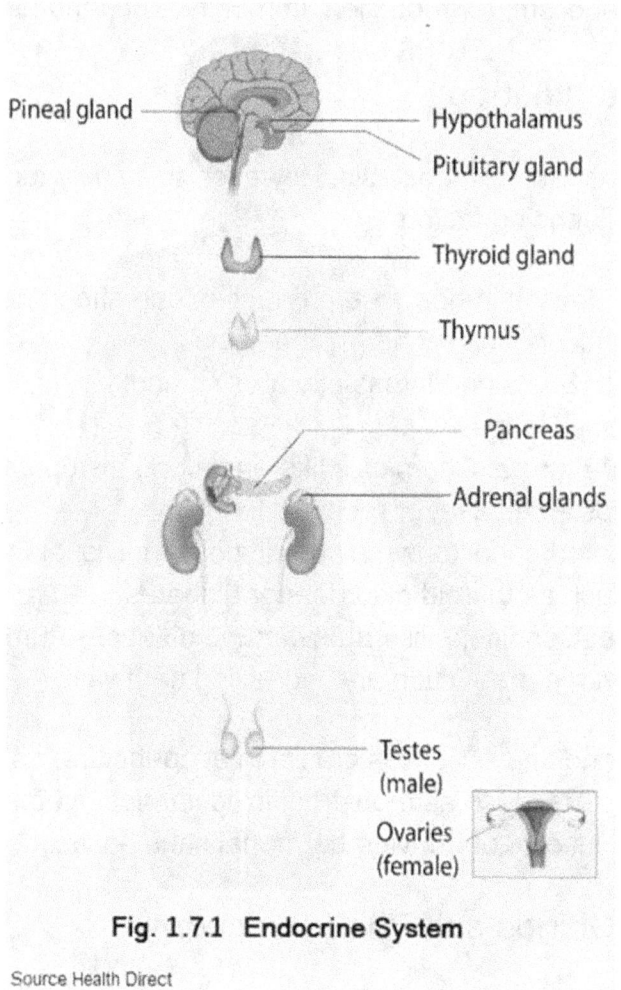

Fig. 1.7.1 Endocrine System

Source Health Direct

The table provides details of the endocrine gland's secreted hormones and their corresponding functions.

Endocrine Gland	Hormone Secreted	Functions
Pituitary	Follicle Stimulating (FSH)	Production of ova and sperm
Pituitary	Luteinizing (LH)	Production of estrogen, testosterone and ovulation
Pituitary	Melatonin	Sleep cycle
Pituitary	Prolactin	Milk production
Pituitary	Oxytocin	Childbirth, lactation and mother-child bonding
Adrenal	Adrenalin	Increases heart rate, blood pressure, metabolism in stress reaction
Adrenal	Aldosterone	Salt and water control
Adrenal	Cortisol	Stress response
Adrenal	Dehydroepiandro-steron Sulphate (DHEA)	Hair growth and body odor
Ovary	Estrogen	Menstrual cycle, pregnancy, production of ova, secondary sex characteristics
Ovary, Testes, Adrenal	Testosterone	Sex drive and secondary sex characteristics in male
Pancreas	Glucagon	Increases blood glucose level
Pancreas	Insulin	Help metabolize blood
Thyroid	Thyroid Hormone	Metabolism and energy level
Para-thyroid	Parathyroid Hormone	Calcium metabolism

Fig. 1.7.2 Hormonal Glands and Their Functions

Clinical Applications: Hormonal Disorders Treated by Acupuncture

Condition	Hormones Affected	Effect of Acupuncture
Stress, Anxiety, Burnout	Cortisol, adrenaline	Reduces cortisol, calms the HPA axis
Polycystic Ovary Syndrome (PCOS)	LH, FSH, testosterone	Normalises LH/FSH ratio, reduces androgen excess
Infertility	Oestrogen, progesterone, LH, FSH	Regulates ovulation, improves endometrial receptivity
Thyroid Disorders	TSH, T3, T4	Modulates thyroid function via the pituitary–thyroid axis
Menopausal Symptoms	Oestrogen, serotonin, beta-endorphins	Reduces hot flashes, mood swings, and insomnia
Diabetes (Type 2)	Insulin, glucagon	Improves insulin sensitivity, stabilises blood glucose
PMS / Menstrual Irregularities	Oestrogen, progesterone	Regulates cycles, reduces pain, and mood-related symptoms

Summary

Acupuncture influences hormones by modulating the neuroendocrine system, restoring balance where there is hyperfunction or hypofunction. Through its effects on the HPA axis, autonomic nervous system, and neurotransmitter pathways, acupuncture serves as a natural regulator for various hormonal disorders, with minimal side effects.

- *Dr. Pardeshi Acupuncture* -

Dr. C Pardeshi MD

1.8 Immune System

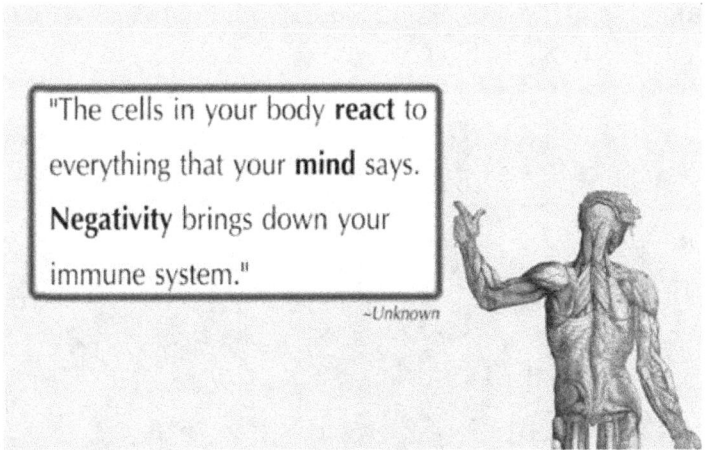

"The cells in your body **react** to everything that your **mind** says. **Negativity** brings down your immune system."

~Unknown

The human body is continuously exposed to various threats, including microorganisms such as bacteria and viruses, toxic substances, and aberrant internal cells. To defend itself, the body is equipped with an extraordinary biological defence network: the immune system. This system, comprising specialized organs, cells, and signalling molecules, protects against infection, supports tissue repair, and maintains internal equilibrium.

Overview

The immune system functions like a multi-tiered fortress:

- **First Line of Defence**: Physical and chemical barriers such as skin and **mucous membranes** prevent the entry of pathogens.
- **Second Line of Defence**: If pathogens breach these barriers, innate immune cells and inflammatory responses are activated to neutralize them.
- **Third Line of Defence**: Adaptive immunity, involving lymphocytes and antibodies, targets specific pathogens precisely and retains memory for future encounters.

Without a functioning immune system, even minor infections could become life-threatening. The immune system is both protective and dynamic, adaptive, and intelligent.

Functions of the Immune System

- **Pathogen Elimination**: Identifies and destroys bacteria, viruses, fungi, and parasites.

- **Immunological Memory**: The system responds more efficiently upon re-exposure to known pathogens through memory cells (primarily B and T lymphocytes).

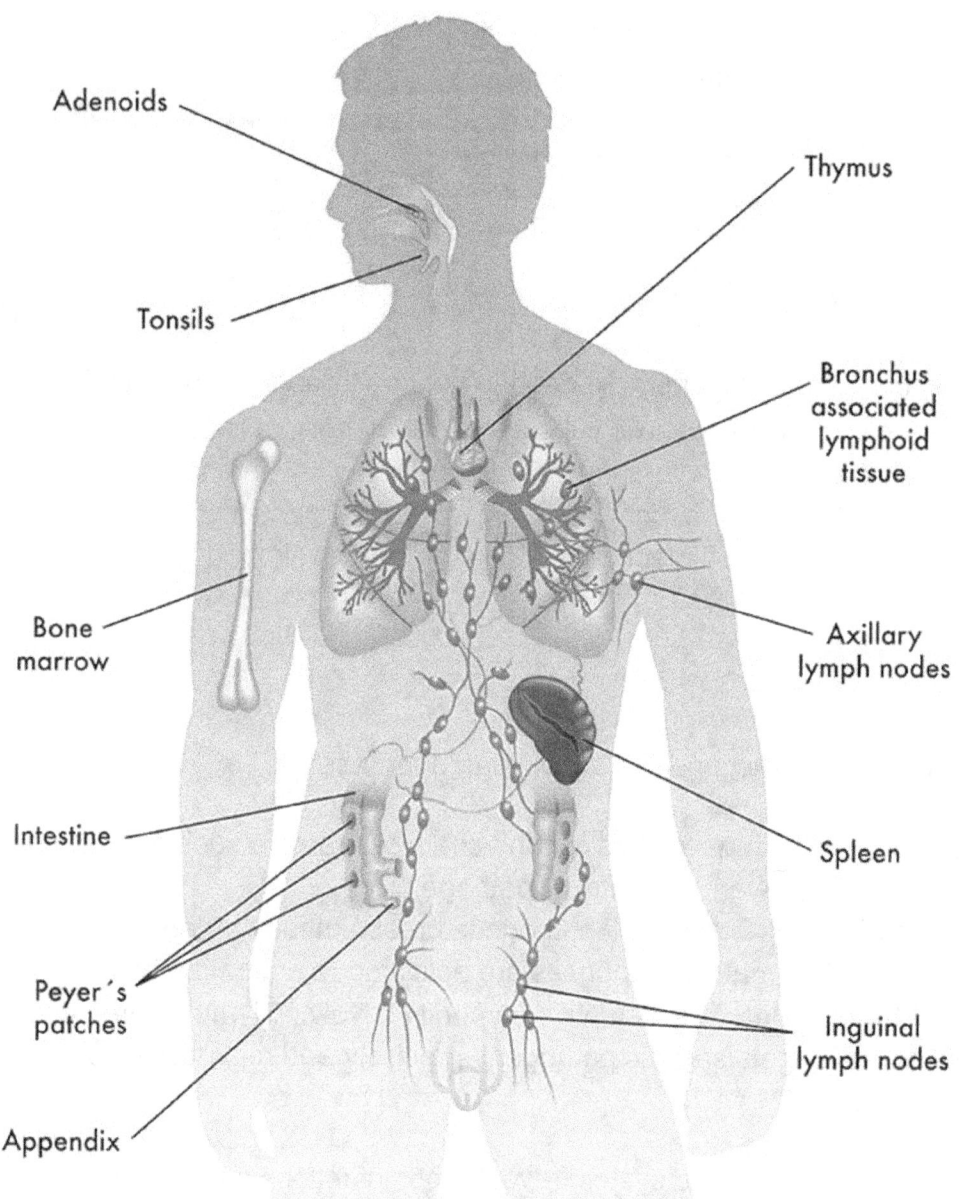

Fig. 1.8 Immune System

Source Health Direct

- **Surveillance and Repair**: Recognizes and removes abnormal or damaged cells, contributing to wound healing.

- **Inflammation Regulation**: Manages pro- and anti-inflammatory responses to maintain tissue health.

Some viral infections, such as influenza and COVID-19, remain recurrent due to frequent mutation and antigenic drift, rendering immune memory partially ineffective.

Notably, acupuncture is known to modulate immune responses, enhance defence mechanisms, and reduce immune hyperactivity. Thus, acupuncturists should possess a solid understanding of immune physiology and pathology.

Components of the Immune System

1. White Blood Cells (Leukocytes)

Produced in the **bone marrow**, white blood cells circulate via blood and lymphatic systems and serve as the core effectors of immunity. They are broadly classified into:

- **Phagocytes**: Engulf and digest pathogens. Subtypes include:
  - **Neutrophils**: Most abundant; first responders against bacterial infection.
  - **Monocytes**: Circulate in blood; mature into macrophages in tissues.
  - **Macrophages**: Phagocytose pathogens and remove cellular debris.
  - **Mast Cells**: Play roles in wound healing and allergic reactions.
- **Lymphocytes**:
  - **B cells**: Produce antibodies; involved in humoral immunity.
  - **T cells**: Include helper (CD4$^+$) and cytotoxic (CD8$^+$) subsets; critical for cellular immunity and immune regulation.
  - **Natural Killer (NK) cells**: Attack virus-infected or cancerous cells.
- **Antibodies (Immunoglobulins)**: Proteins secreted by B cells that recognize specific **antigens** on pathogens and tag them for destruction.

2. Lymphatic Organs

- **Spleen**: Filters blood, removes pathogens, and destroys aged red blood cells. It is a site of immune cell activation and antibody production.
- **Thymus**: Located in the upper chest; it is the maturation site for T-lymphocytes and crucial for early-life immune development.
- **Lymph Nodes**: Filter lymph and house lymphocytes. They act as checkpoints for immune surveillance and activation.

Immune System Disorders

Immune dysfunction can manifest as either deficiency or hyperactivity, both of which can be addressed, to varying extents, through acupuncture-mediated modulation.

1. Immunodeficiency

Occurs when part of the immune system is missing or inactive. Causes include:

- **Primary (Inherited)**: e.g., Severe Combined Immunodeficiency (SCID)
- **Secondary (Acquired)**: e.g., HIV/AIDS, chemotherapy, malnutrition

2. Hypersensitivity and Allergic Conditions

An overactive immune response to harmless substances (allergens), resulting in:

- Allergic rhinitis, asthma, food allergies
- Urticaria, eczema, atopic dermatitis

Allergic disorders often respond favourably to acupuncture by modulating immune reactivity and reducing inflammation.

3. Autoimmune Diseases

Here, the immune system attacks the body's cells. Examples include:

- **Rheumatoid Arthritis**
- **Systemic Lupus Erythematosus**
- **Type 1 Diabetes Mellitus**
- **Autoimmune Thyroid Disease (e.g., Hashimoto's, Graves')**
- **Multiple Sclerosis**

Acupuncture has shown promise in managing symptoms and improving quality of life in autoimmune conditions through immunoregulatory effects.

Clinical Applications in Immune-Related Conditions

Condition	Immune Effect of Acupuncture
Allergic Rhinitis / Asthma	Reduces IgE, stabilises mast cells, and modulates Th2 response.
Rheumatoid Arthritis / SLE	Downregulates pro-inflammatory cytokines, improves joint function.
Chronic Fatigue / ME	Boosts NK cell function, improves energy, and resilience.
Cancer Support (Immunomodulation)	Enhances immune surveillance, alleviates chemo-induced immunosuppression
Recurrent Infections	Increases WBC and antibody production
Post-viral Syndrome / Long COVID	Regulates inflammation, restores immune balance
Skin Conditions (e.g., eczema)	Reduces inflammatory cytokines, stabilises skin immune response

Summary

Acupuncture offers significant immunoregulatory benefits by enhancing the body's natural defence mechanisms and restoring balance in cases of immune dysfunction. It is especially effective in managing chronic inflammation, immune deficiencies, allergies, and autoimmune conditions, providing a systemic, drug-free therapeutic approach.

In conclusion, the immune system is a complex and dynamic network essential for maintaining health and survival. A solid understanding of its physiological functions equips acupuncturists to treat various immune-related disorders, including infections, hypersensitivity reactions, and autoimmune diseases, with greater precision and confidence.

-Dr. Pardeshi Acupuncture-

1.9   Lymphatic System

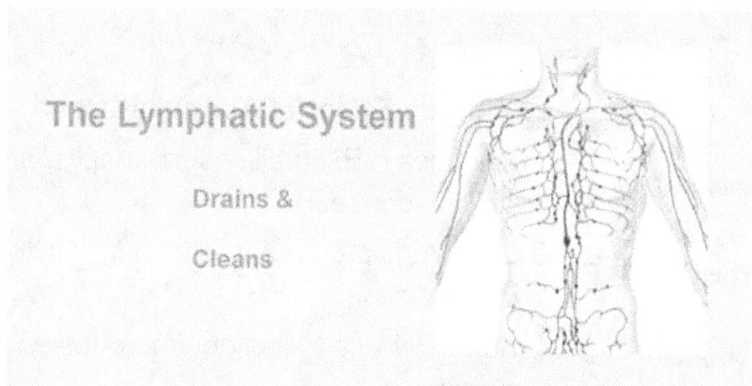

The lymphatic system is essential to the body's circulatory and immune systems. It serves as both a drainage network and an immunological defence mechanism. The lymphatic system transports lymph, a clear fluid derived from interstitial (extracellular) fluid, back into the bloodstream while also playing a vital role in immune surveillance and fat absorption.

Structure and Components

The lymphatic system comprises an extensive network of lymphatic vessels, lymph nodes, and lymphoid organs, including:

- **Bone marrow**
- **Thymus**
- **Spleen**
- **Tonsils**
- **Gut-associated lymphoid tissue (GALT)**
- **Interstitial tissue**

Lymphoid organs are broadly classified as:

- **Primary Lymphoid Organs** – Sites of lymphocyte maturation:
  - **Bone marrow**: Origin and maturation site of B lymphocytes.
  - **Thymus**: Site where T lymphocytes differentiate and mature.
- **Secondary Lymphoid Organs** – Sites of lymphocyte activation and response:
  - **Lymph nodes**
  - **Spleen**
  - **Mucosa-associated lymphoid tissue (MALT)**

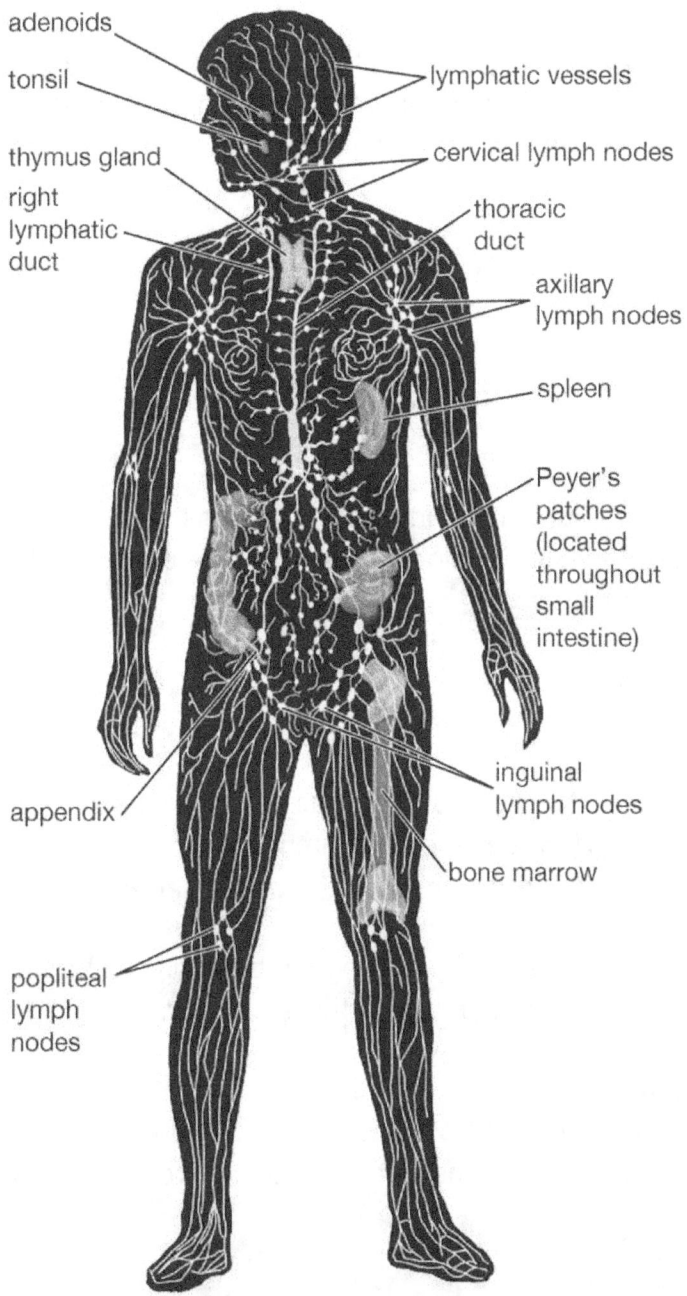

adenoids

tonsil

thymus gland

right lymphatic duct

lymphatic vessels

cervical lymph nodes

thoracic duct

axillary lymph nodes

spleen

Peyer's patches (located throughout small intestine)

appendix

inguinal lymph nodes

bone marrow

popliteal lymph nodes

Fig. 1.9 Lymphatic System

Source: Encyclopedia Britanica Inc

Physiological Role

The lymphatic system closely mirrors the circulatory system in structure and purpose, but operates independently from the heart-driven vascular circuit. It maintains fluid homeostasis by collecting excess tissue fluid (interstitial fluid) that escapes from capillaries and returning it to the bloodstream via lymphatic vessels.

- **Interstitial Fluid Formation**: As blood circulates, plasma leaks through capillary walls into tissues, carrying oxygen, nutrients, and signalling molecules. Most of this fluid is reabsorbed, but a portion remains in the extracellular space.
- **Lymph Formation and Transport**: This leftover fluid, along with cellular debris, proteins, and foreign substances, is collected by lymphatic capillaries and transported as **lymph**.

Functions of the Lymphatic System

The lymphatic system performs **three primary functions**:

1. **Fluid Homeostasis**
   It removes excess fluid (including water, proteins, and waste products) from tissues and returns it to the bloodstream. Failure of this function leads to **oedema** or fluid accumulation.

2. **Immune Defence**
   The lymphatic system facilitates the production, maturation, and deployment of:

   - **B lymphocytes** (antibody-producing cells)
   - **T lymphocytes** (cell-mediated immunity)
   - **Plasma cells**, **monocytes**, and **macrophages**

   These immune cells encounter pathogens primarily in lymph nodes, where antigen presentation and immune activation occur.

2. **Fat Absorption**
   Specialized lymphatic vessels in the small intestine, known as **lacteals**, absorb dietary fats as **chyle** and transport them to the circulatory system.

Clinical Applications

Acupuncture has shown benefit in various clinical situations where lymphatic dysfunction or fluid imbalance plays a role. by enhancing circulation and promoting immune regulation, acupuncture supports acute and chronic conditions.

1. Lymphedema (post-mastectomy or post-surgical)
Acupuncture can reduce limb swelling, improve mobility, and relieve heaviness or tightness. Commonly used points include SP 9, ST 36, CV 9, and local ashi points. Combining acupuncture with gentle cupping or tuina massage may enhance drainage.

2. Chronic infections and immune deficiency

In recurrent infections or sluggish immune response cases, acupuncture strengthens lymphatic filtering and antigen processing. It supports lymph node function through LI 11, ST 36, and UB 13.

3. Inflammatory conditions

acupuncture may help resolve chronic inflammation where lymphatic flow is impaired, such as in rheumatoid arthritis, sinusitis, or inflammatory skin conditions. points like SP 10, LI 4, and GB 34 aid in reducing cytokine overload and lymph congestion.

4. Detoxification and fluid retention

for patients with generalised swelling, fatigue, or a sensation of heaviness, acupuncture assists in fluid mobilisation and toxin clearance. acupuncture at CV 9, SP 6, and ST 28 supports urinary excretion and interstitial fluid regulation.

5. Post-surgical recovery

after trauma or surgery, acupuncture helps reduce lymphatic pooling and scar tissue formation, promoting faster healing. Points near the surgical site and distal tonifying points may accelerate lymphatic clearance and tissue repair.

-Dr. Pardeshi Acupuncture-

1.10 Digestive System and Abdomen

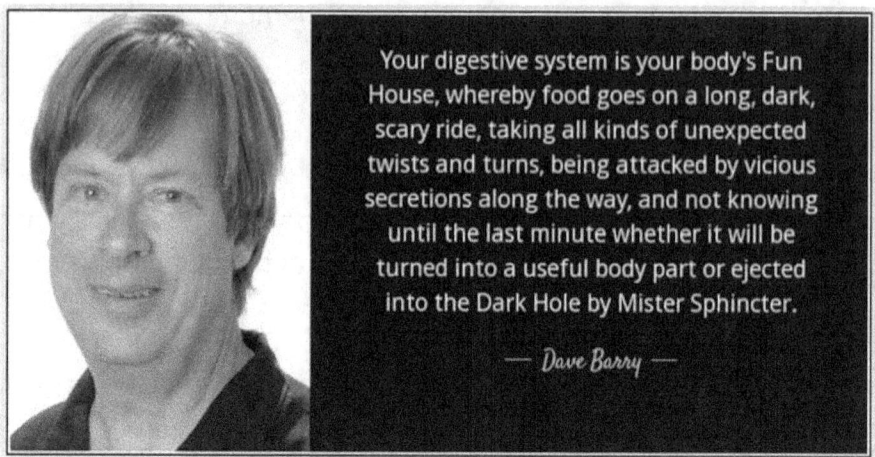

Your digestive system is your body's Fun House, whereby food goes on a long, dark, scary ride, taking all kinds of unexpected twists and turns, being attacked by vicious secretions along the way, and not knowing until the last minute whether it will be turned into a useful body part or ejected into the Dark Hole by Mister Sphincter.

— Dave Barry —

The digestive system plays a fundamental role in breaking down food, absorbing nutrients, and eliminating waste. Its efficient function is vital to maintaining energy levels, metabolic balance, and immune health. However, this complex system is vulnerable to disruption by various factors, including diet, stress, infection, and systemic diseases. Common digestive disorders include gastroesophageal reflux disease (GERD), irritable bowel syndrome (IBS), constipation, nausea and vomiting, and abdominal pain.

Acupuncture offers an effective complementary therapy for many gastrointestinal conditions. Targeting specific meridian points can modulate neural, hormonal, and immunological activity to improve digestive function.

Key Abdominal Organs and Their Functions

Stomach

- A thick-walled muscular organ located in the left upper abdomen.
- Divided into four regions: cardia, fundus, body, and pylorus.

Functions:

- Mechanical mixing of food with gastric secretions to form chyme.
- Secretion of hydrochloric acid (for antimicrobial action) and pepsin (for protein digestion).
- Regulation of gastric emptying through the pyloric sphincter.
- Absorption of limited substances (e.g., water, alcohol, and some lipid-soluble drugs).

- Facilitates iron solubilisation and intrinsic factor production for vitamin B_{12} absorption.

Liver

- The largest internal organ, located in the right upper quadrant beneath the diaphragm.
- Dual blood supply: oxygenated blood from the hepatic artery; nutrient-rich blood from the portal vein.

Functions:

- Production of bile for fat digestion.
- Metabolism of carbohydrates, fats, proteins, hormones, and drugs.
- Detoxification of metabolic byproducts and xenobiotics.
- Storage of glycogen, iron, and fat-soluble vitamins.
- Synthesis of plasma proteins (e.g., albumin, clotting factors).
- Breakdown of red blood cells and bilirubin processing.

Gall Bladder

- Small, pear-shaped organ beneath the liver.
- Stores, concentrates, and releases bile into the duodenum via the bile duct for fat emulsification.

Pancreas

- A retroperitoneal gland with exocrine and endocrine functions.
- Produces digestive enzymes (amylase, lipase, proteases) and hormones (insulin and glucagon) for glucose regulation.

Small Intestine

- Consists of three sections: duodenum, jejunum, and ileum.
- Main site for enzymatic digestion and nutrient absorption.

Functions:

- Absorption of amino acids, sugars, fatty acids, vitamins, and minerals.
- Continued digestion of macronutrients.

- Facilitates water and electrolyte absorption.

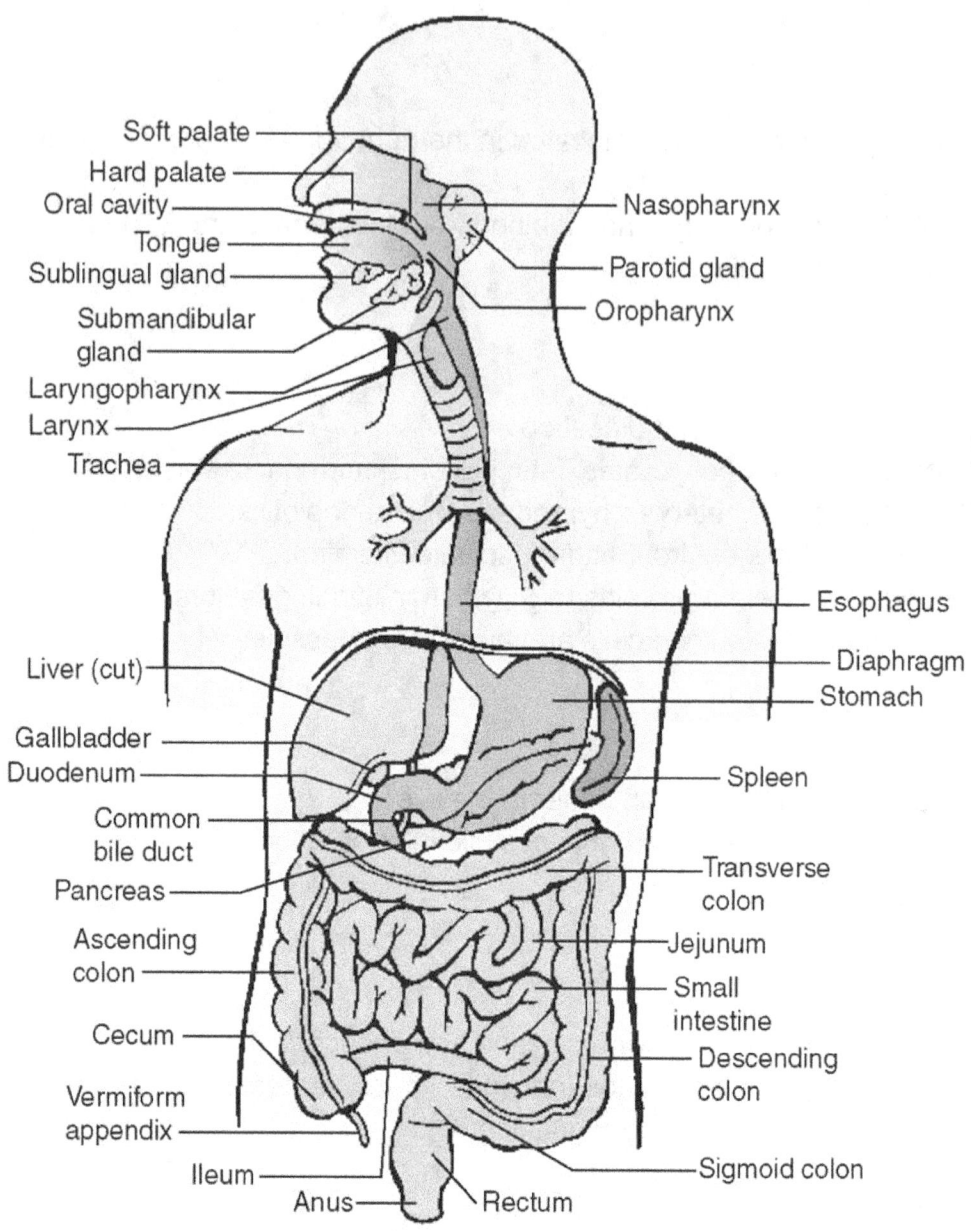

Fig. 1.10.1 Digestive System

Source: Clevland Clinic

Large Intestine

- Comprises caecum, colon (ascending, transverse, descending, sigmoid), rectum, and anal canal.

Functions:

- Absorption of water, electrolytes, and vitamins (especially K and folic acid).
- Storage and controlled expulsion of faeces.
- Hosts beneficial gut microbiota that synthesise essential vitamins.

Spleen

- Located in the left upper abdomen.
- Although not a digestive organ, it is intimately related to abdominal and immune function.
- Filters blood, recycles aged red blood cells, and stores lymphocytes and platelets.

Kidneys

- Paired retroperitoneal organs are positioned on either side of the spine.
- Regulate fluid and electrolyte balance, remove metabolic waste via urine, and contribute to acid–base homeostasis.
- Associated with the adrenal glands, which secrete aldosterone, adrenaline, and noradrenaline hormones.

An in-depth understanding of abdominal organ functions and pathologies enhances the acupuncturist's diagnostic precision and point selection, especially when treating digestive, metabolic, and systemic complaints.

Clinical Applications

1. Functional gastrointestinal disorders (FGIDs)
Conditions like irritable bowel syndrome (IBS), functional dyspepsia, and bloating respond well to acupuncture. Points such as ST 36, CV 12, and SP 4 are commonly used to relieve pain, regulate motility, and reduce visceral hypersensitivity.

2. Nausea and vomiting
Acupuncture at PC 6 is especially effective for treating nausea caused by pregnancy, chemotherapy, or post-operative recovery. It reduces activity in brain areas related to nausea perception and promotes gastric emptying.

3. Acid reflux and gastritis
Points like CV 12, ST 36, and PC 6 reduce acid production, improve gastric lining repair, and lower inflammation. Acupuncture is often used in conjunction with dietary changes to manage reflux and upper gastrointestinal distress.

4. constipation and diarrhoea

Acupuncture restores intestinal rhythm and improves stool frequency and consistency. ST 25, ST 37, and SP 15 are commonly selected for regulating the bowel. It is effective in both spastic and sluggish bowel states.

5. Inflammatory bowel disease (IBD)

In conditions such as ulcerative colitis or Crohn's disease, acupuncture can help reduce mucosal inflammation, immune overactivity, and abdominal cramping. It may be used as an adjunct to medical treatment to promote remission and improve quality of life.

6. Liver and gallbladder dysfunction

Acupuncture influences bile secretion and liver enzyme activity, and it is beneficial in conditions such as gallbladder stasis, fatty liver disease, or hepatic detoxification imbalance. Points such as LV 3, GB 34, and ST 25 help promote the smooth flow of liver qi and digestion.

- Dr. Pardeshi Acupuncture -

1.11 Respiratory System

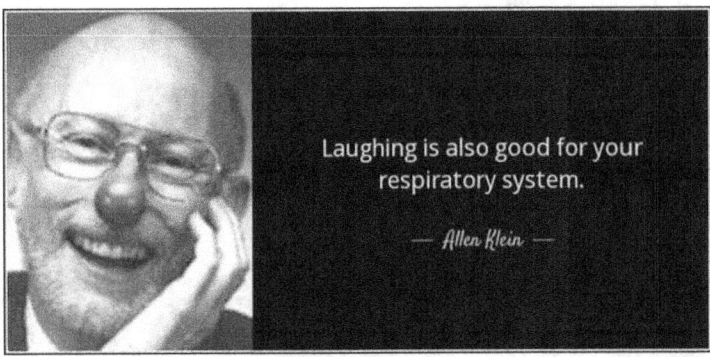

The respiratory system is responsible for exchanging gases essential for life, absorbing oxygen, and eliminating carbon dioxide. It comprises the nasal cavity, pharynx, larynx, trachea, bronchi, lungs, and alveoli. Air enters the body as the diaphragm contracts and the chest expands, creating negative pressure that draws air into the lungs via the trachea.

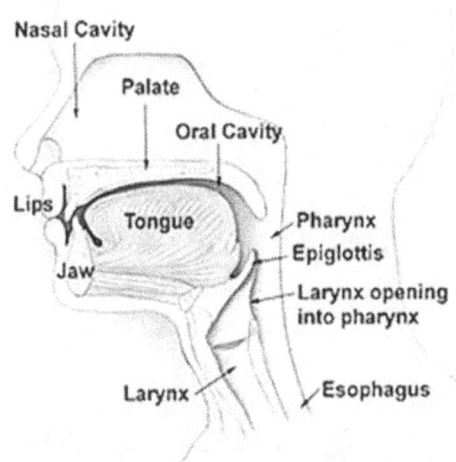

Fig. 1.11.1 Upper Respiratory Tract

As inhaled air passes through the upper respiratory tract, it is filtered, humidified, and warmed to near body temperature. This conditioning process primarily occurs in the nasal cavity, where the nasal mucosa and paranasal sinuses moisten and warm the air. Nasal hairs (vibrissae) trap large particles, while sneezing is a protective reflex to expel irritants. The nose also contributes to speech articulation through nasalisation, and the sinuses function as resonating chambers that modify vocal quality. However, sneezing may aerosolise infectious droplets, facilitating disease transmission.

The pharynx, situated in the throat, serves as a crucial anatomical junction between the respiratory and digestive systems. It connects the mouth to the oesophagus and the nasal cavity to the trachea. The nasopharynx connects the upper throat to the nasal cavity, and the Eustachian tubes link it to the middle ears, facilitating pressure regulation. The larynx, or voice box, contains the vocal cords and the epiglottis, which prevent aspiration of food and liquid during swallowing. In children, the subglottic larynx is the narrowest portion of the upper airway and is a critical site in paediatric airway assessment. The tonsils and adenoids, composed of lymphoid tissue, form part of the immune system, providing early defence against airborne pathogens.

The lungs are the primary organs of respiration. Air reaches them through progressively branching airways: the trachea, bronchi, bronchioles, alveolar ducts, and alveoli. The lungs contain an estimated 2,400 km of airways and 300–500 million alveoli—tiny air sacs where gas exchange occurs. Oxygen from inhaled air diffuses across the alveolar membrane into capillaries, while carbon dioxide and water vapour pass from the blood into the alveoli to be exhaled.

Pulmonary circulation is unique:

- **Deoxygenated blood** from the right side of the heart is transported to the lungs.
- After gas exchange, **oxygenated blood** returns to the left side of the heart and is pumped to the rest of the body.
- The lungs also receive a separate **bronchial blood supply** to nourish their tissues.

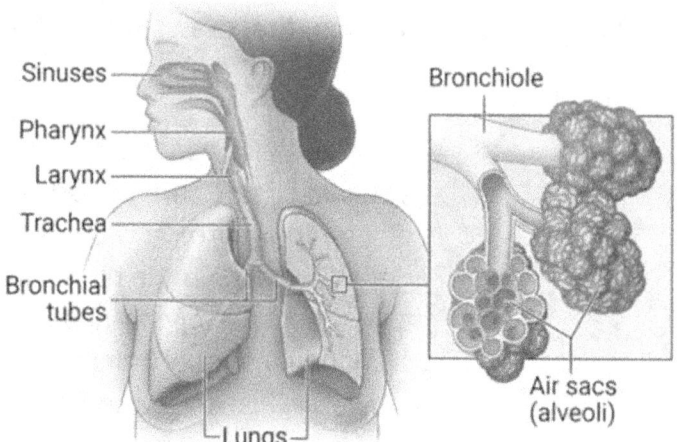

Fig. 1.11.2 Structure Of Lung of Lungs

This continuous exchange supports homeostasis, maintaining the body's internal balance of oxygen and carbon dioxide.

Beyond respiration, the system serves other vital roles:

- **Phonation** (voice production) via the vocal cords
- **Olfaction** (sense of smell) through receptors in the nasal cavity
- **Reflex protection** via sneezing and coughing to expel irritants
- **Air filtration** using mucous and ciliated epithelium, which trap and remove particulates before they reach the alveoli

In acupuncture, respiratory disorders such as asthma, bronchitis, allergic rhinitis, and chronic cough are often addressed through targeted stimulation of points that influence autonomic tone, bronchial dilation, and immune response.

Clinical indications and point examples

Condition	Common Points Used	Clinical Effect
Asthma	LU 1, LU 5, UBL 13, Dingchuan (EX-B1), ST 36	Reduces bronchospasm, improves breathing
Allergic rhinitis	LI 20, LI 4, GV 23, Yintang, Bitong	Relieves nasal blockage and sneezing
Chronic bronchitis / COPD	LU 7, ST 36, BL 13, CV 17	Improves oxygenation and immune resilience
Acute upper respiratory infection	LI 4, LU 7, LI 11, GB 20	Shortens the duration and intensity of symptoms
Sinusitis	LI 20, Bitong, Yintang, ST 8, LI 4	Relieves sinus congestion and pressure
Post-COVID recovery	ST 36, LU 9, CV 17, SP 6	Enhances lung repair and energy restoration

Summary

Acupuncture is an effective and holistic tool for treating respiratory conditions. Addressing the symptoms and underlying physiological dysfunctions, such as inflammation, immune imbalance, and autonomic dysregulation, offers a valuable complementary approach to managing a wide range of pulmonary disorders.

-Dr. Pardeshi Acupuncture-

1.12 Reproductive System

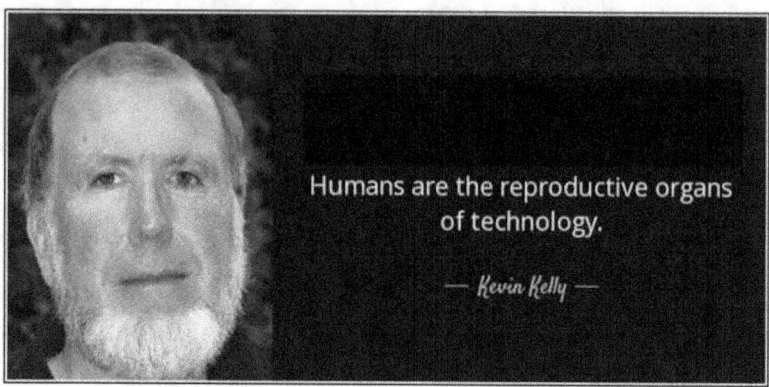

Humans are the reproductive organs of technology.

— *Kevin Kelly* —

The reproductive system ensures the continuation of human life by producing, transporting, and uniting gametes and supporting the development of offspring. It comprises a coordinated network of primary and secondary reproductive organs, along with complex hormonal regulation.

Core Functions of the Reproductive System

1. **Hormone Production**
   The ovaries in females and the testes in males secrete essential reproductive hormones. These hormones regulate sexual development, gamete production, the menstrual cycle, and secondary sexual characteristics.
2. **Gamete Production**
   - **Ovaries** produce ova (eggs), the female gametes.
   - **Testes** produce spermatozoa (sperm), the male gametes.
3. **Gamete Transport**
   Secondary structures, such as the fallopian tubes and vas deferens, act as conduits, transporting gametes toward fertilization sites.
4. **Support of Offspring Development**
   The uterus provides an ideal environment for the fertilised ovum to implant and develop into a foetus. It supplies nutrients, protection, and structural support throughout pregnancy.

Male Reproductive System

The field of andrology deals with male reproductive health, analogous to gynaecology in females. Male reproductive organs are predominantly external and include:

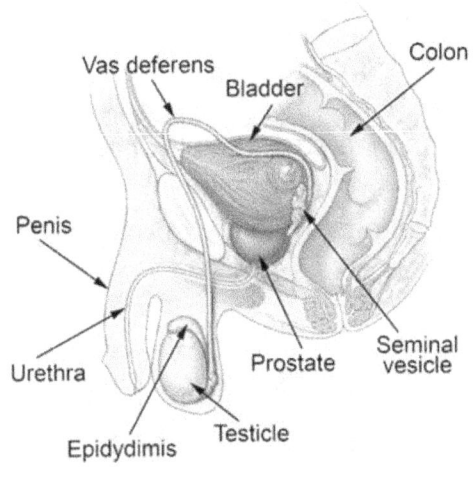

Fig. 1.12.1 Male Reproductive Organs

External Organs:

o **Penis**: Also, part of the urinary system, it delivers sperm during ejaculation.
o **Scrotum**: Encloses and protects the testes, maintaining optimal temperature for spermatogenesis.
• **Internal Organs**:
o **Testes**: Produce sperm and testosterone.
o **Epididymis**: Stores and matures sperm.
o **Vas deferens**: Transports sperm to the ejaculatory ducts.
o **Seminal vesicles**, **prostate**, and **bulbo-urethral glands**: Secrete seminal fluid, which nourishes and protects sperm.

Female Reproductive System

Internal Reproductive Organs:

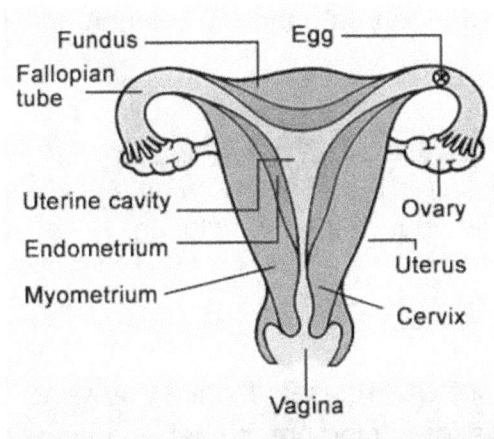

Fig. 1.12.2 Female Reproductive Organs

Ovaries: Release ova and secrete oestrogen and progesterone.

• **Fallopian tubes**: Transport ova toward the uterus and serve as the site of fertilisation.
• **Uterus**: Supports implantation and foetal development.
• **Vagina**: Muscular canal for intercourse and childbirth.
• **Placenta** (during pregnancy): Facilitates nutrient and gas exchange between mother and foetus.

External Reproductive Organs:

• **Vulva**: External genitalia including the labia and vestibule.
• **Clitoris**: The Erectile tissue involved in sexual arousal.

Acupuncture may be integrated into both male and female fertility protocols, as well as in the management of reproductive disorders such as dysmenorrhoea, endometriosis, erectile dysfunction, and hormonal imbalance.

Clinical applications

1. Infertility (female and male)
Acupuncture improves ovulation, enhances egg quality, and increases the likelihood of successful implantation. It is often used alongside assisted reproductive technologies (ART) like IVF. In men, it enhances sperm count, motility, and morphology. Commonly used points include ST 36, SP 6, CV 4, KI 3, and LV 3.

2. Menstrual disorders
Acupuncture regulates the menstrual cycle and relieves pain in conditions such as dysmenorrhoea, amenorrhoea, and irregular periods. Specific points, including SP 6, CV 3, ST 29, and LI 4, regulate uterine blood flow and hormonal balance.

3. Polycystic ovary syndrome (PCOS)
Acupuncture helps restore ovulation, reduce androgen excess, and improve insulin sensitivity. Frequent points include SP 6, ST 25, CV 6, and UB 23, often used in combination with electroacupuncture.

4. Menopause and perimenopause
Acupuncture alleviates hot flashes, night sweats, mood swings, and insomnia without hormone replacement therapy. Points such as KI 3, SP 6, GV 20, and HT 7 nourish kidney yin and calm the mind.

5. Sexual dysfunction
For conditions like erectile dysfunction, premature ejaculation, or low libido, acupuncture improves pelvic blood flow, testosterone levels, and nervous system regulation. Common points include CV 4, ST 36, SP 6, and UB 52.

6. Pregnancy support
Acupuncture is used to manage early pregnancy symptoms (nausea, fatigue), prevent miscarriage, and prepare for labour. It is also effective for turning breech babies using point UB 67 and promoting cervical ripening near term.

-Dr. Pardeshi Acupuncture-

1.13 Urinary System

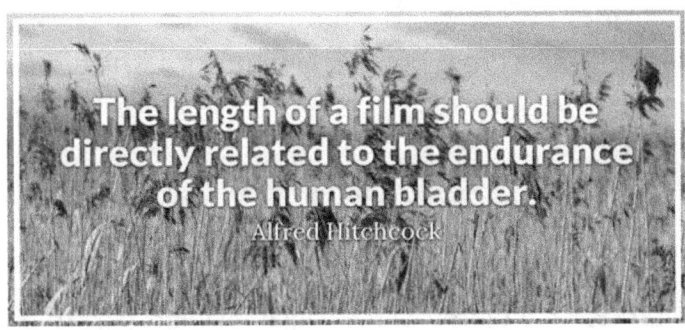

The urinary system plays a vital role in maintaining the body's internal environment. It eliminates waste products, regulates fluid and electrolyte balance, and maintains acid–base homeostasis. This system comprises the kidneys, ureters, bladder, and urethra, functioning together in a tightly regulated sequence.

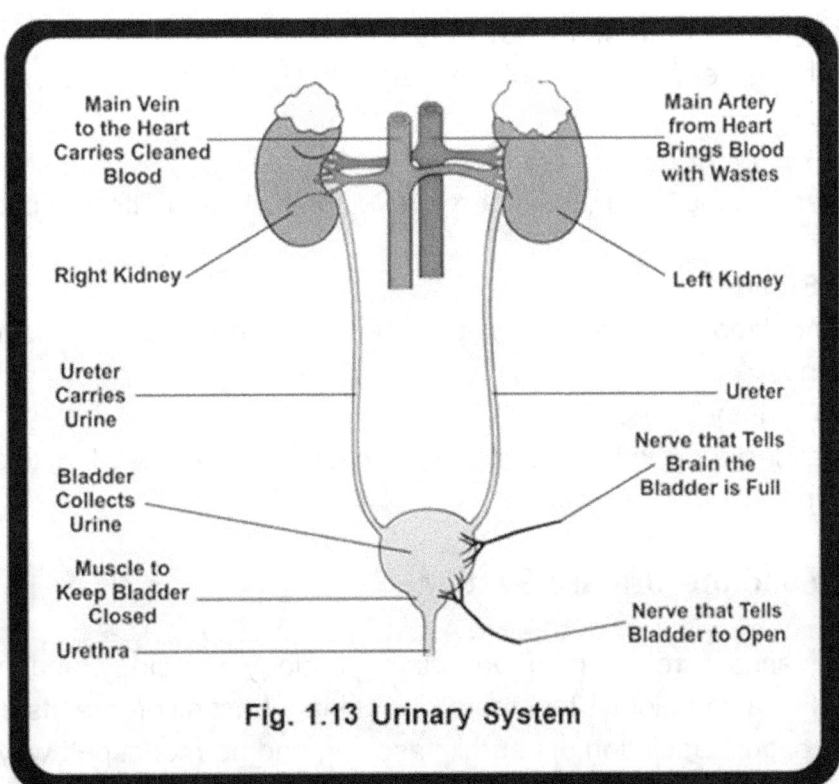

Fig. 1.13 Urinary System

Core Functions of the Urinary System

1. **Filtration of Blood**
   The **kidneys** act as the body's filtration units. They remove metabolic waste,

excess electrolytes, and surplus water from the bloodstream while preserving essential substances.

2. **Formation of Urine**
   Filtered waste and water are processed into **urine**, which reflects the body's waste load and hydration status.
3. **Urine Transport**
   Ureters, muscular tubes, transport urine from each kidney to the **urinary bladder**.
4. **Urine Storage**
   The **bladder** temporarily stores urine until it is voluntarily released.
5. **Urine Elimination**
   During **micturition**, urine exits the body through the **urethra**, regulated by involuntary and voluntary sphincters.

Common Disorders of the Urinary System

- **Urinary Tract Infections (UTIs)**
  Caused by bacterial invasion of the urinary tract, commonly affecting the bladder or urethra.
- **Urinary Incontinence**
  Involuntary leakage of urine is more prevalent in older adults and postpartum females.
- **Kidney Stones**
  Crystalline deposits formed from concentrated minerals, often causing severe flank pain.
- **Chronic Kidney Disease (CKD)**
  A gradual decline in kidney function over time, potentially leading to end-stage renal failure.

Acupuncture and the Urinary System

Although not a standard treatment modality in nephrology or urology, acupuncture has shown potential as a complementary therapy in urinary tract disorders. Its effects may be mediated through modulation of neural, vascular, and hormonal pathways.

1. Pain Relief

Acupuncture effectively manages renal colic, pelvic pain, and discomfort associated with urinary tract infections (UTIs) by stimulating the release of endorphins and modulating nociceptive transmission.

2. Urinary Incontinence

Clinical studies indicate that acupuncture may improve urge and stress incontinence by influencing detrusor muscle tone, sphincter function, and autonomic nerve regulation.

3. Kidney Function Support

In early-stage chronic kidney disease (CKD), acupuncture may promote renal perfusion and reduce inflammatory mediators, potentially slowing disease progression.

4. Stress Reduction and Autonomic Balance

Stress, a known contributor to urinary dysfunction, can be effectively managed with acupuncture, promoting parasympathetic tone and aiding in bladder control.

As acupuncture is increasingly integrated into integrative medicine frameworks, understanding the physiology and pathophysiology of the urinary system enhances the clinician's ability to select appropriate acupuncture points and track patient outcomes effectively.

-Dr. Pardeshi Acupuncture-

1.14 Integumentary System

**The Best Foundation You Can Wear
Is Glowing Healthy Skin**

The integumentary system is the body's outermost protective covering, comprising the skin, hair, nails, sweat glands, and sebaceous glands. It serves as a critical barrier against environmental hazards, including pathogens, ultraviolet radiation, and physical injury. Beyond protection, the system plays vital roles in regulating body temperature, excreting waste products, synthesizing vitamin D, and enabling sensory perception through nerve endings. The skin itself is a dynamic organ composed of distinct layers, including the epidermis, dermis, and hypodermis, each contributing to its structure and function. The integumentary system reflects overall health and is essential to maintaining homeostasis, making it fundamental to human physiology and medicine.

Core Functions of the Integumentary System

1. **Protection**
   The skin acts as a physical and immunological barrier, shielding the body from mechanical trauma, microbial invasion, chemical exposure, and harmful ultraviolet (UV) radiation.
2. **Thermoregulation**
   Sweat glands and cutaneous blood vessels help regulate body temperature through evaporation and vasodilation/constriction, maintaining thermal balance.
3. **Sensation**
   The skin houses numerous sensory receptors that detect touch, pressure, pain, temperature, and vibration. These receptors allow interaction with the environment and facilitate protective reflexes.
4. **Vitamin D Synthesis**
   Exposure to sunlight triggers the conversion of 7-dehydrocholesterol in the skin to vitamin D_3, essential for calcium metabolism and bone health.
5. **Excretion**
   The skin excretes waste products, such as urea, ammonia, and salts, through sweat, which assists in waste removal and cooling.

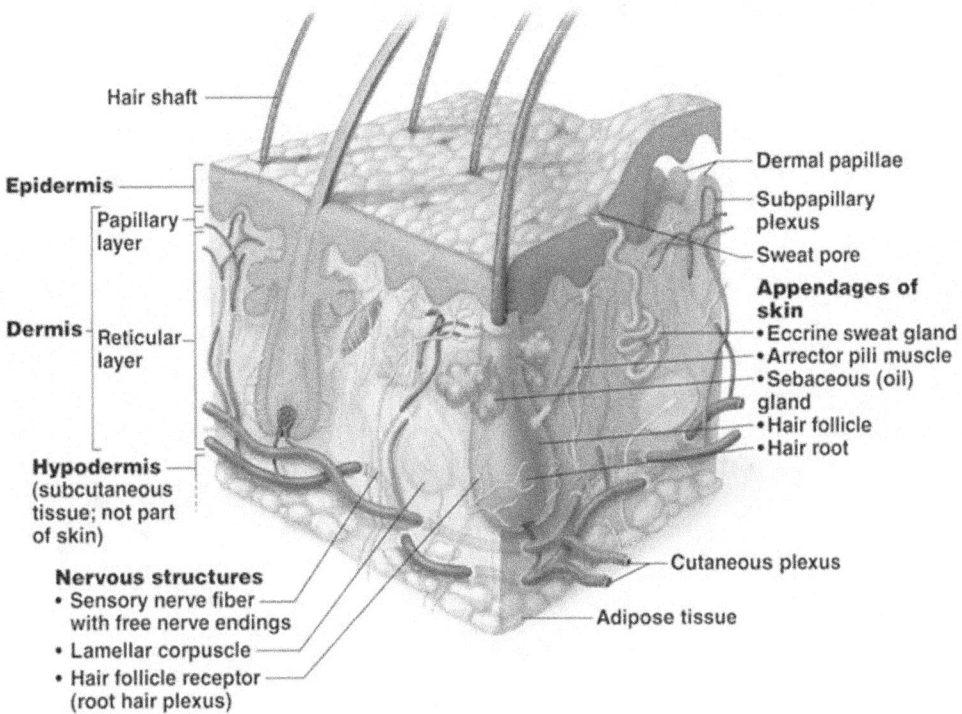

Fig. 1.14 Integumentary System

Acupuncture and the Integumentary System

Acupuncture, traditionally used to maintain systemic balance and alleviate pain, is now being investigated for its potential impact on skin health, inflammatory modulation, and pain perception. Emerging research suggests several potential benefits:

1. Management of Dermatological Conditions

Acupuncture may be beneficial in conditions such as acne, eczema, psoriasis, and urticaria. It may modulate immune and inflammatory responses, improve local circulation, and promote skin healing.

2. Pain Relief in Skin and Musculoskeletal Disorders

Chronic conditions affecting skin and connective tissue (e.g., postherpetic neuralgia, neuropathic pain, fibromyalgia) often respond to acupuncture via the modulation of nociceptive pathways and endogenous opioid release.

3. Stress and Psycho-dermatology

Psychological stress is known to exacerbate many skin conditions. Acupuncture's stress-reducing and anxiolytic effects may support dermatological health indirectly by regulating neuroendocrine responses.

Understanding the structure and function of the integumentary system enables acupuncturists to appreciate skin-related manifestations of systemic imbalance more effectively and design effective treatment strategies for dermatological and pain syndromes.

-Dr. Pardeshi Acupuncture-

1.15 Cardiovascular System

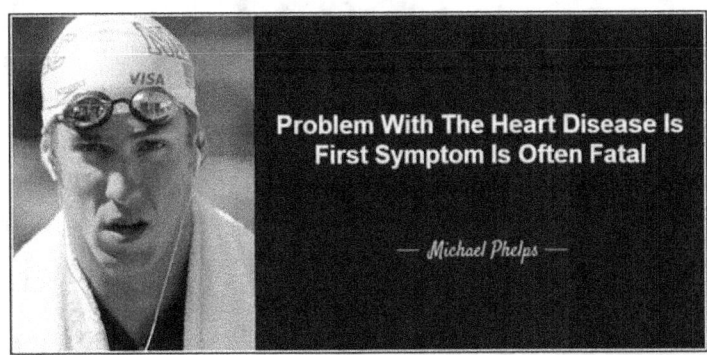

The cardiovascular or circulatory system transports vital substances throughout the body. It comprises the heart, blood vessels (including arteries, veins, and capillaries), and blood, and is closely integrated with the lymphatic system.

Structure and Components

- **Heart**: A muscular organ that serves as the central pump, propelling blood throughout the body.
- **Blood Vessels**:
  - **Arteries** carry oxygenated blood away from the heart.
  - **Veins** return deoxygenated blood to the heart.
  - **Capillaries** facilitate the exchange of gases, nutrients, and waste at the tissue level.
- **Blood**: A fluid connective tissue composed of plasma, red blood cells (erythrocytes), white blood cells (leukocytes), and platelets (thrombocytes).
- **Lymphatic System**: Although structurally separate, the lymphatic system complements the cardiovascular system by draining interstitial fluid, facilitating immune responses, and transporting lipids.

Types of Circulation

1. **Pulmonary Circulation**
   Carries deoxygenated blood from the heart to the lungs for oxygenation and returns oxygen-rich blood to the heart.
2. **Systemic Circulation**
   Distributes oxygenated blood from the heart to all body tissues, and returns deoxygenated blood to the heart.
   - **Macro-circulation**: Involves major arteries and veins.

- ○ **Micro-circulation**: Involves arterioles, capillaries, and venules where exchange occurs.

The human cardiovascular system is closed; blood remains within vessels at all times. Exchange with tissues occurs via diffusion through capillary walls into the interstitial fluid, which bathes and nourishes cells.

In contrast, the lymphatic system is an open system that collects and returns interstitial fluid to the bloodstream, serving critical immune functions.

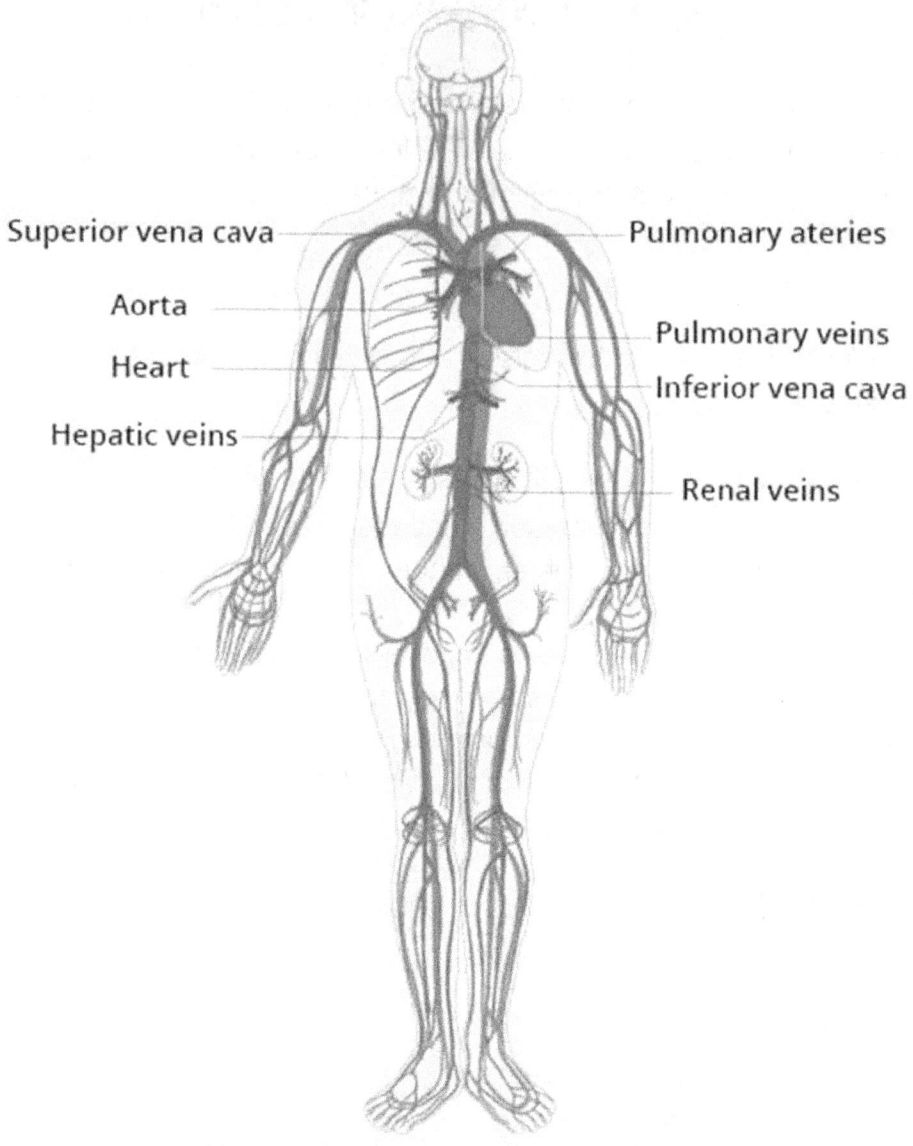

Fig. 1.15 Cardio-Vascular System

Blood Volume and Composition

- The average adult circulates 4.7 to 5.7 litres of blood, roughly **7%** of body weight.
- Blood consists of:
  - **Plasma**: The liquid matrix, transporting dissolved substances.
  - **Red blood cells**: Carry oxygen via haemoglobin.
  - **White blood cells**: Defend against infection.
  - **Platelets**: Facilitate clotting and wound repair.

Functions of the Cardiovascular System

- **Transport**: Delivers oxygen, carbon dioxide, nutrients, hormones, and metabolic waste.
- **Protection**: White blood cells and immune proteins defend against infection.
- **Regulation**:
  - Maintains pH and electrolyte balance.
  - Distributes heat to regulate body temperature.
  - Maintains fluid balance and blood pressure.
  - Aids wound healing and homeostasis post-injury.

Acupuncture and the Cardiovascular System

Acupuncture has a well-documented impact on the cardiovascular system through its effects on autonomic regulation, vascular tone, cardiac rhythm, and blood pressure. It influences both central and peripheral circulation, offering therapeutic benefits in the treatment of hypertension, arrhythmias, angina, and heart failure.

Autonomic modulation

Acupuncture helps balance the sympathetic and parasympathetic nervous systems. Stimulation of specific points such as PC 6, HT 7, and ST 36 activates brain regions like the hypothalamus and medulla, which regulate cardiac output and vascular resistance. This modulation reduces heart rate, improves variability, and improves autonomic balance in stress-induced or functional cardiac disorders.

Regulation of blood pressure

Acupuncture has antihypertensive effects mediated by decreased sympathetic outflow, improved baroreceptor sensitivity, and increased nitric oxide release. Studies have shown that regular acupuncture at points such as LI 11, ST 36, and KI 3 lowers systolic and diastolic blood pressure in patients with mild to moderate hypertension.

Improvement of cardiac function

In conditions like ischemic heart disease or heart failure, acupuncture may improve myocardial perfusion and reduce cardiac workload. PC 6 is commonly used to alleviate chest pain, calm palpitations, and reduce anxiety associated with angina. Electroacupuncture can further enhance these effects by stimulating vagal tone.

Circulatory and microvascular effects

Acupuncture enhances peripheral circulation and microvascular perfusion. It dilates arterioles and improves capillary blood flow, which helps treat conditions like Raynaud's phenomenon, diabetic microangiopathy, or chronic venous insufficiency. Points such as SP 6, ST 36, and UB 17 support blood flow and vessel integrity.

Anti-inflammatory and antithrombotic effects

Acupuncture may reduce systemic inflammation and platelet aggregation, contributing to cardiovascular protection. These effects are beneficial in preventing atherosclerosis and thrombosis. Anti-inflammatory cytokine modulation and improved lipid metabolism have been observed in clinical trials with regular acupuncture treatment.

Psycho-cardiological relevance

Given the strong link between emotional stress and cardiovascular disease, acupuncture's calming effect on the central nervous system reduces anxiety, insomnia, and sympathetic overactivity. This contributes indirectly to better cardiac outcomes, particularly in stress-related hypertension and arrhythmias.

Summary

Acupuncture offers a multidimensional approach to cardiovascular health. By modulating autonomic tone, improving circulation, lowering blood pressure, and calming the mind, it serves as a valuable complementary therapy in both the prevention and management of heart and vascular conditions.

-Dr. Pardeshi Acupuncture-

2 Human Surface Anatomy

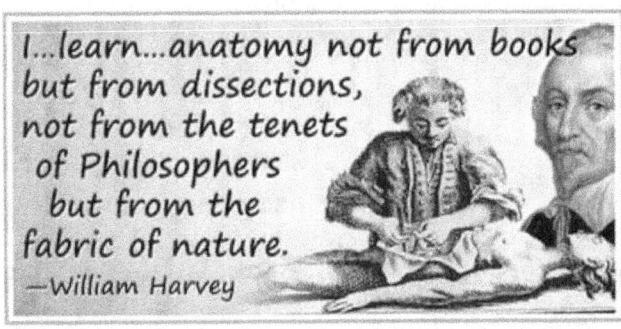

Surface anatomy, also called superficial or visual anatomy, involves studying external body features that are visible or easily felt without dissection. This includes structures like muscles, bones, and blood vessels. Understanding surface anatomy gives acupuncturists a basic map of internal structures, improving diagnostic precision and treatment effectiveness.

Importance of Surface Anatomy in Acupuncture

- **Precise Point Location**: Surface landmarks guide acupuncturists in accurately identifying acupuncture points.
- **Comprehending Deeper Relationships**: Many surface features correspond to internal organs, facilitating an understanding of the effects of stimulation.
- **Clinical Collaboration**: A shared understanding of surface anatomy facilitates effective communication among healthcare providers.

Proficiency in surface anatomy allows acupuncturists to ensure consistency in anatomical descriptions.

- Develop keen observational skills for identifying anatomical landmarks.
- Understand the interrelationship between external and internal structures.
- Perform needling safely and effectively to achieve optimal therapeutic benefits.

Anatomical Position Fig 2.1

The standard anatomical position is a universally accepted reference posture used in anatomy to ensure clear and consistent descriptions of body structures and their locations. In this position, the individual stands upright with the body facing forward, feet flat and slightly apart, arms at the sides, and palms turned forward. The head is level, and the eyes are directed straight ahead. This orientation provides a common framework for anatomical terminology, allowing directional terms such as "anterior," "posterior," "medial," and "lateral" to be used without ambiguity, regardless of the subject's actual body position during observation or dissection.

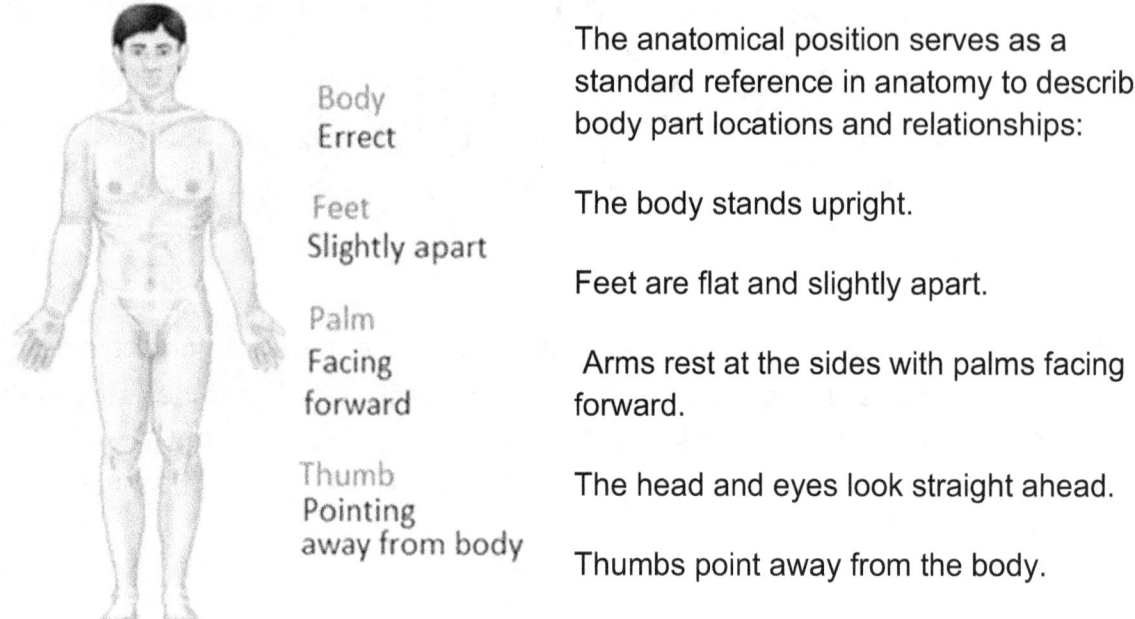

The anatomical position serves as a standard reference in anatomy to describe body part locations and relationships:

Body Errect

The body stands upright.

Feet Slightly apart

Feet are flat and slightly apart.

Palm Facing forward

Arms rest at the sides with palms facing forward.

Thumb Pointing away from body

The head and eyes look straight ahead.

Thumbs point away from the body.

Fig. 2.1 Anatomical Position

This position forms the basis for all directional terms in anatomy, such as *anterior* (front), *posterior* (back), *medial* (toward the midline), and *lateral* (away from the midline). It also serves as a foundational reference in acupuncture for precisely locating meridians and points, enabling uniformity in teaching, practice, and research.

Anterior and Posterior Landmarks

Practitioners can achieve precise localization of meridians and points across varied body types by relying on these stable structures.Accurate identification enhances reproducibility, reduces treatment variability, and improves clinical outcomes. Thorough knowledge of surface anatomy ensures that needling remains effective and safe, whether referencing bony prominences or muscle borders.

Anterior (Front) Landmarks (Fig. 2.2)

Anterior landmarks are located on the front surface of the body and are frequently used to locate points on the Conception Vessel, Stomach, Spleen, Lung, and Heart meridians. Key anterior landmarks include:

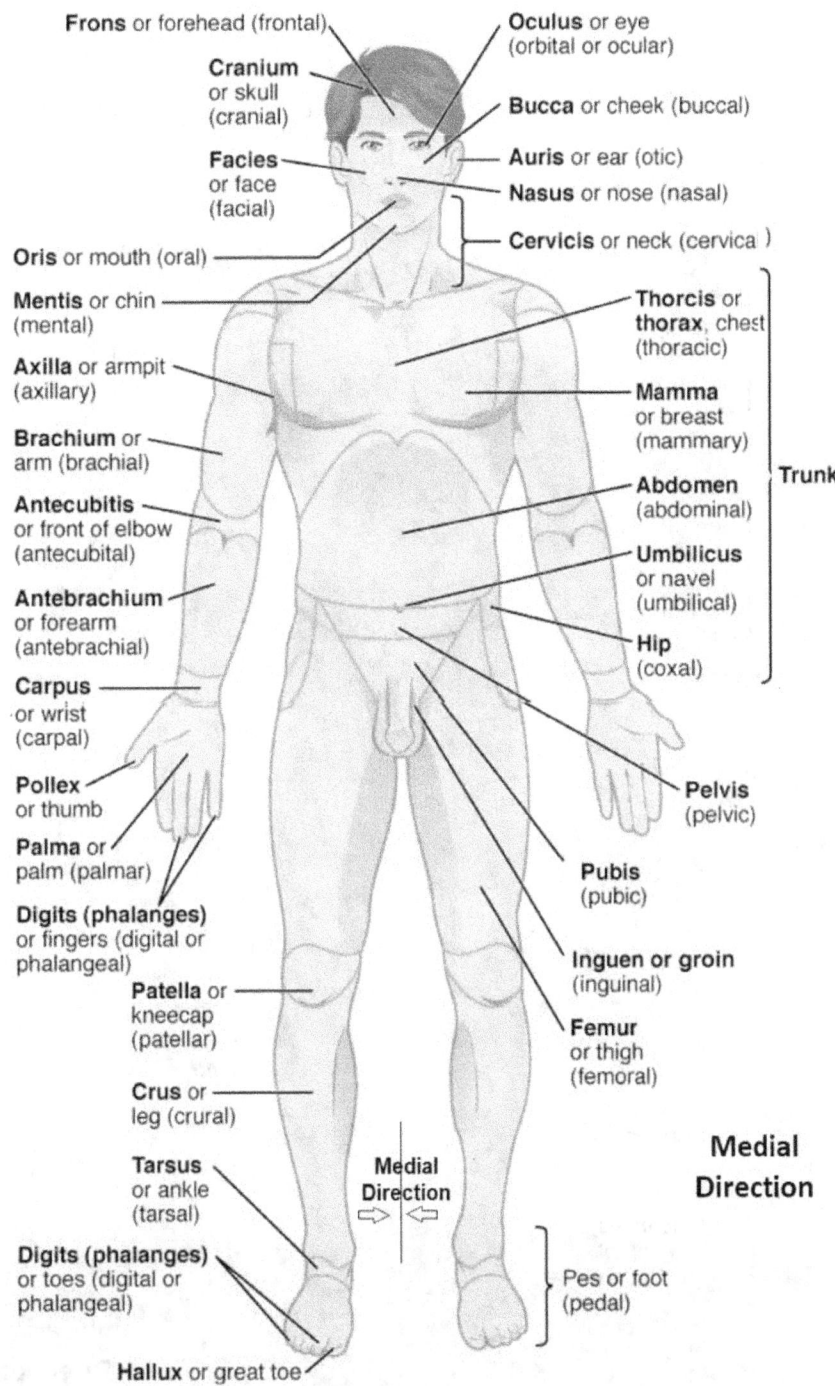

Frons or forehead (frontal)

Cranium or skull (cranial)

Facies or face (facial)

Oris or mouth (oral)

Mentis or chin (mental)

Axilla or armpit (axillary)

Brachium or arm (brachial)

Antecubitis or front of elbow (antecubital)

Antebrachium or forearm (antebrachial)

Carpus or wrist (carpal)

Pollex or thumb

Palma or palm (palmar)

Digits (phalanges) or fingers (digital or phalangeal)

Patella or kneecap (patellar)

Crus or leg (crural)

Tarsus or ankle (tarsal)

Digits (phalanges) or toes (digital or phalangeal)

Hallux or great toe

Oculus or eye (orbital or ocular)

Bucca or cheek (buccal)

Auris or ear (otic)

Nasus or nose (nasal)

Cervicis or neck (cervica)

Thorcis or thorax, chest (thoracic)

Mamma or breast (mammary)

Abdomen (abdominal)

Umbilicus or navel (umbilical)

Hip (coxal)

Trunk

Pelvis (pelvic)

Pubis (pubic)

Inguen or groin (inguinal)

Femur or thigh (femoral)

Medial Direction

Medial Direction

Pes or foot (pedal)

Fig. 2.2 Anterior Surface Anatomy

Source OpenStax

Posterior (Back) Landmarks Fig. 2.3

- **Interscapular Region**: Between the scapulae; includes the rhomboids, trapezius, and levator scapulae.
- **Infra-scapular Region**: Below the scapula and lateral to the vertebral column.

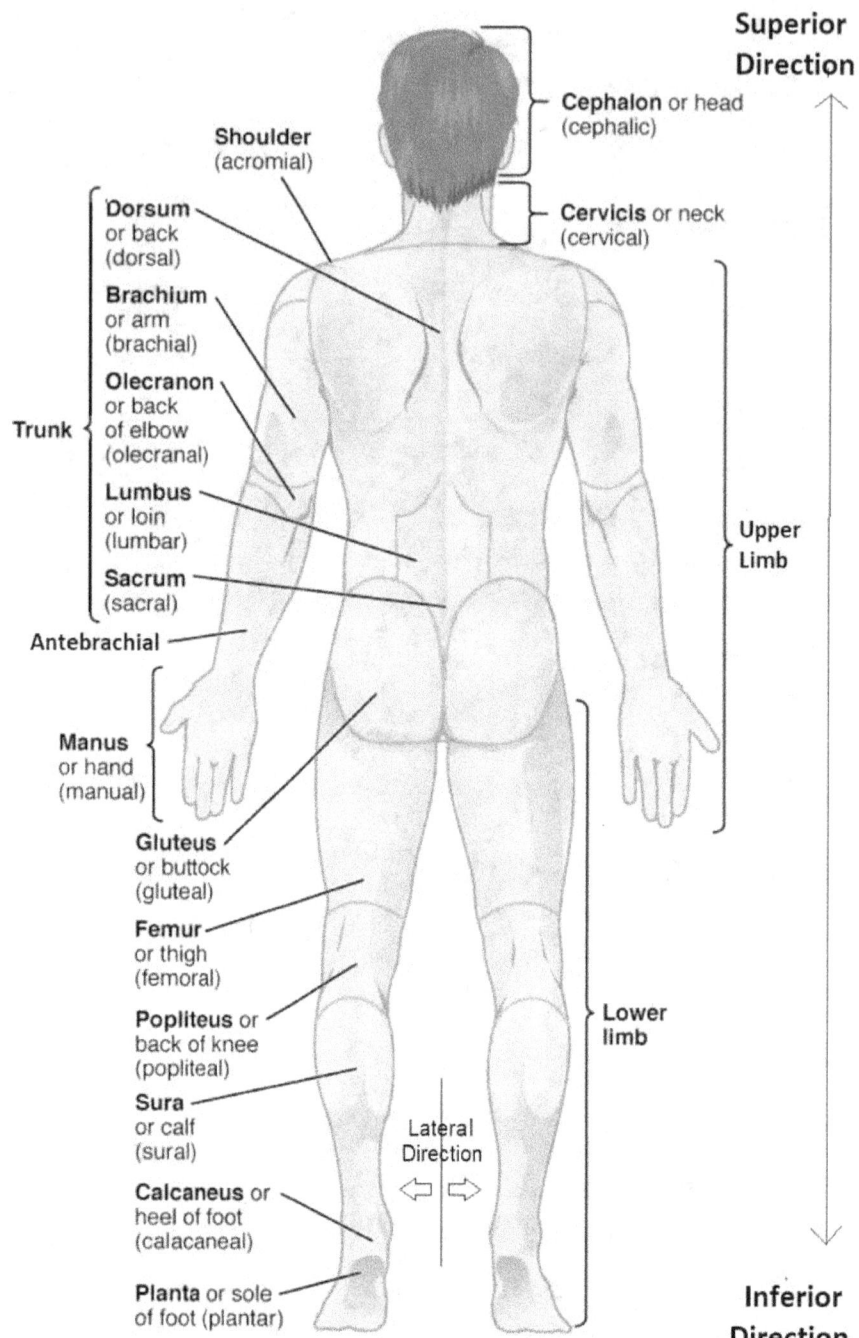

Fig. 2.3 Landmarks on Posterior Surface of Body

- **Sacral Region**: Covers the sacrum (S1–S5), a triangular bone at the spine's base.
- **Gluteal Region**: Located over the buttocks, includes major nerves like the superior and inferior gluteal nerves.

- **Perineal Region**: The diamond-shaped surface between the pubic symphysis and coccyx, essential for urogenital and GI function.
- **Vertebral Region**: Comprises cervical (C1–C7), thoracic (T1–T12), and lumbar (L1–L5) vertebrae, with sacrum and coccyx forming the terminal end. (See Chapter 1.4)

Posterior landmarks are found on the back of the body and are key to locating points on the Urinary Bladder, Governing Vessel, and Small Intestine meridians. These include:

- **External occipital protuberance (inion)** – helps locate GV 16
- **Spinous processes of vertebrae** – used to trace segmental levels (e.g., GV 14 at C7, BL 13 at T3)
- **Inferior angles of the scapula** – typically aligned with the T7 vertebra
- **Iliac crests** – level with L4, useful in lumbar and sacral point location

Clinical Importance of Acupuncture

- These landmarks help translate textbook descriptions into practice by providing consistent palpation points.
- They are crucial for scanning and needling safely, especially near vital structures (e.g., lungs, kidneys).
- They assist in aligning the patient's body symmetrically, ensuring proper meridian tracing.
- Familiarity with bony and soft tissue landmarks enhances both manual palpation and visual inspection, allowing confident identification of Ashi points and trigger zones.

Spinal Landmarks Fig 2.4

This illustration presents the posterior anatomical framework of the human torso, highlighting the spinal column as a central reference axis and delineating muscular, bony, and soft tissue zones that guide acupuncture and clinical assessment.

The vertical alignment of the spine, from the cervicothoracic junction to the sacrum, provides key orientation for vertebral-level acupuncture points (especially along the Governing Vessel and Urinary Bladder meridians). Each spinous process, from C7 to S2, acts as a tactile landmark for locating associated internal organ segments and cutaneous innervation zones (dermatomes).

Laterally, the image distinguishes between various scapular subdivisions and paraspinal reference lines, forming a grid essential for symmetrical palpation, especially when needling bilateral points, such as BL 13 (Lung Shu) or BL 23 (Kidney Shu). The 12th rib and iliac crest help define the lumbar border, beyond which the sacral foramina and posterior superior iliac spine (PSIS) guide deep pelvic and sacral treatments.

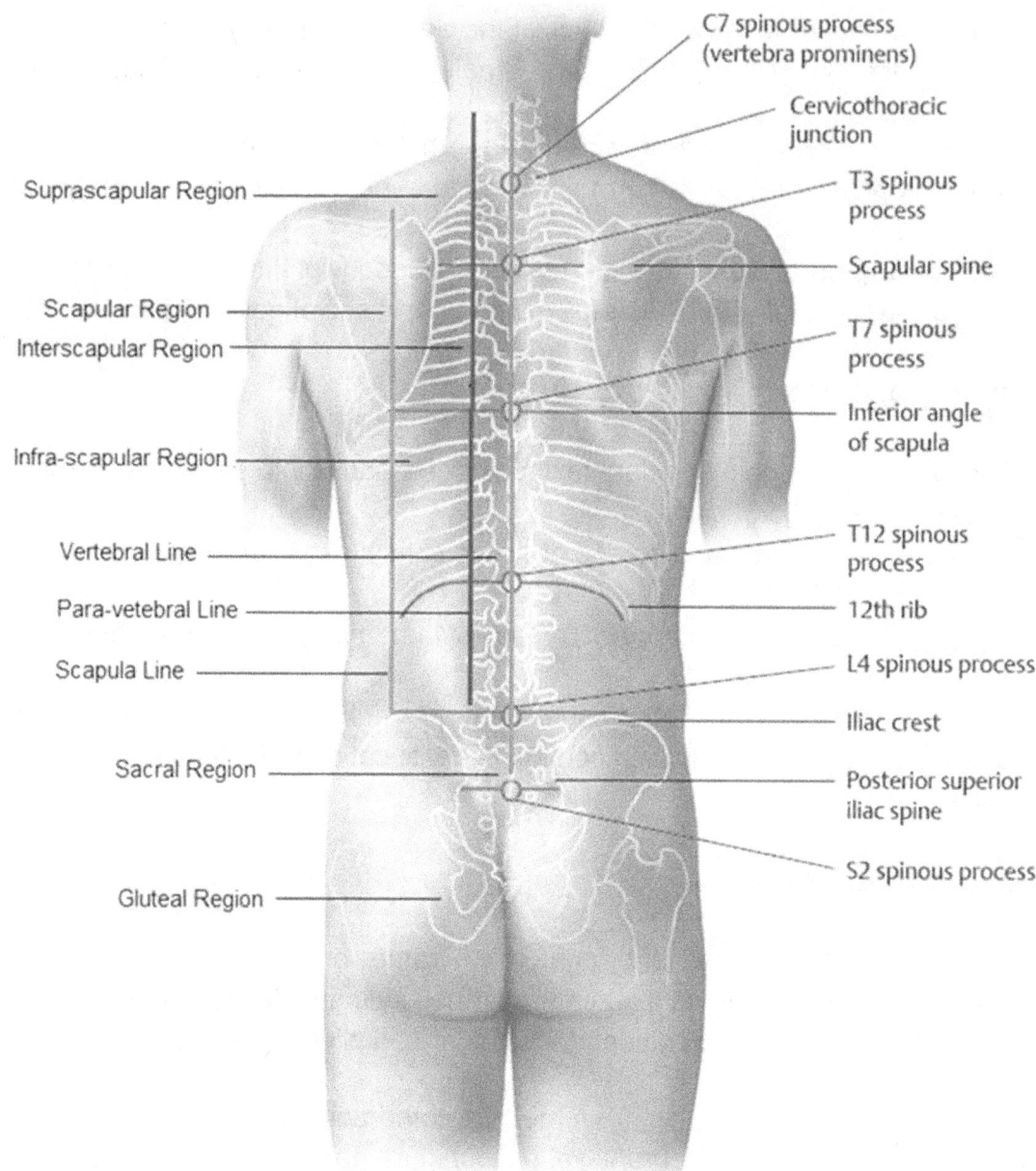

Fig. 2.4 Dorsal Trunk Landmarks

Clinically, this view supports precise localisation of:

- Shu points on the Urinary Bladder channel
- Sacral acupuncture for pelvic and genitourinary disorders
- Trigger point and myofascial work in the scapular and gluteal zones

Given its proximity to the lungs, kidneys, and neurovascular bundles, the image provides anatomical orientation and safe needle depth estimation.

Abdominal Quadrants and Regions (Fig. 2.5)

The abdomen is divided into specific regions to standardize the description of organ locations, improve clinical diagnosis, and guide procedures such as acupuncture, palpation, and surgery.

While the *four-quadrant system* (RUQ, LUQ, RLQ, LLQ) is commonly used in clinical settings, the nine-region system offers greater precision, particularly in identifying acupuncture point relations and internal organ mapping.

Division Method

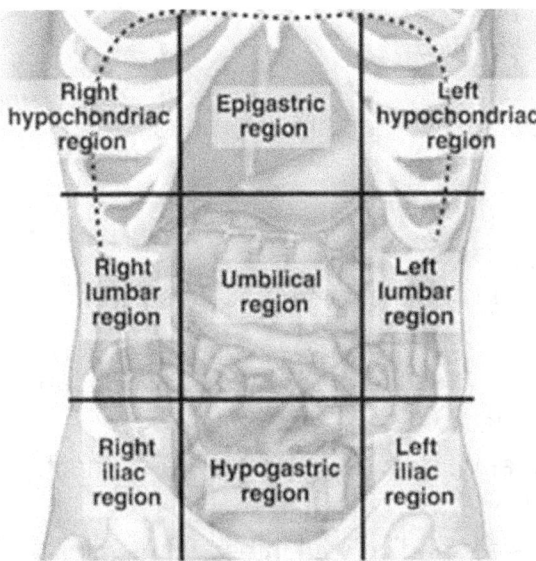

The **nine regions** are created using:

Two vertical lines (parasagittal planes) – These pass through the midpoints of the clavicles (midclavicular lines).

Two horizontal lines:

The subcostal plane is just below the rib cage (usually through the L2 vertebra).

Trans-tubercular plane – through the iliac tubercles (approx. at L5 level).

Fig. 2.5 Regions of Abdomen

Nine Abdominal Regions and Key Organs

Region	Location	Major Organs Contained
Right Hypochondriac	Upper right	Liver, gall bladder, right kidney

Region	Location	Major Organs Contained
Epigastric	Upper central	Stomach, liver, pancreas, duodenum
Left Hypochondriac	Upper left	Spleen, stomach, pancreas tail, left kidney
Right Lumbar	Mid right	Ascending colon, right kidney
Umbilical	Centre (around the navel)	Duodenum, jejunum, ileum, transverse colon
Left Lumbar	Mid left	Descending colon, left kidney
Right Iliac (Inguinal)	Lower right	Appendix, caecum, right ovary in females
Hypogastric (Pubic)	Lower centre	Bladder, uterus, sigmoid colon
Left Iliac (Inguinal)	Lower left	Sigmoid colon, descending colon, and left ovary in females

Relevance to Acupuncture and Clinical Practice

- Acupuncture points on the **abdomen** treat digestive, urinary, reproductive, and energy-regulating disorders.
- These regions help correlate symptoms with underlying organs, e.g.:
    - Pain in the right iliac region may suggest appendicitis.
    - Tenderness in the epigastric region could relate to stomach ulcers or liver conditions.
- Many abdominal points along the Conception Vessel (REN), Stomach (ST), and Spleen (SP) meridians lie within these regions.
    - E.g., REN 12 (Zhongwan) lies in the epigastric region, over the stomach and pancreas.
    - ST 25 lies in the umbilical region, corresponding with intestinal functions.

Summary

The nine-region division of the abdomen enhances diagnostic accuracy, supports safe acupuncture point location, and improves communication across medical disciplines. Acupuncturists benefit from knowing these internal-organ-to-surface correspondences to apply effective and targeted treatment protocols.

Surface Anatomy of Internal Organs, Their Nerve Roots, and Clinical Utility: Fig. 2.6

Two Anatomical Reference Lines

- **Left Side (Blue)**: Denotes the level of the **middle of vertebral bodies** (e.g., T12 body).
- **Right Side (Red)**: Denotes the level of the **spinous processes** (e.g., T12 spinous process is lower than T12 body due to spinal angulation).

Surface Anatomy and Corresponding Vertebral Levels

Here's how this helps with diagnostic and treatment relevance:

Thoracic Organs

Organ/Structure	Vertebral Level	Nerve Root (Dermatome/Myotome)
Tracheal bifurcation	T4-T5	T2–T4
Heart	T5–T7	T1–T5 (cardiac plexus)
Lungs	T2–T6	T2–T6
Esophagus	T6–T10	T6–T10 (Vagus + sympathetic)

Spinal nerves emerge from specific vertebral segments:

- **C1–C8 (Cervical)**: Neck, shoulders, upper limbs.
- **T1–T12 (Thoracic)**: Chest and abdominal wall.
- **L1–L5 (Lumbar)**: Lower abdomen, groin, thighs.
  S1–S5 (Sacral): Posterior thighs, legs, feet.
- **Co1 (Coccygeal)**: Coccyx region.

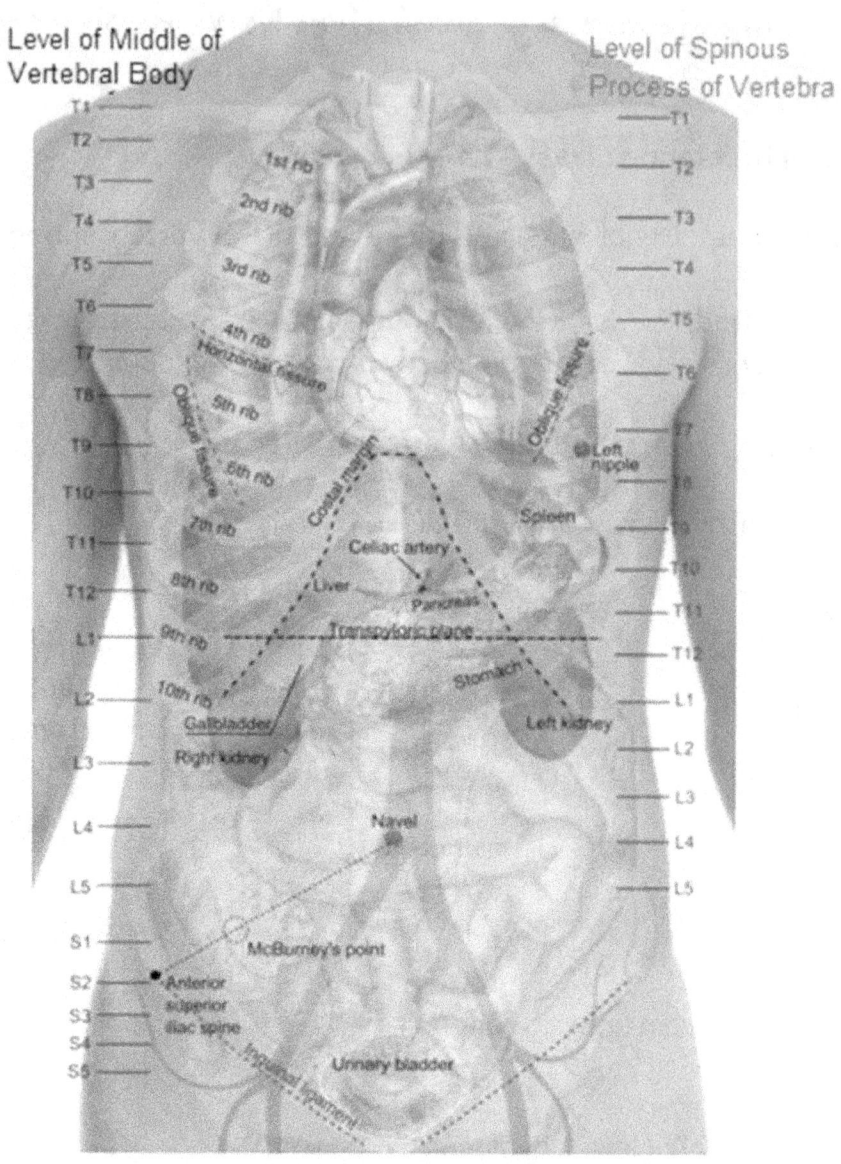

Fig. 2.6 Surface Anatomy
of Internal Organs and their Levels

Abdominal Organs

Organ	Vertebral Level	Nerve Root
Stomach	T9–T12	T6–T9
Liver	T8–T11	T6–T9 (right phrenic + lower thoracic splanchnic)
Pancreas	T11–L1	T5–T11
Kidneys	T11–L2	T10–L1
Spleen	T10	T6–T8

Pelvic Organs

Organ	Vertebral Level	Nerve Root
Urinary Bladder	S2–S4	Parasympathetic S2–S4, sympathetic T11–L2
Uterus/Ovaries	T10–L1 (ovaries), S2–S4 (uterus)	Related pelvic splanchnic nerves

Clinical Relevance to Acupuncture and Diagnosis

- **Spinous Process Palpation**: Identifying vertebral landmarks helps localise acupuncture points for internal disorders.
- **Segmental Innervation**: Visceral pain is often referred to the dermatome corresponding to its spinal level. Example:
    - **Umbilicus** at **T10**: Pain in appendicitis starts here.
    - **Gallbladder** at **T7–T9**: Referred pain to right scapula via **phrenic nerve (C3–C5)**.
- **Transverse Plane**: Lines like the **transpyloric plane** (L1) help locate key structures: pylorus, pancreas neck, duodenum, and kidneys.

Key Takeaway

This figure aids:

1. Precise surface localisation of internal organs.
2. Matching visceral complaints with spinal levels and dermatomes.
3. Targeted needling or electroacupuncture by correlating vertebral landmarks with organ dysfunction or referred pain.

Body Lines and Areas on the Trunk Fig. 2.7

These are imaginary vertical or horizontal lines that act as anatomical reference planes. They are instrumental in acupuncture, surgery, and physical examination.

Anterior Body Lines (Frontal View)

1. Midsternal Line *(red)*

- Passes through the middle of the sternum.

- Used as a median reference line in the thorax.
- Important in locating:
  - REN (Conception Vessel) acupuncture points (e.g., REN 17 at the sternal angle).
  - Auscultation of heart sounds (2nd ICS—Right of this line is the aortic area).

2. Parasternal Line

- Just lateral to the edge of the sternum.
- **Follows the costal cartilage line**.
- Helpful in:
  - Locating points like KI 22–KI 27.
  - Needle insertion with caution due to proximity to the pleura.

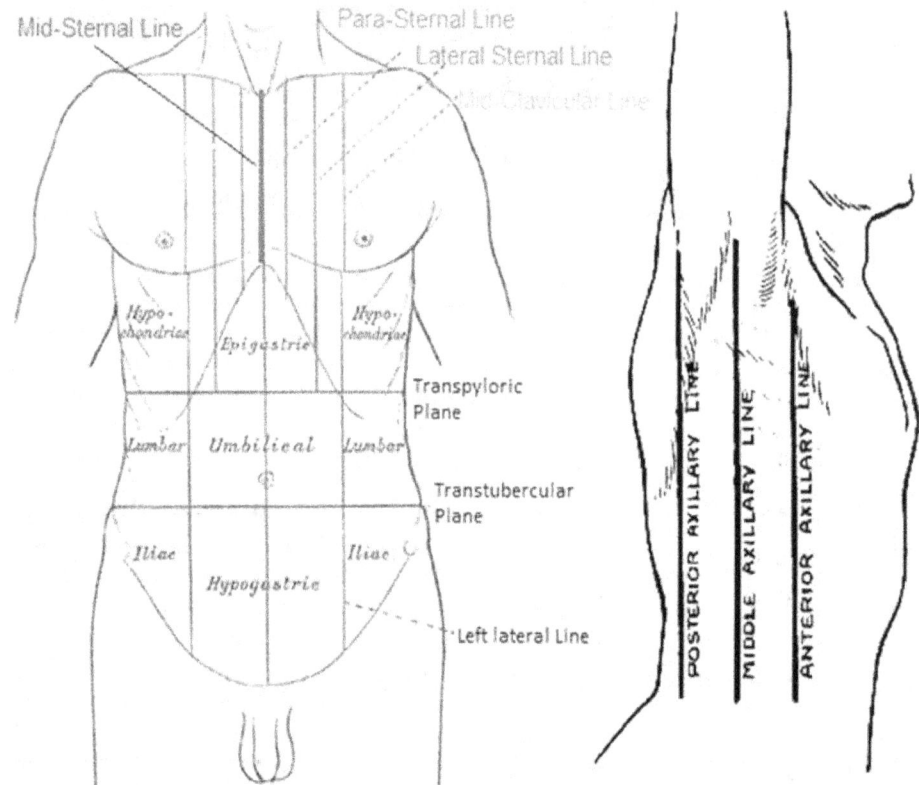

Fig. 2.7 Body Lines and Areas on Trunk

3. Lateral Sternal Line

- Further lateral than the parasternal line.

- It is not always used in clinical acupuncture, but it helps identify intercostal spaces.

4. Midclavicular Line *(blue)*

- Passes vertically through the midpoint of the clavicle.
- Vital for:
  - Defining the cardiac apex beat (5th ICS, left side).
  - Locating ST 13 to ST 18 and SP 17 to SP 21.
  - Liver and gallbladder surface projections.

Abdominal Reference Planes (Transverse)

5. Transpyloric Plane

- Horizontal line halfway between the suprasternal notch and the pubic symphysis (~L1).
- Crosses:
  - Pylorus of the stomach
  - Duodenum, pancreas neck
  - Gallbladder fundus

6. Trans tubercular Plane

- Passes through the iliac tubercles (~L5).
- Helps mark the lower border of the lumbar region and divide the abdominal quadrants.

Vertical Trunk Lines on Abdomen

- **Midclavicular Lines** again divide the abdomen into:
  - Epigastric, Umbilical, and Hypogastric regions (midline)
  - Hypochondriac, Lumbar, Iliac/Inguinal regions (sides)
- Useful in:
  - Locating ST, SP, LR, and GB meridian points.
  - Diagnosing regional abdominal tenderness or organomegaly.

Lateral Body Lines (Side View)

These run vertically down the lateral chest and help locate acupuncture points and auscultation zones.

Line	Location	Clinical Use
Anterior Axillary Line	Anterior fold of the axilla	Important for HT and LU meridians
Mid-Axillary Line	Middle of the axilla	Surface projection of the heart and lungs
Posterior Axillary Line	Posterior axillary fold	Locates scapular and dorsal points

Key Meridian Pathways and Their Surface Reference Lines with Representative Points

Meridian	Reference Line	Points Example
REN	Midsternal Line	REN 12 (Zhongwan), REN 17 (Shanzhong)
Stomach (ST)	2 cun from midline (~midclavicular)	ST 19–ST 30
Spleen (SP)	4 cun from midline	SP 13–SP 15
Gallbladder (GB)	Lateral side, mid-axillary	GB 22 (Yuan Ye), GB 24 (Riyue)

Clinical Relevance to Acupuncture

- These body lines standardise point location and organ mapping.
- Understanding them enables accurate diagnosis, safe needling, and effective treatment.
- They are the acupuncture equivalent of "longitude and latitude" on the human body.

Relative Anatomical Directions are standard directional terms used in acupuncture: Fig. 2.9

Anterior (Ventral): Toward the front. **Posterior (Dorsal)**: Toward the back.

Superior (Cephalad): Above. **Inferior (Caudad)**: Below.

Medial: Toward the midline. **Lateral**: Away from the midline.

Proximal: Near the trunk. **Distal**: Far from the trunk.

Plantar: Sole. **Dorsal**: Top of the foot or back of the hand.

Radial: Thumb side of the forearm. **Ulnar**: Little finger side of the forearm.

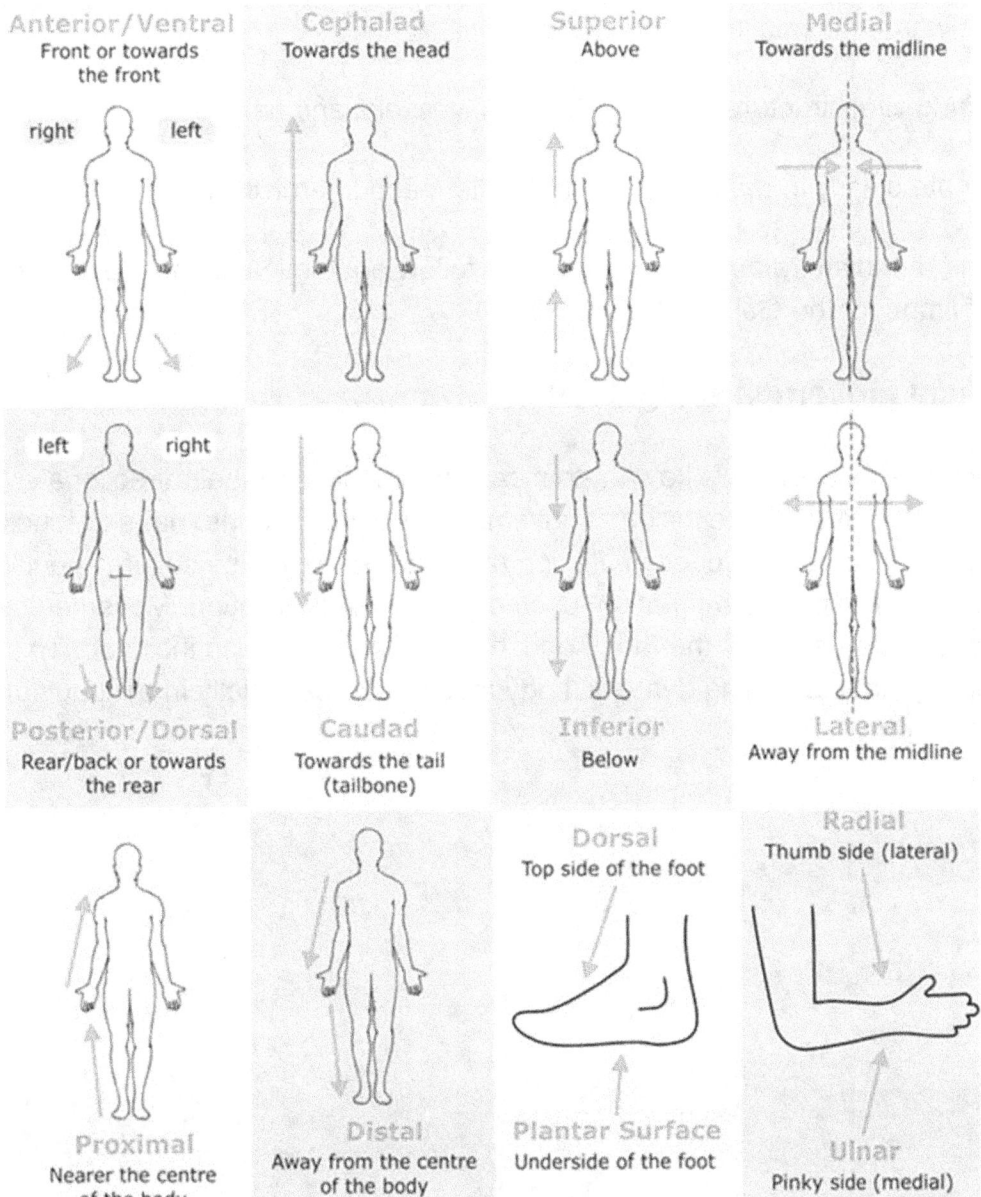

Fig. 2.9 Anatomical Directions

Clinical Significance of Anatomical Directions

Accurate understanding of anatomical directions allows practitioners to:

Locate points precisely when they lie between structures (e.g., muscle borders or bones).

Adjust needle angle and depth according to the directional anatomy (e.g., oblique insertion towards the midline for ST 12).

Avoid injuring vital structures, such as organs, vessels, and nerves.

Communicate clearly in teaching, documentation, and interdisciplinary settings.

Understand meridian trajectories, which often follow anatomical planes (e.g., the lateral surface of limbs for the Gall Bladder meridian).

Anatomical Movements Fig. 2.10

The following table overviews key anatomical movements and their directional characteristics. With clear definitions, movements are grouped into pairs or functional sets (e.g., abduction and adduction, flexion and extension). It also covers specialised actions such as pronation, supination, circumduction, and deviation. Movements unique to specific regions—such as the foot, hand, or mandible—are also included. This table is essential for understanding dynamic body mechanics, especially in acupuncture and physical therapy.

Movement	Direction	Movement	Direction
Abduction	Moving away from the midline	Medial rotation	Spiral movement towards the midline
Adduction	Moving towards the midline	Lateral (external) rotation	Spiral movement away from the midline
Flexion	Decreasing the angle between two structures	Extention (trunk)	Bending backward
Extension	Increasing the angle between the two structures	Pronation	Medial rotation of the radius, resulting in the palm facing posteriorly (if in anatomical position) or inferiorly (if the elbow is flexed)
Plantar-flexion	Flexion of the plantar (underside) part of the foot	Supination	Lateral rotation of the radius, resulting in the palm facing anteriorly (if in anatomical position) or superiorly (if the elbow is flexed)
Dorsi-flexion	Flexion of the dorsum (top) part of the foot	Circumduction	A combined movement starting with flexion, then abduction, extension, and ending with adduction
Retrusion	Moving backward (tongue, mandible)	Deviation	Movement of the wrist joint towards the radial or ulnar sides (radial deviation, ulnar deviation)
Protraction	Moving forwards and laterally simultaneously	Opposition	Touching the pad of any one of your fingers with the thumb of the same hand
Retraction	Moving backward and medially simultaneously	Reposition	Separating the pad of any of your fingers from the thumb of the same hand
Depression	Moving downwards	Inversion	The plantar side of the foot is moved towards the median plane
Elevation	Moving upwards	Eversion	The plantar side of the foot is moved away from the median plane

Fig. 2.10 Anatomical Body Movements

Clinical Relevance of Anatomical Movements

- Movements help expose tendons, muscle bellies, and joint spaces where points are located.
- Certain points are easier to locate or needle when the joint is in a specific position (e.g., ST 38 with shoulder movement for frozen shoulder).
- Assessing limited or painful movement guides point selection, especially in musculoskeletal disorders and rehabilitation.
- Dynamic palpation during movement helps identify trigger points and tissue resistance that may not be obvious at rest.

Anatomical Planes: Body planes aid orientation: Fig. 2.8

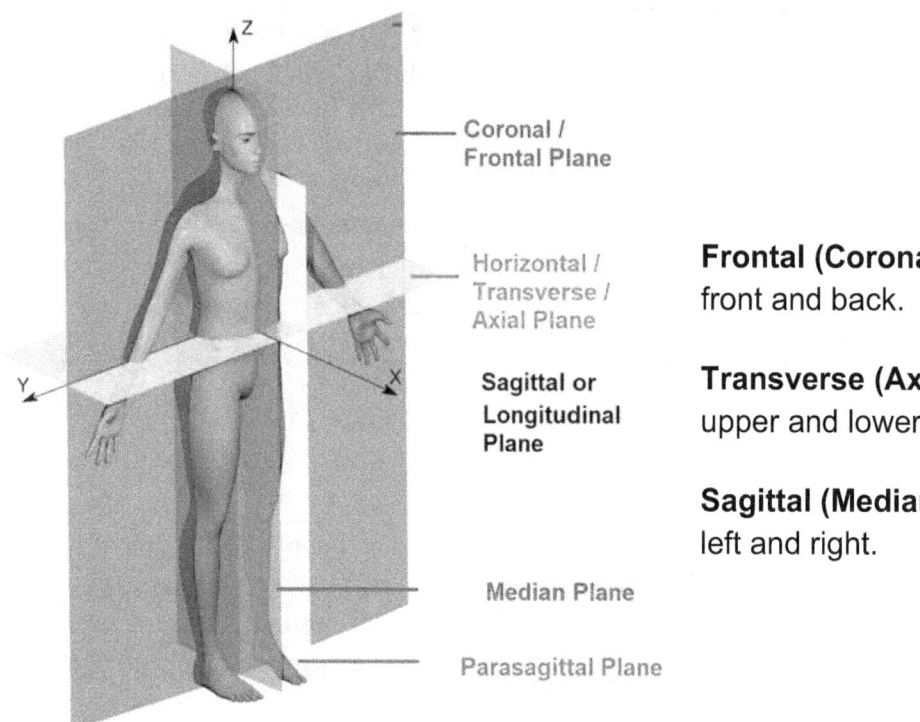

Coronal / Frontal Plane

Horizontal / Transverse / Axial Plane

Sagittal or Longitudinal Plane

Median Plane

Parasagittal Plane

Fig. 2.8 Body Planes

Frontal (Coronal) Plane: Divides front and back.

Transverse (Axial) Plane: Divides upper and lower.

Sagittal (Median) Plane: Divides left and right.

Section II - Acupuncture Therapy

3 An Introduction to Acupuncture

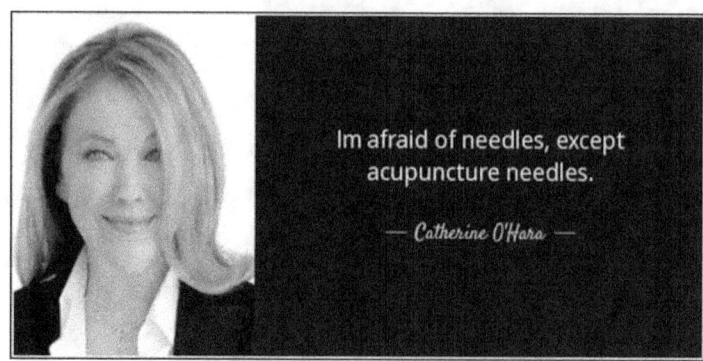

Im afraid of needles, except acupuncture needles.

— Catherine O'Hara —

Acupuncture is a medical therapy that involves the insertion of thin, flexible, sterile, and atraumatic needles at specific points on the human body to relieve pain and manage various health conditions. Rooted in centuries-old tradition, acupuncture has served millions as a cost-effective and minimally invasive treatment. In modern medicine, it is increasingly recognised as a viable first-line therapy for several diseases. Its applications span from musculoskeletal pain and neurological symptoms to psychological stress and internal organ dysfunction. Originating in China over 2000 years ago, acupuncture has stood the test of time as a drugless, safe, and essentially painless modality in experienced hands.

Traditional Chinese Medicine (TCM) Foundations: According to TCM philosophy, human beings are said to mirror the universe in terms of structure and function. This concept posits that natural laws govern human health, with wellness achieved through a state of balance and equilibrium. The opposing yet interdependent forces—Yin and Yang- are central to this idea. Harmony between these forces ensures health, while imbalance leads to disease.

Disease causation in TCM includes Yin-Yang imbalance, external environmental factors, improper diet, overwork or underactivity, phlegm accumulation, and injuries. Vital energy—called Qi (also spelled Chi or Chee)—is the life force that animates the body. It flows through a network of meridians, or channels. When Qi is obstructed, illness arises. Restoring the smooth flow of Qi by needling specific acupuncture points along these meridians restores health.

Meridians (Channels) Meridians are conceptual pathways that transport Qi throughout the body and link internal organs. There are fourteen principal meridians:

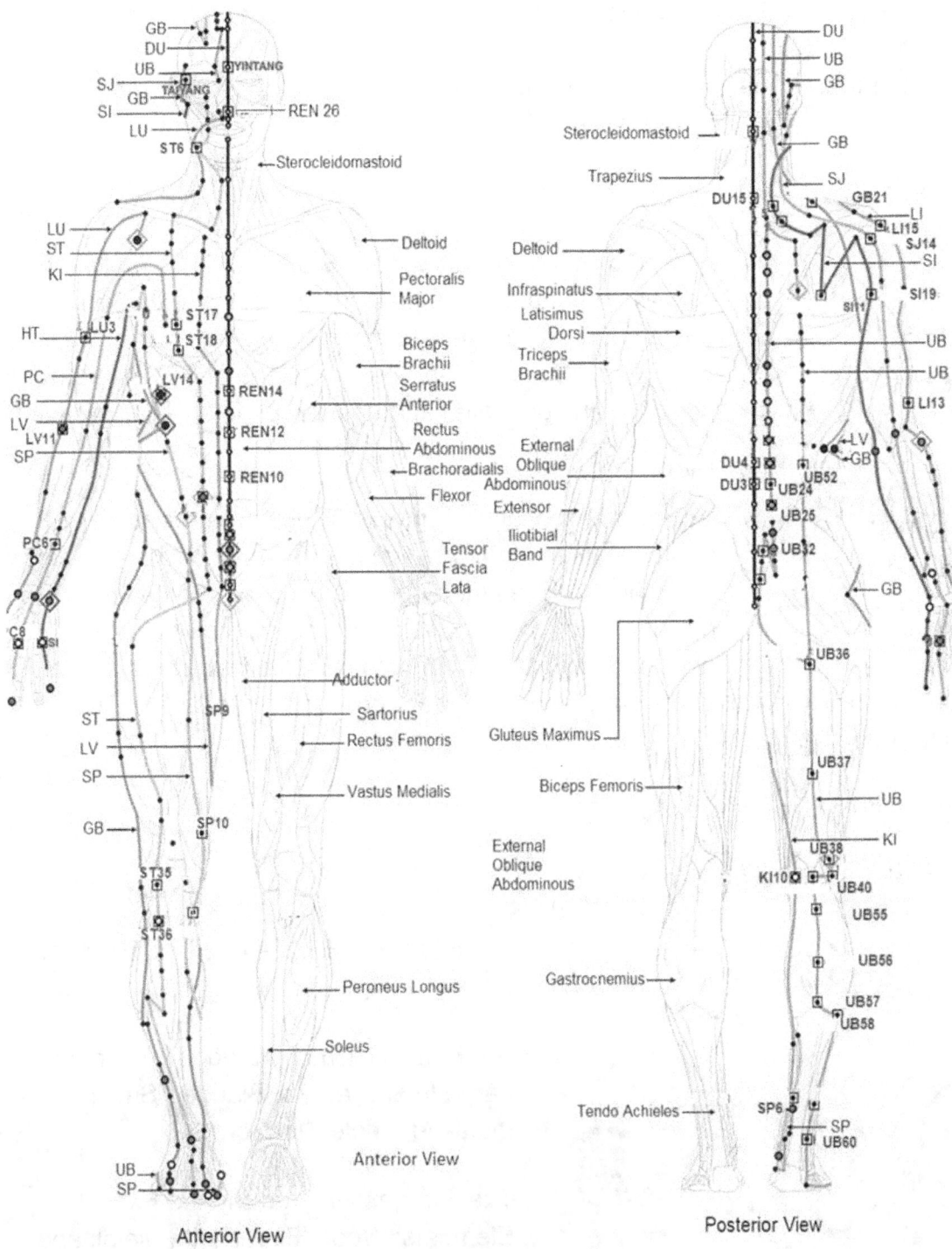

Fig. 3.2 Acupuncture Channels

- **Arm Yin Meridians**: Lung, Pericardium, Heart – originate from the chest and run to the hand.
- **Arm Yang Meridians**: Large Intestine, Small Intestine, Triple Warmer – travel from the hand to the face.

- **Leg Yang Meridians**: Stomach, Urinary Bladder, Gall Bladder – run from the face to the foot.
- **Leg Yin Meridians**: Spleen, Liver, Kidney – start at the foot and ascend to the chest.

Additionally:

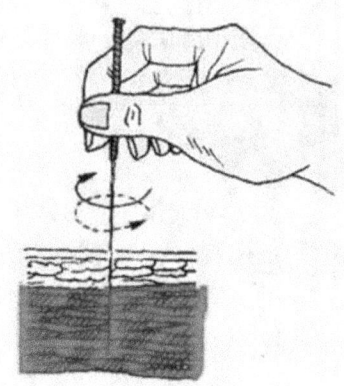

Fig. 3.1 Acupuncture Points and Needling

- **DU (Governing Vessel)**: Begins at DU 1 (between coccyx and anus) and runs along the spine to the head, ending at DU 28 in the upper labial frenulum.
- **REN (Conception Vessel)**: Starts at REN 1 (between the anus and genitalia) and travels up the anterior midline to REN 24 in the mento-labial groove.

Acupuncture Points Fig. 3.1: These are precise anatomical landmarks on the body's surface where needle insertion produces therapeutic effects. Needling is performed to remove Qi stagnation and restore physiological balance. Additional systems include the Tung, scalp, auricular, abdominal, and extra points, which are not rooted in classical TCM but are clinically effective.

TCM Organs and Five Elements.

TCM classifies internal organs into:

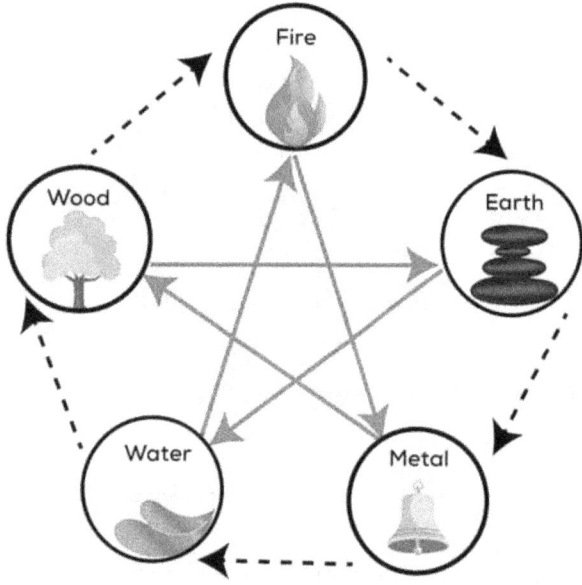

Fig. 3.5 Inter-relations of Five Elements

Zang (solid): Heart, Pericardium, Liver, Spleen, Lung, Kidney.

Fu (hollow): Urinary Bladder, Stomach, Large Intestine, Gall Bladder, Small Intestine, Triple Warmer.

These organs interact via the Five Elements: Wood, Fire, Earth, Metal, and Water. Each element corresponds with personality traits, physiological functions, and disease tendencies:

Wood (Liver, Gall Bladder): Athletic, anxious, prone to migraines.

Fire (Heart, SI, Pericardium, TW): Passionate, irritable, insomnia-prone.

Earth (Stomach, Spleen): Nurturing, worrisome, digestive issues.

Metal (Lung, Large Intestine): Honest, melancholic, allergy-prone.

Water (Kidney, UB): Wise, fearful, susceptible to urinary and back disorders.

Qi (Chi or Chee) Fig. 3.4 Qi is the fundamental life energy that flows along meridians, maintaining internal organ function and overall health. Comparable to the Indian concept of 'prāṇa,' Qi symbolises air, life force, or vital energy. Its unobstructed flow is essential for health.

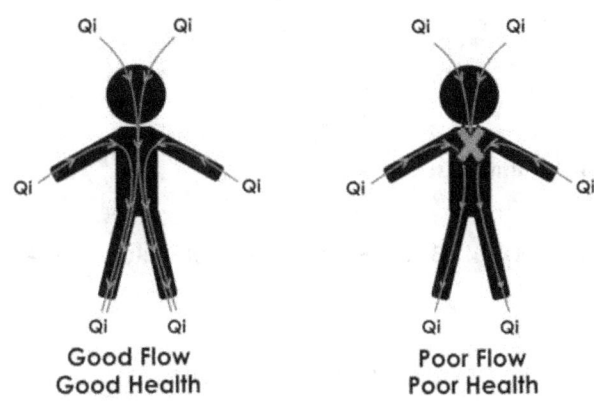

Good Flow
Good Health

Poor Flow
Poor Health

Fig. 3.4 Flow of Qi and Health

Deqi Sensation Fig. 3.3 Deqi (pronounced "day-chee") is a distinctive sensory response elicited during needle manipulation. Patients may experience aching, tingling, or fullness, while practitioners sense tightness or tension around the needle insertion site. Deqi is essential for therapeutic effectiveness and is a marker of correct point stimulation.

Diagnostic Methods in TCM Diagnosis in TCM is based on:

- **Inquiry**
- **Inspection (particularly of the tongue)**
- **Auscultation**
- **Olfaction**
- **Palpation (particularly the pulse)**

Treatment plans are determined based on the overall pattern derived from these observations.

Cun: A Unit of Measurement Fig. 3.6. Cun is a proportional body-based measurement unit used in traditional Chinese medicine, specifically acupuncture. It varies between individuals:

- 1 cun = width of the thumb at the knuckle
- 1.5 cun = width of index and middle fingers
- 3 cun = width of four fingers together

This relative system allows consistent point location across different body sizes and shapes.

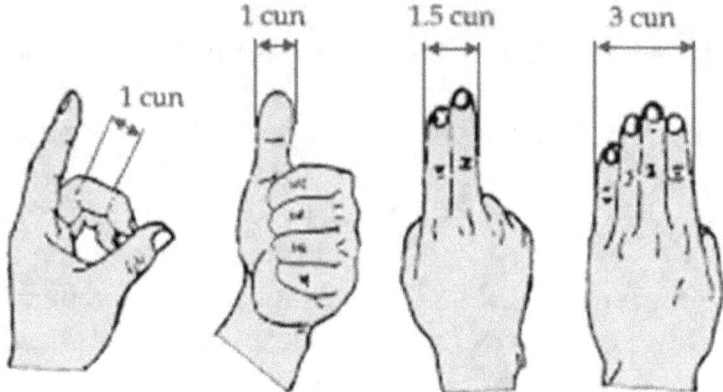

Fig. 3.6 Measurement unit of CUN

Bonus Effects of Acupuncture Fig. 3.7: Many patients undergoing acupuncture for a specific issue often report additional benefits:

Pain Relief: Due to the endogenous release of opioids and serotonin

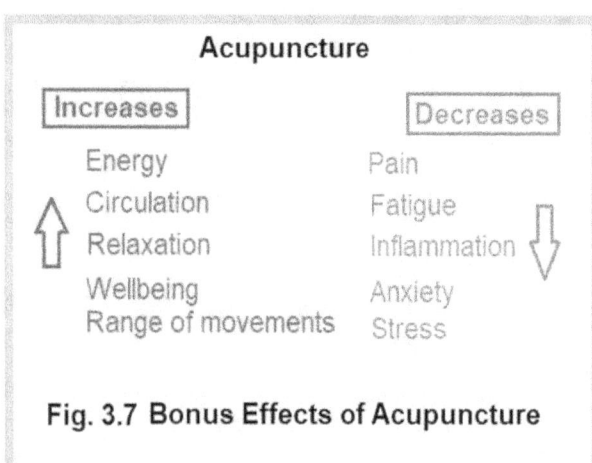

Fig. 3.7 Bonus Effects of Acupuncture

- **Improved Sleep**: Via limbic system modulation
- **Metabolic Support**: Enhanced glycaemic control, skin improvement
- **Enhanced Immunity**: Strengthened resistance to infections
- **Increased Energy and Calmness**: Via nervous system balance
- **Improved Digestion and Sexual Function**

Clinical Utility Acupuncture effectively manages musculoskeletal and neuropathic pain, obstetric discomfort, post-surgical recovery, and immunity-related disorders. It can replace anaesthesia in minor procedures and support mental health and preventive care.

Challenges and Criticisms: Early Chinese pioneers developed acupuncture without the aid of scientific tools, guided by observational insight. Yet modern critics challenge TCM:

- **No anatomical or physiological evidence** for meridians or specific acupuncture points.
- TCM organ definitions do not align with biomedical understanding.
- Diagnostic methods (e.g., tongue inspection, pulse reading) are seen as subjective.
- Clinical trials often struggle to prove point specificity due to effects at non-specific (sham) points.

Despite this, acupuncture's practical success has led to the development of diverse systems, including Tung, scalp, and auricular acupuncture. While TCM provides the historical framework, modern practice increasingly demands integration with anatomy, neurophysiology, and evidence-based research.

Moving forward, it is crucial to bridge ancient traditions with scientific principles. Acupuncture has demonstrated efficacy in numerous conditions, providing an affordable and side-effect-free complement to mainstream medicine. Rigorous study and open-minded integration can significantly enrich healthcare systems worldwide.

-Modern Acupuncture-

4 Modes of Action of Acupuncture

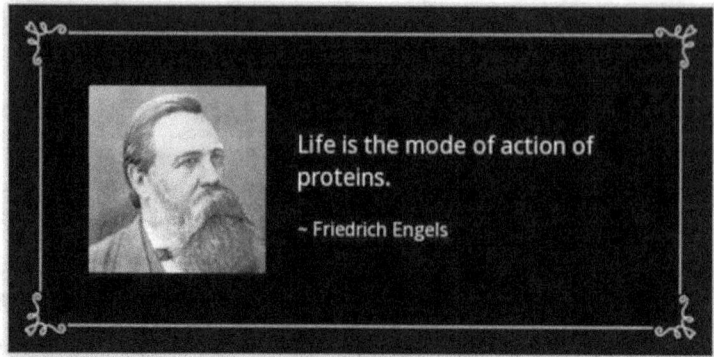

Life is the mode of action of proteins.

~ Friedrich Engels

Despite its profound clinical efficacy, the exact mechanism by which acupuncture exerts its therapeutic effects has long remained enigmatic. Over the decades, numerous scientific investigations have sought to elucidate the biological and neurological basis of acupuncture. While the complete picture is still evolving, current evidence supports several plausible mechanisms by which acupuncture influences the body. These include local, spinal, supraspinal, neuroendocrine, and emotional pathways, as well as traditional theoretical explanations.

Local Action

Acupuncture stimulates peripheral structures, tiny myelinated Aδ nerve fibres in the skin and muscles. It also activates connective tissue, nerve endings, periosteum, and fascia, triggering several local physiological responses:

- Release of neuropeptides such as enkephalins, beta-endorphins, and dynorphins.
- Increased local blood flow.
- Reduction in oedema and inflammation.
- Promotion of tissue repair.

These local effects are particularly beneficial for treating pain, non-healing wounds, and internal inflammatory conditions, such as retroocular oedema.

Spinal Cord Mechanism: Gate Control Theory.

When an acupuncture needle stimulates Aδ fibres, collateral branches of these nerves synapse in the dorsal horn of the spinal cord. Here, interneurons, particularly in the substantia gelatinosa, release enkephalins, which inhibit the transmission of pain signals to higher centres. This neuro-modulatory process effectively "closes the gate" to pain transmission, producing lasting analgesic effects.

Midbrain Activation: Descending Inhibitory Control.

Acupuncture activates descending inhibitory pain pathways in the midbrain, particularly in the periaqueductal grey (PAG) region. The PAG modulates pain through serotonergic and noradrenergic pathways that descend to the spinal cord. This central mechanism significantly reduces the perception of pain independently of peripheral stimulation.

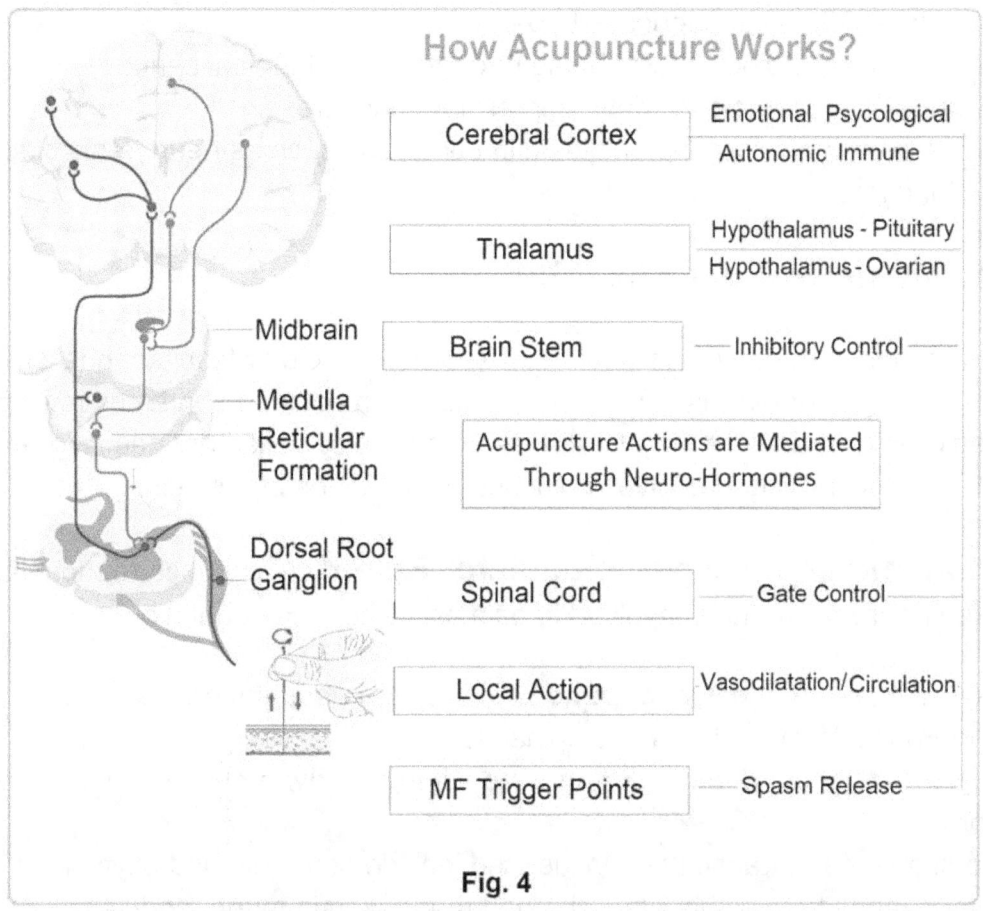

Fig. 4

Neuroendocrine Regulation

Acupuncture influences several hormonal axes:

- **Hypothalamic-pituitary-adrenal (HPA) Axis:** This axis stimulates the release of adrenocorticotropic hormone (ACTH) and beta-endorphins, contributing to analgesia and anti-inflammatory responses.

- **Hypothalamic-pituitary-ovarian (HPO) Axis:** This axis affects the release of gonadotropin-releasing hormone (GnRH), modulating female reproductive hormones. This mechanism underlies the use of acupuncture in managing menstrual irregularities, infertility, and menopausal syndromes.

Limbic System and Brain Function

The limbic system, which regulates emotional responses, mood, and behavioural patterns, is significantly influenced by acupuncture. The stimulation:

- Modulates affective responses to pain.
- Promotes psychological well-being through neurochemical changes.
- Reduces symptoms of anxiety, depression, and stress.
- Alters autonomic responses, aiding in conditions such as neurogenic bladder dysfunction.

Myofascial Trigger Points (MTrPs):

MTrPs are hyperirritable nodules within taut skeletal muscle or fascia bands, typically formed due to injury or overuse. They are painful upon palpation and may refer pain to distant regions. Acupuncture targeting these points—also called dry needling—relieves muscular tension and often resolves pain instantly, with lasting effects.

Neurotransmitter and Neuromodulator Release

Acupuncture modulates several key neurotransmitters involved in pain and emotional regulation:

- **Low-frequency electroacupuncture** induces release of enkephalins and beta-endorphins from the brain and spinal cord.
- **High-frequency electroacupuncture** stimulates dynorphin release in the spinal cord.
- Additional neurotransmitters influenced include serotonin and oxytocin, which may contribute to analgesia, improved mood, and immune modulation.

Traditional Chinese Medicine (TCM) Perspective.

From a classical TCM viewpoint, acupuncture regulates the flow of Qi (life force) through the meridians. Its actions are classified based on the clinical syndrome:

- **Tonification**: Strengthens Qi and body resistance in deficiency syndromes.
- **Sedation**: Dispels pathogenic factors and stagnation in excess syndromes.

- **Warming effect**: Warms meridians and Yang Qi, resolving cold-induced obstructions.
- **Clearing heat**: Eliminates internal heat and pathogenic fire.
- **Raising Qi**: Promotes the upward flow in cases of organ prolapse.
- **Descending Qi**: Controls rebellious Qi in conditions like cough or vomiting.

Conclusion: Acupuncture's mechanisms are multifaceted, involving both peripheral and central nervous system structures, neurochemical mediators, and traditional concepts of energy flow. While modern science continues to uncover its physiological basis, evidence-based studies increasingly support acupuncture's therapeutic efficacy. Understanding its scientific and traditional foundations enables more precise application and broader acceptance of acupuncture in contemporary healthcare.

Why do acupuncturists need to know the modes of action of acupuncture?

Understanding the modes of action of acupuncture is essential for practitioners to apply treatments with greater precision, confidence, and clinical effectiveness. It bridges the gap between traditional theory and modern biomedical science, allowing acupuncturists to explain their interventions in terms understandable to both patients and healthcare professionals.

Knowledge of how acupuncture works—through mechanisms such as neural modulation, neurohormonal regulation, immune system activation, and microcirculatory improvement—helps in rational point selection, appropriate needling techniques, and setting realistic treatment goals. It also aids in tailoring protocols for specific conditions, such as pain, hormonal imbalance, organ dysfunction, or psychological disorders.

Furthermore, awareness of acupuncture's physiological effects supports informed consent, enhances communication with integrative medical teams, and strengthens the credibility of acupuncture within the scientific and medical communities. For educators and researchers, it forms the foundation for clinical study design and evidence-based practice.

Knowing the modes of action empowers acupuncturists to elevate their practice from an intuitive skill to a scientifically grounded healthcare approach, thereby improving outcomes and enhancing their professional standing.

-Modern Acupuncture-

5A: Techniques of Acupuncture

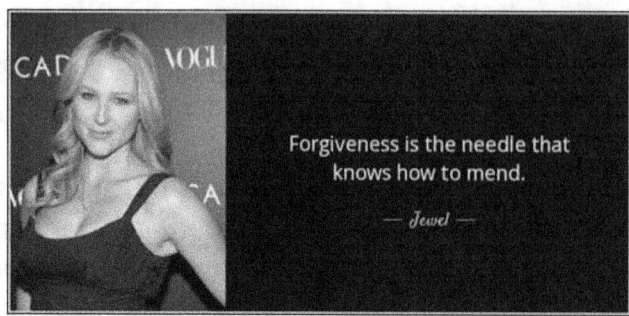

Precise needling technique lies at the heart of effective acupuncture therapy. Success depends on accurate point selection and skilful needle handling tailored to different anatomical sites and clinical conditions. A systematic and rational approach from patient preparation to post-treatment care ensures safe, effective, and consistent outcomes.

Preparation for Needling

- **Patient Counselling**: Explain the procedure, expected sensations, needle retention time, and number of sessions. Obtain informed consent and clarify treatment costs.
- **Environment**: The treatment room should be clean, well-ventilated, and illuminated.
- **Patient Comfort**: Patients should wear loose clothing and be positioned comfortably to expose the treatment area. For female patients, a female attendant should be present.
- **Practitioner Hygiene**: The acupuncturist must wash hands thoroughly and maintain aseptic technique. The first session should be conducted on a bed to manage any potential syncope.

Specifications of Needles Fig 5.1

- **Quality**: Use disposable, pre-sterilized, flexible needles. Tubed needles are preferred for their precision and reduced pain.
- **Diameter and Length**: Choose diameter (0.14–0.50 mm; usually 0.25 mm) and length (13 mm–150 mm) based on anatomical location. For example, GB 30 requires 75–150 mm; flat tibial surfaces, on the other hand, need only 13 mm.
- **Surface Texture**: Rougher surfaces offer greater stimulation than highly polished ones.
- **Sterility**: Needles must be used once. If reusing (where legally permitted), follow strict sterilisation protocols (see Chapter 53).

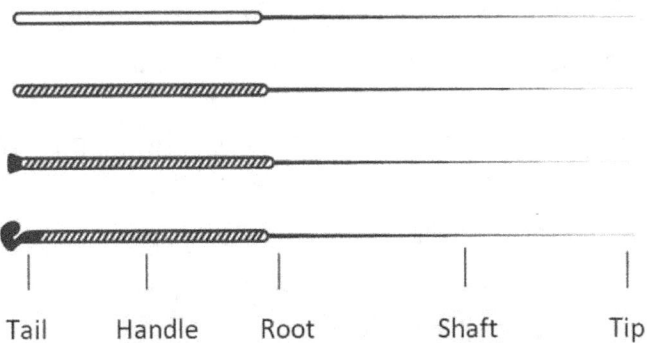

Fig.5.1 Parts of Acupuncture Needle

Tail Handle Root Shaft Tip

Ear Needles Fig 5.2:

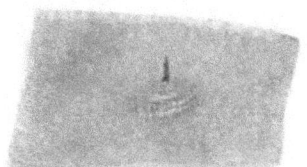

In auricular acupuncture, tiny needles or ear tacks stimulate specific points.

Fig. 5.2 Ear Needles

Needle Insertion Techniques Fig 5.3

General Guidelines: Ensure correct patient and practitioner positioning. Avoid antiseptic solutions before needling to preserve neurological sensitivity. However, antiseptics should be used after the bleeding has stopped.

With the Tube: Palpate the point, place the tube, and tap the needle through the skin with a swift, finger-stroke motion.

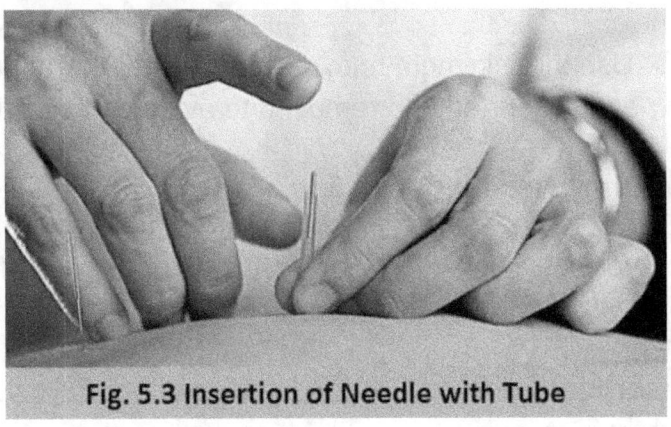

Fig. 5.3 Insertion of Needle with Tube

Deeper insertion is performed gradually, taking into account anatomical considerations. If needed, pre-bend the needle slightly for directional control.

Without the Tube, Fig. 5.4: Hold the needle between the thumb and fingers. Insert swiftly to minimise pain. Accuracy and patient preparation are critical. Observe the patient's response and adjust the angle as necessary.

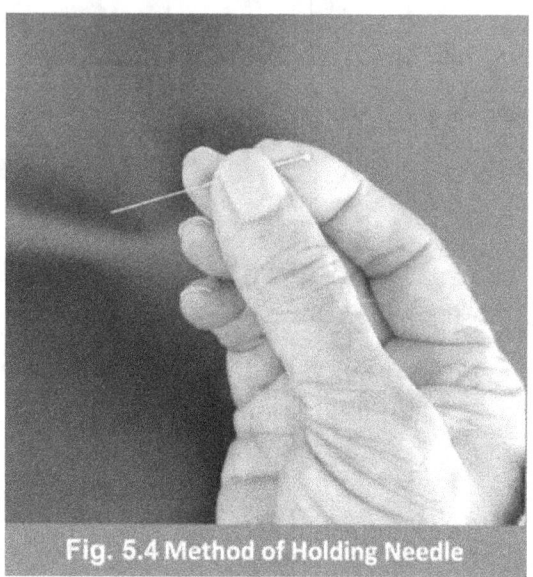

Fig. 5.4 Method of Holding Needle

Arrival of Qi (Deqi)

- After insertion, rotate the needle slightly and observe for Qi sensation. The ideal clinical response is warmth or heat.
- **Other Sensations**: Tingling, numbness, heaviness, dull ache, or radiating sensation. These should be explained as typical signs of Qi activation.
- **Techniques to Induce Qi**: If Deqi is absent, adjust the needle angle obliquely or alter the depth. Experience and anatomical knowledge guide effective adjustment.

Number of Needles: Use the minimum number required for therapeutic effect—usually 3 to 5. Record each needle inserted and removed to avoid complications.

Pain Management During Needling, Fig. 5.5

Pain on Insertion: Typically caused by poor technique or the use of blunt needles. It can be minimised by swift, controlled insertion.

Pain After Insertion: Often caused by deep insertion or excessive manipulation. Withdraw slightly to relieve.

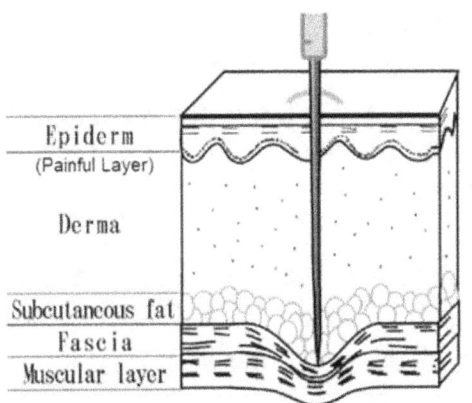

Fig. 5.5 Common Tissues of Insertions

Directing Energy to the Affected Area: Encourage patients to move the affected part during or after treatment, such as walking for knee pain. In cases where movement is impossible, focus the patient's attention mentally on the target area to stimulate the cortical response.

Manual Stimulation Fig. 5.6

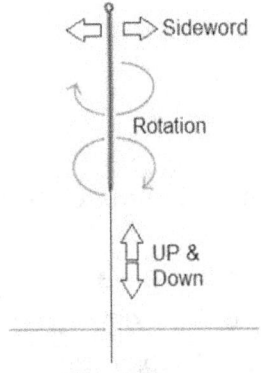

Stimulate the needle every five minutes using flicking, rotation, or vertical movements. This prevents tissue adaptation.

- Retain needles for 30–40 minutes.
- For electroacupuncture, see Chapter 15.

**Fig. 5.6
Manual Stimulation**

Removal of Needles

- Use a cotton swab to hold the skin. Remove the needle in the reverse direction without touching the shaft.
- Discard immediately in a sharp box.
- Massage the point post-removal to prevent soreness. Please allow the patient to rest for 5–10 minutes before moving or leaving the clinic.

Complications and Their Management

- **Stuck Needle**: This may occur due to muscle spasm or rotation in a single direction. Rotate in reverse, massage, or allow your muscles to relax.
- **Broken Needle**: This is rare with high-quality needles. If breakage occurs, avoid movement. Remove with forceps if visible; surgical removal may be necessary if the object is embedded.

Sharp Disposal Protocol: Used needles are hazardous waste. Dispose of them in a biohazard-labelled sharp container. Account for every needle used. Sharps include hypodermic needles, blades, glass, and other sharp, penetrating items.

Assessment and Follow-Up

- **Immediate Relief**: Seen in 10–15% of musculoskeletal cases. Reassess after three days.
- **Partial Relief**: 60–65% show 25–40% improvement. Continue treatment as indicated.
- **No Relief**: About 15% show no response. Evaluate thoroughly before continuing.
- Long-term conditions require periodic evaluation to guide the treatment plan.

Treatment Schedule

- **Initial Phase**: Daily for the first three sessions.
- **Intermediate Phase**: Alternate-day sessions for 1 week.
- **Maintenance**: Twice weekly until optimal results are achieved.
- If no effect is seen in 7 sessions, reassess the appropriateness of acupuncture.

Individualised Approach Acupuncture remains a partly empirical, individualised therapy. While the above protocol reflects the author's experience and the existing literature, clinicians should adapt it based on rational, evidence-based reasoning tailored to each patient.

5B Side Effects and Emergencies in Acupuncture

Acupuncture is generally safe when performed by a trained and experienced practitioner. Side effects are rare, mild, and typically self-limiting. However, awareness of possible adverse effects and emergencies is essential for safe practice.

Common Side Effects of Acupuncture

1. Soreness
Mild soreness may occur at needling sites, particularly on the hands and feet (e.g., LI 4). If a trigger or Ashi point is released, soreness may be felt in the surrounding muscles. Gentle massage post-treatment is often sufficient to alleviate discomfort. Typically, soreness resolves within 24 hours but may last longer following deep trigger point release.

2. Aggravation of Symptoms
Occasionally, acupuncture may temporarily exacerbate existing symptoms. This reaction is more common in hypersensitive individuals or when overstimulation occurs. Patients should be reassured, and treatment should be withheld until symptoms subside. Subsequent sessions should begin with mild stimulation to assess individual response.

3. Muscle Twitching
Muscle twitching may occur during or after acupuncture, particularly with electroacupuncture. It reflects peripheral stimulation and is typically harmless.

4. Emotional Release
Some patients experience emotional release post-treatment, such as euphoria, laughter, or crying. These responses are attributed to central nervous system modulation and usually subside quickly.

5. Minor Bleeding
Slight bleeding may occur at needle removal. Applying firm pressure for a few minutes is usually sufficient to control it.

6. Fatigue
Some patients feel drowsy or fatigued after treatment. This reaction indicates the need for rest. Caution should be exercised if patients plan to drive after the session.

7. Bruising:

Occasional bruising results from puncturing small subcutaneous vessels. It poses no medical concern but may cause temporary aesthetic discomfort. Patients on anticoagulants should be identified beforehand.

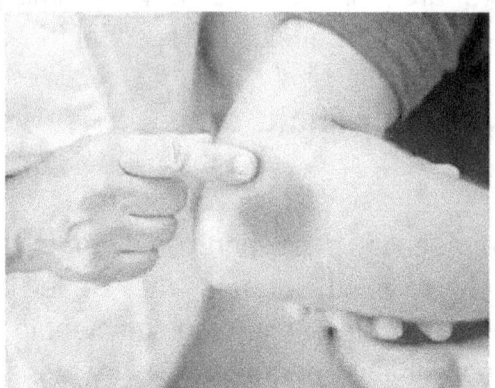

Fig. 5.7 Bruising

8. Light-headedness and Fainting

Rarely, patients may experience light-headedness or syncope, especially when rising suddenly. A few minutes of rest after treatment mitigates this risk.

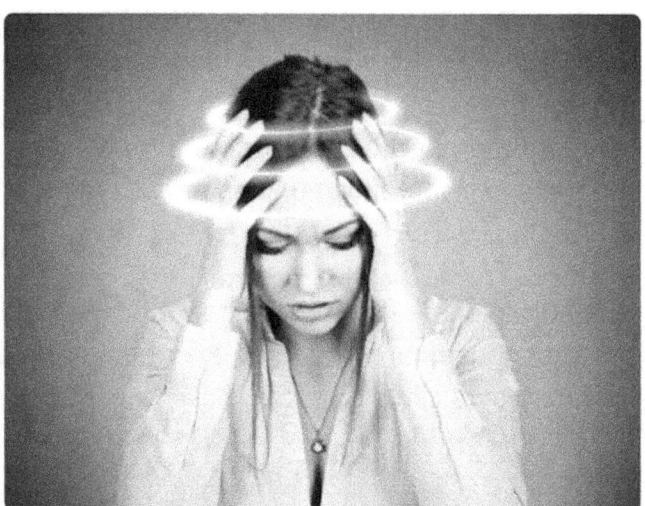

Fig. 5.8 Light Headedness

Emergencies in Acupuncture

1. Syncope (Vasovagal Reaction)

Syncope is the most frequent emergency in acupuncture and results from transient cerebral hypoperfusion, often triggered by anxiety, pain, or fear.

Warning Signs:

- Pallor, sweating, nausea, and dizziness
- Gradual loss of consciousness
- Brief seizure-like jerks without postictal confusion
- Rapid recovery

Differential Diagnosis:

Distinguish syncope from seizures:

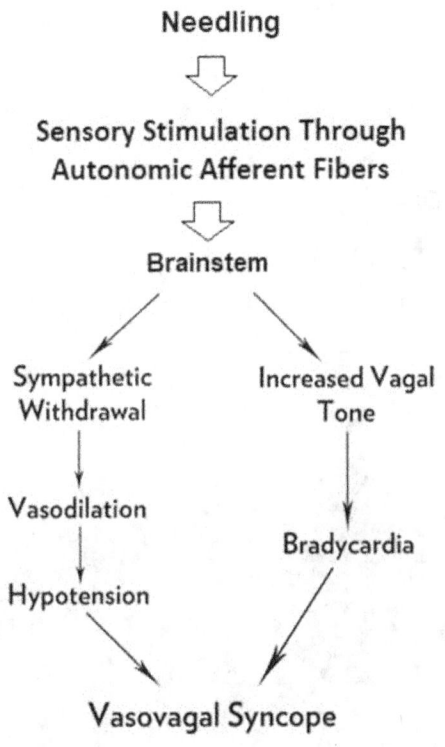

Fig. 5.9 Vasovagal Syncope Dynamics

- Syncope is often preceded by prodrome (nausea, sweating), brief, and followed by full awareness.
- Seizures may present with aura, prolonged unconsciousness, confusion, incontinence, or injury.

Management:

- Remove needles immediately
- Lay patient supine with legs elevated (Trendelenburg position)
- Ensure airway patency
- Encourage leg movement if semiconscious
- Observe for signs of seizure, cardiac, or metabolic causes
- Call for emergency help if recovery is delayed

Prevention:

- Take a thorough history, including cardiac conditions and prior syncope
- Begin the first treatment on a bed

- Avoid sudden or intense stimulation, especially at the neck or in anxious patients
- Distract and prepare patients verbally
- Keep an emergency kit and referral network ready
- Train clinic staff in basic emergency protocols

2. Pneumothorax

Pneumothorax is a rare but serious complication, resulting from pleural puncture, usually when needling the thoracic region.

Symptoms:

- Sudden, one-sided chest pain
- Shortness of breath
- Diminished breath sounds and hyperresonance on percussion

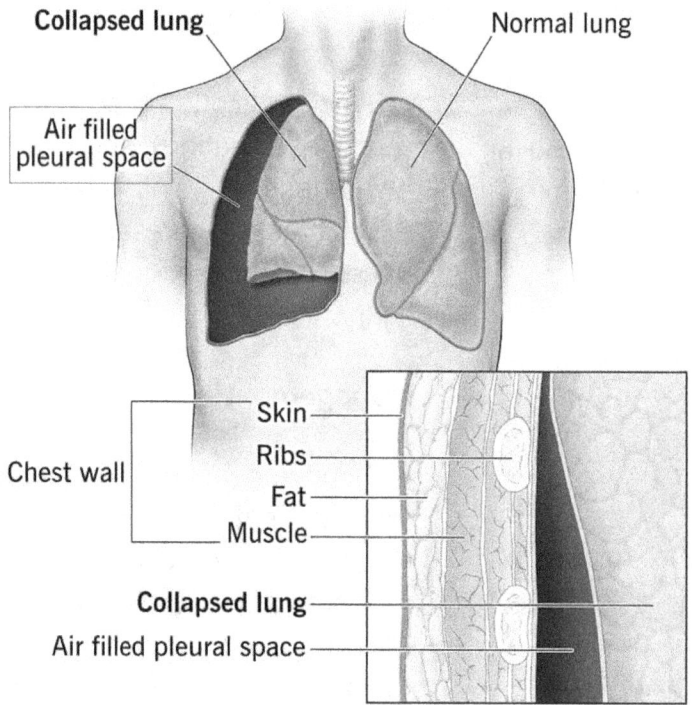

Fig. 5.10 Pneumothorax

Diagnosis and Management:
Most small pneumothoraxes resolve spontaneously in healthy individuals. Large or symptomatic cases may require observation, needle aspiration, or chest tube insertion.

Prevention:

- Use shallow, oblique insertion on the thorax
- Avoid deep needling near the clavicle, scapula, or suprascapular fossa
- Avoid needling over thin bone or near apices of lungs
- Exercise caution in frail or elderly patients

Comment:

The risk of pneumothorax from acupuncture is often exaggerated. Evidence from the British Acupuncture Council reports an extremely low incidence, despite millions of treatments being administered yearly. Pneumothorax more commonly results from trauma, COPD, or mechanical ventilation, not acupuncture.

3. Other Rare but Serious Injuries

- **Cardiac tamponade:** From vertical needling over the sternum with an abnormal foramen
- **Vascular injury:** Large vessels near the trachea, groin, or arms may be punctured
- **CNS injury:** Deep needling near C1 can damage central structures
- **Abdominal organ damage:** Avoid deep needling without palpation
- **Skull defects:** Avoid scalp needling over open fontanelle or post-surgical defects
- **Electroacupuncture contraindications:** Avoid in patients with pacemakers or implanted electronics

Summary of Safety Principles

- Avoid acupuncture in patients with known bleeding disorders or active skin infections
- Do not apply electroacupuncture across the thorax or in those with pacemakers
- Complications are exceedingly rare with properly trained acupuncturists
- There are no absolute contraindications when anatomical safety, patient condition, and rational technique are respected

'Modern Acupuncture' emphasises evidence-informed practice and anatomical safety. With proper precautions, acupuncture remains one of the safest therapeutic interventions in healthcare.

-Dr. Pardeshi Acupuncture-

6. Channels and Acupuncture Points

6.1 Lung Channel (LU)

The Lung channel, also known as the Hand Tai Yin channel, originates at LU 1, establishing an internal connection with the Liver channel. It runs along the anterior-medial aspect of the upper limb, passing through the cubital region (LU 5), the forearm, and the wrist. It traverses the thenar eminence of the palm and ends at the radial side of the thumb's tip (LU 11), where it externally connects with the Large Intestine channel.

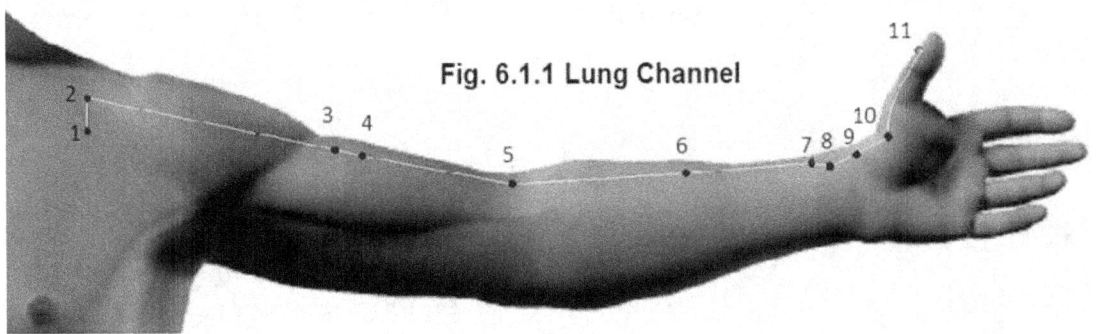

Fig. 6.1.1 Lung Channel

This channel is central to respiratory, throat, and upper limb disorders. The key acupuncture points, LU 1, 5, 6, 7, 8, 9, 10, and 11, are described below.

LU 1 – Zhongfu (Middle Palace)

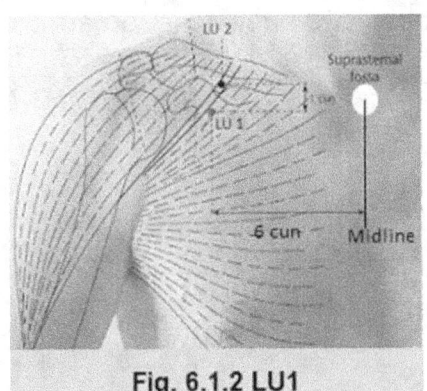

Fig. 6.1.2 LU1

Location:
Six cun are lateral to the anterior midline (REN channel) in the first intercostal space, and one cun is inferior to LU 2.

Needling Technique:
Insert obliquely or laterally 0.5–0.8 cun. Avoid deep or perpendicular insertion to prevent pneumothorax.

Indications:
Cough, wheezing, asthma, chest congestion, shoulder and back pain, vomiting.

LU 5 – (Cubit Marsh)

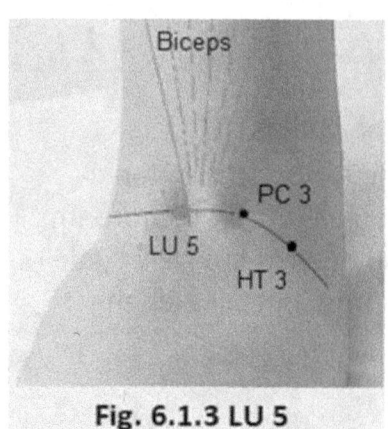

Fig. 6.1.3 LU 5

Location:
On the cubital crease, in the depression lateral to the biceps brachii tendon, the elbow is slightly flexed.

Needling Technique:
Perpendicular insertion, 0.5–1 cun. Avoid the cubital vein.

Indications:
Cough, asthma, sore throat, chest fullness, mastitis, arm pain, and elbow pain.

LU 6 – (Maximum Opening)

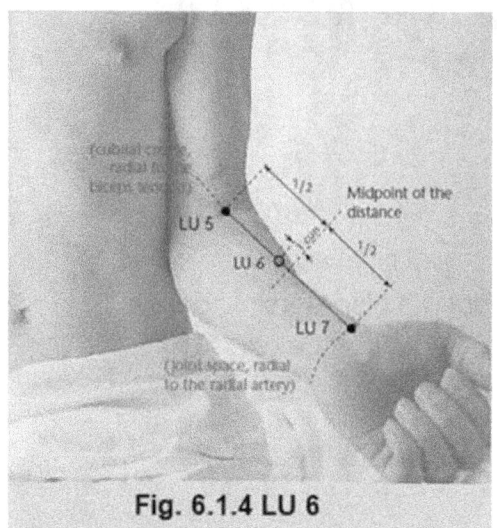

Fig. 6.1.4 LU 6

Location:
On the flexor aspect of the forearm, seven cun proximal to LU 9, on the line joining LU 9 and LU 5. Alternatively, in palpable depression, one cun above the midpoint between LU 5 and LU 7.

Needling Technique:
Perpendicular or oblique insertion, 0.5–1.5 cun.

Indications:
Acute cough, pain in the chest, asthma, sore throat, pain in the elbow, and pain in the forearm.

LU 7 – (Broken Sequence)

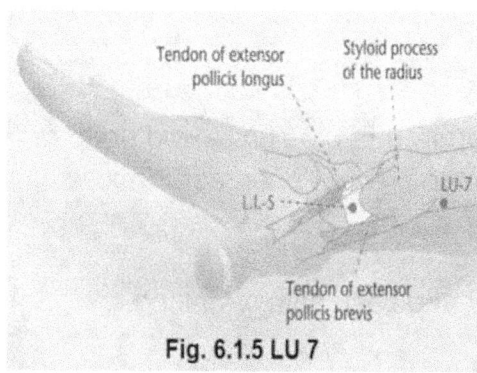

Fig. 6.1.5 LU 7

Location:
1.5 cun proximal to LI 5, in the cleft between the tendons of the brachioradialis and abductor pollicis longus, just proximal to the styloid process of the radius.

Needling Technique:
Pinch the skin and insert the needle transversely, 0.5–1 cun, in a proximal or distal direction. Avoid the cephalic vein.

Indications:
Headache, neck stiffness, cough, asthma, sore throat, facial paralysis, toothache, wrist pain, and weakness.

LU 8 – (Channel Gutter)

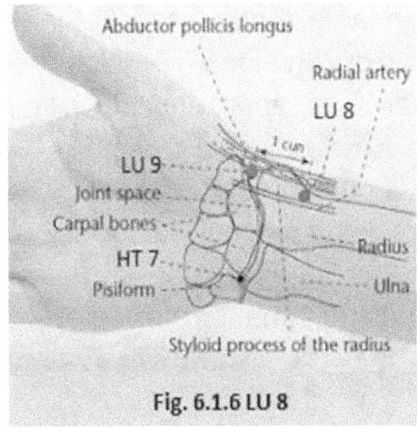

Fig. 6.1.6 LU 8

Location:
1 cun proximal to the wrist crease, in the depression lateral to the radial artery.

Needling Technique:
Perpendicular insertion, 0.1–0.2 cun. Avoid the radial artery.

Indications:
Cough, asthma, fever, sore throat, chest pain, wrist pain.

LU 9 – (Supreme Abyss)

Location:
At the wrist joint, in the depression between the radial artery and the tendon of the abductor pollicis longus, on the same level as HT 7 (at the lower border of the pisiform bone).

Needling Technique:
Perpendicular insertion, 0.3–0.5 cun. Take care to avoid the radial artery.

Indications:
Cough, asthma, sore throat, palpitations, pain in the chest, wrist, and forearm.

LU 10 – (Fish Border)

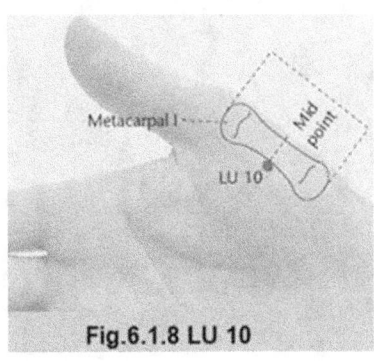

Fig.6.1.8 LU 10

Location:
On the thenar eminence, in the depression between the midpoint of the first metacarpal bone's shaft and the thenar muscles.

Needling Technique:
Perpendicular insertion, 0.5–1 cun, close to the metacarpal bone.

Indications:
Throat disorders, hoarseness, fever, and sensations of heat in the palms.

LU 11 – (Lesser Shang)

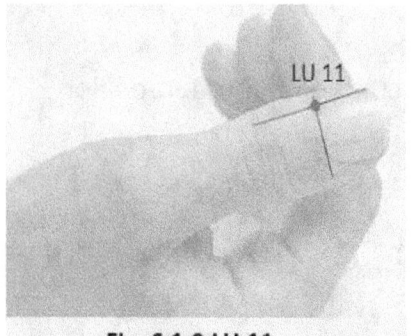
Fig. 6.1.9 LU 11

Location: LU 11 is located on the extensor aspect of the thumb, at the junction of lines drawn along the radial border of the nail and the nail base, approximately 0.1 cun from the corner.
Needling Technique: LU 11 is punctured at a perpendicular or oblique direction proximally 0.1 to 0.2 cun or pricked to bleed.
Indications: Sore throat, cough, asthma, epistaxis, fever, loss of consciousness, and thumb pain.

Clinical Significance of Lung Channel

LU 1 and LU 7 are commonly used for external respiratory conditions, while LU 9, the Yuan-Source point, is clinically significant for chronic lung and cardiac complaints. LU 11 is crucial in resuscitation protocols and the treatment of acute tonsillar infections. The Lung channel governs respiration and controls Qi and body fluids. It is essential for maintaining the body's defensive Qi (Wei Qi), which protects against external pathogens. Clinically, it is often used to treat respiratory system disorders, such as cough, asthma, bronchitis, sore throat, and shortness of breath.

In addition to respiratory issues, the Lung channel plays a crucial role in regulating skin and water metabolism, including spontaneous sweating, dryness, edema, and certain skin disorders. Emotional imbalances, such as grief and sadness, which are associated with Lung function, are also addressed through this channel.

-Modern Acupuncture-

6.2 Large Intestine Channel (LI)

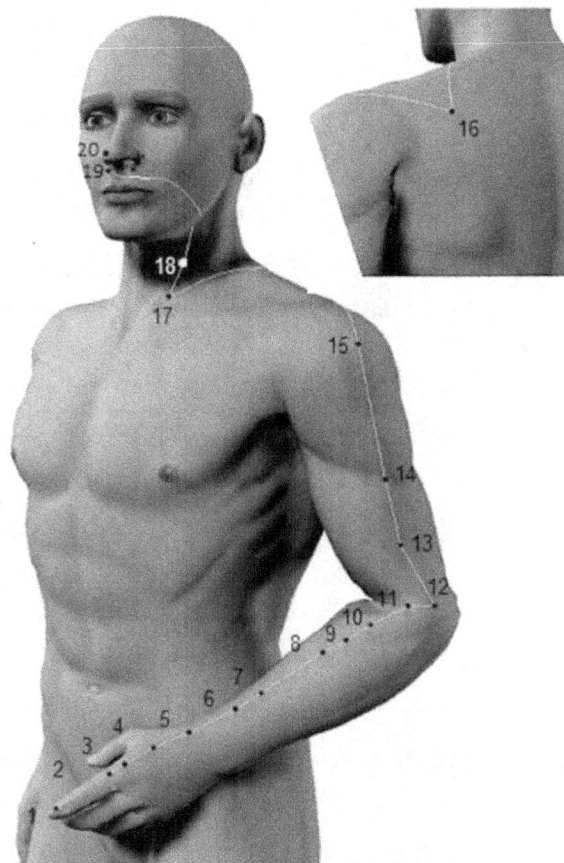

The Large Intestine channel, the Hand Yang Ming channel, begins at the radial side of the index finger (LI 1), following its internal linkage with the Lung channel. It ascends along the radial aspect of the index finger, passes through the first and second metacarpal interspace (LI 4), and continues along the lateral aspect of the forearm and upper arm to the shoulder (LI 15). From there, it traverses the supraclavicular fossa (LI 16), ascends the neck and cheek, curves around the upper lip, and crosses the midline at the philtrum to terminate beside the nose at LI 20, where it connects to the Stomach channel.

As outlined below, key acupuncture points along this meridian include LI 1, 2, 3, 4, 5, 10, 11, 12, 14, 15, 18, and 20.

Fig. 6.2.1 Large Intestine Channel

LI 1 – (Metal Yang)

Location:

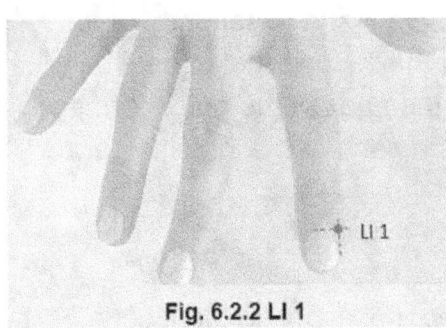

Fig. 6.2.2 LI 1

On the dorsal aspect of the index finger, at the junction of the radial nail border and the base of the nail, approximately 0.1 cun from the nail corner.
Needling Technique:
Perpendicular or oblique proximal insertion 0.1–0.2 cun, or prick to bleed.
Indications:
Toothache, sore throat, submandibular swelling, and numbness of fingers.

LI 2 – (Second Space)

Location:

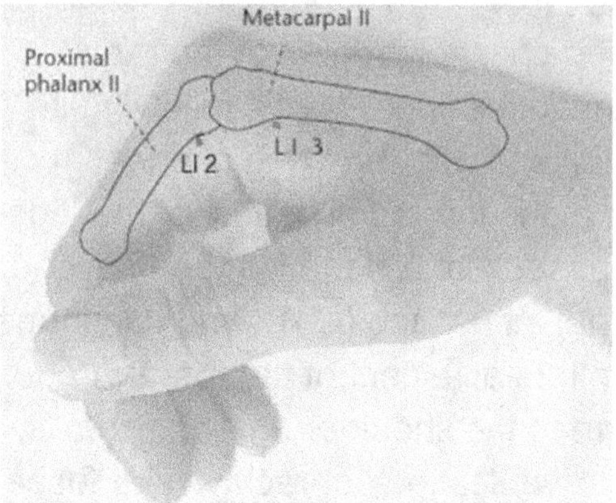

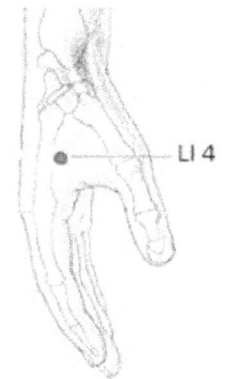

Metacarpal II
Proximal phalanx II
LI 2 LI 3

Fig. 6.2.3 LI 2, 3

On the radial border of the index finger, in the depression distal to the metacarpophalangeal joint. Best located with the finger slightly flexed.
Needling Technique:
Oblique insertion proximal or distal 0.2–0.3 cun, or oblique-perpendicular insertion toward the palm up to 0.5 cun.
Indications:
Epistaxis, fever, toothache, sore throat.

LI 3 – (Third Space)

Location:
In the depression, it is proximal to the head of the second metacarpal bone, on the radial side. Best located when the hand is loosely clenched.
Needling Technique:
Perpendicular insertion 0.5–2 cun, directed toward SI 3. Maintain correct hand position to avoid over-penetration.
Indications:
Toothache, eye pain, sore throat, swelling, and redness of the fingers and hand dorsum.

LI 4 – (Joining Valley)

Location:

LI 4

Fig. 6.2.4 LI 4

On the dorsum of the hand, between the first and second metacarpal bones, at the midpoint of the second metacarpal bone, close to its radial border. Located at the apex of the bulge formed when the thumb is pressed against the base of the index finger.
Needling Technique:
Perpendicular or oblique insertion 0.5–1 cun.
Indications:
Headache, eye and face pain/swelling, nasal obstruction, sore throat, toothache, deafness, facial paralysis, fever, abdominal pain, dysentery, constipation, delayed labour, amenorrhoea, and paralysis of the upper limb.

LI 5 – (Yang Stream)

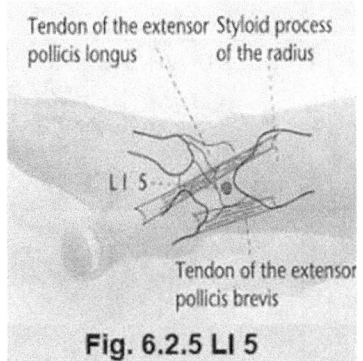

Tendon of the extensor pollicis longus
Styloid process of the radius
LI 5
Tendon of the extensor pollicis brevis

Fig. 6.2.5 LI 5

Location:
On the radial side of the wrist, in the depression between the extensor pollicis longus and brevis tendons.
Needling Technique:
Perpendicular insertion 0.3–0.5 cun.
Indications:
Wrist pain, headache, sore throat, redness and swelling of the eyes, and toothache.

LI 10 – (Arm Three Miles)

Location:

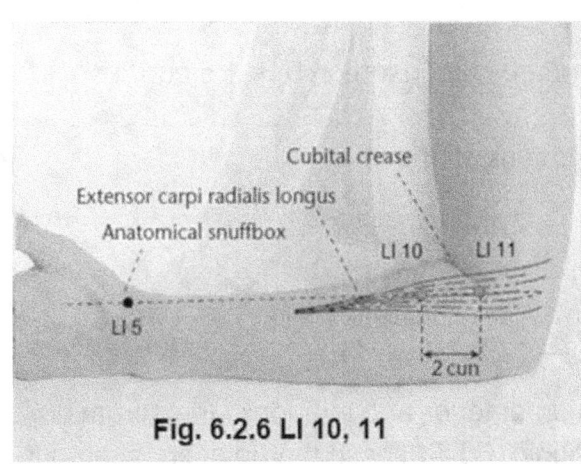

Cubital crease
Extensor carpi radialis longus
Anatomical snuffbox
LI 10   LI 11
LI 5
2 cun

Fig. 6.2.6 LI 10, 11

On the radial side of the forearm, two cun distal to LI 11, on the line joining LI 11 and LI 5. Best located with the elbow flexed and arm supinated.
Needling Technique:
Perpendicular or oblique insertion 0.5–1.5 cun.
Indications:
Abdominal pain, diarrhoea, swelling of the cheek, motor impairment of the upper limbs, shoulder and back pain.

LI 11 – (Pool at the Crook)

Location:
At the lateral end of the transverse cubital crease, midway between LU 5 and the lateral epicondyle of the humerus, with the elbow flexed.
Needling Technique:
Perpendicular insertion 1–1.5 cun.
Indications:
High fever, sore throat, urticaria, vomiting, diarrhoea, redness and pain in the eyes, and upper limb paralysis.

LI 12 – (Elbow Seam)

Location:
With the elbow flexed, one cun proximal and 1 cun lateral to LI 11, just above the lateral epicondyle of the humerus.
Needling Technique:
Perpendicular insertion 0.5–1 cun.
Indications:
Pain, numbness, or stiffness of the elbow and upper arm.

LI 14 – (Upper Arm)

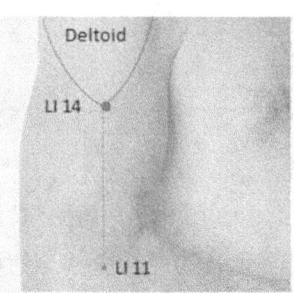

Fig. 6.2.8 LI 14

Location:
On the lateral side of the upper arm, on the line connecting LI 11 and LI 15, 7 cun above LI 11, at the insertion of the deltoid muscle.
Needling Technique:
Perpendicular or upward oblique insertion 0.8–1.5 cun.
Indications:
Shoulder and arm pain, neck stiffness.

LI 15 – (Shoulder Bone)

Location:

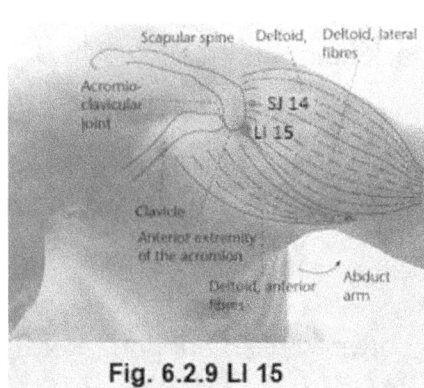

Fig. 6.2.9 LI 15

In the depression anterior and inferior to the acromion, at the deltoid origin. SJ 14 lies in the adjacent posterior-inferior depression. Both are more palpable with arm abduction.
Needling Technique:
Perpendicular insertion 1–1.5 cun (arm abducted) toward the axilla, or transverse-oblique insertion 1.5–2 cun toward the elbow.
Indications:
Shoulder pain, motor impairment of the upper limbs.

LI 18 – (Support the Prominence)

Location:
On the lateral side of the neck, level with the tip of the laryngeal prominence, between the sternal and clavicular heads of the sternocleidomastoid muscle. May be ~3 cun

lateral to the midline.
Needling Technique:
Perpendicular insertion 0.3–0.5 cun or oblique insertion 0.5–0.8 cun.
Caution:
Deeper needling may risk puncture of the carotid artery or jugular vein.
Indications:
Cough, asthma, sore throat, sudden loss of voice.

LI 20 – (Welcome Fragrance)

Location:

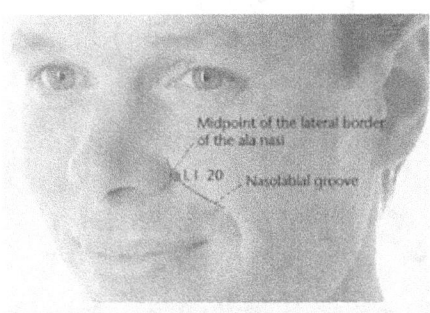

Fig. 6.2.11 LI 20

In the nasolabial groove, at the level of the midpoint of the lateral border of the ala nasi.
Needling Technique:
Transverse insertion medio-superiorly 0.3–0.5 cun, or connect with M-HN-14 at the highest point of the groove.
Indications:
Nasal obstruction, rhinorrhoea, epistaxis, facial swelling, deviation of the mouth, and itching of the face.

Large Intestine Channel – Clinical Significance

As it passes through these regions, the large intestine channel is commonly used to treat disorders of the head, face, and sensory organs. It benefits conditions such as toothache, facial pain, sinusitis, nasal congestion, sore throat, and eye irritation. One of its most essential points, LI 4, is widely used for relieving pain, reducing inflammation, and treating febrile conditions.

The channel also regulates bowel movements and helps treat digestive issues, including constipation, diarrhea, and abdominal discomfort. As an organ paired with the Lung in the interior-exterior relationship, it helps clear external pathogenic factors, making it useful for symptoms such as fever, chills, and the early stages of respiratory infections.

On a psychological level, the Large Intestine is associated with the ability to let go, both physically and emotionally. It is often involved in treatments for emotional rigidity, obsessive thoughts, and unresolved grief.

-Modern Acupuncture-

6.3 Stomach Channel (ST)

The Stomach Channel, also known as the Foot Yang Ming Channel, begins at ST 1, located between the eyeball and the infraorbital ridge, directly below the pupil. After linking with the Large Intestine channel, it descends along the lateral aspect of the nose to the mouth corner, curves around the mandible, ascends anterior to the ear and hairline to ST 8 at the forehead. From there, it descends along the throat to the supraclavicular fossa (ST 11), continuing down the chest and abdomen along the mammillary line. It reaches the inguinal region (ST 30), then travels down the anterior thigh, passing through the knee (ST 35), the anterior aspect of the leg, and finally reaches the lateral side of the tip of the second toe at ST 45, where it connects with the Spleen channel.

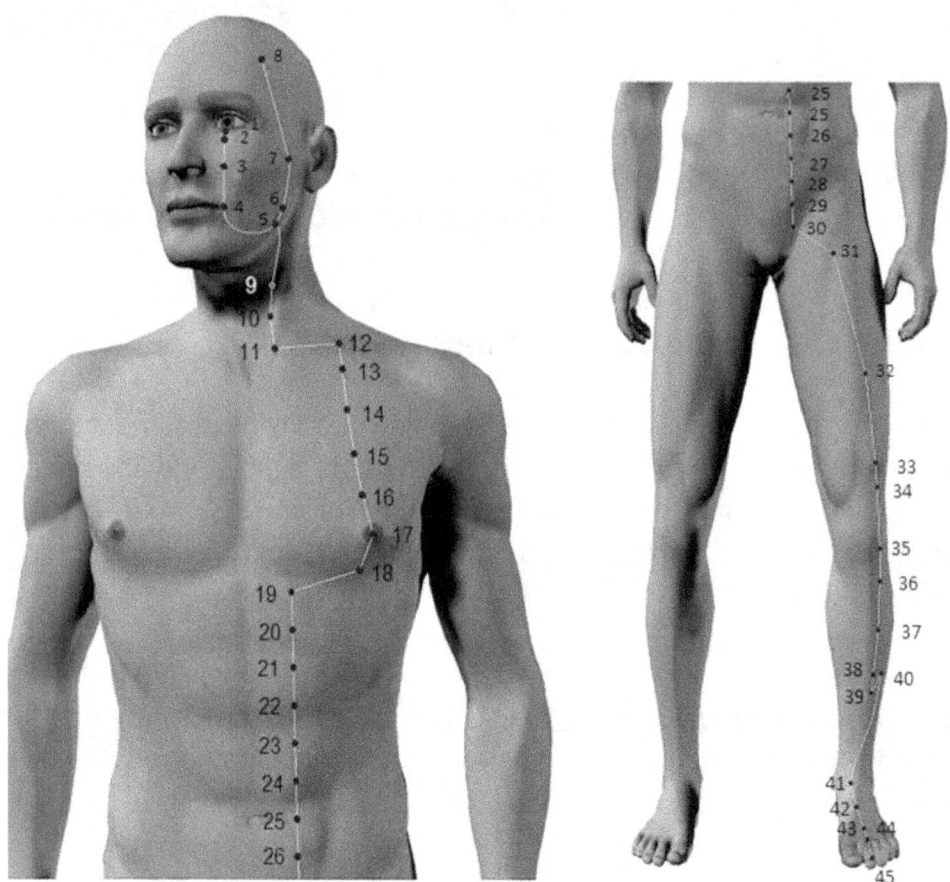

Fig. 6.3.1 Stomach Channel

Below are detailed descriptions of key points along the Stomach Channel:

ST 3 "Great Crevice"

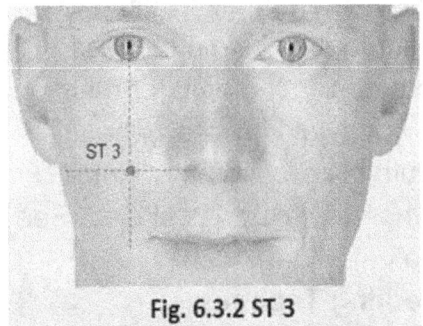

Fig. 6.3.2 ST 3

Location: Directly below the pupil, at the ala nasi's lower border on the nasolabial groove's lateral side.
Needling Technique: Perpendicular insertion 0.3 to 0.4 cun, followed by transverse direction to connect with ST 4 and SI 18.
Indications: Facial paralysis, twitching of eyelids, epistaxis, toothache, swelling of lips and cheeks.

ST 4 "Earth Granary"

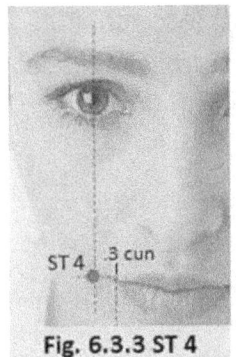

Fig. 6.3.3 ST 4

Location: Directly below the pupil, lateral to the corner of the mouth.
Needling Technique: Subcutaneous insertion 1 to 1.5 cun with the needle tip directed toward ST 6.
Indications: Deviation of the mouth, salivation, twitching of eyelids.

ST 6 "Jawbone"

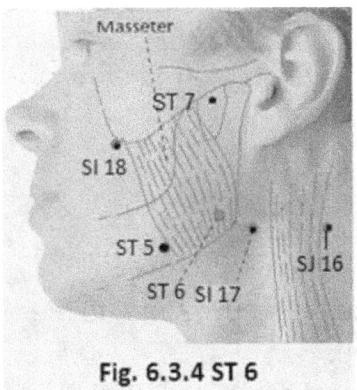

Fig. 6.3.4 ST 6

Location: At the prominence of the masseter muscle, approximately one fingerbreadth anterior and superior to the angle of the jaw when the teeth are clenched.
Needling Technique: Perpendicular insertion 0.5 cun, then transverse toward ST 4, ST 5, or ST 7.
Indications: Facial paralysis, toothache, swelling of the cheek and face, mumps, locked jaw.

ST 7 "Below the Joint"

Location: At the lower border of the zygomatic arch, in the depression anterior to the condyloid process of the mandible. Although this point is palpated with the

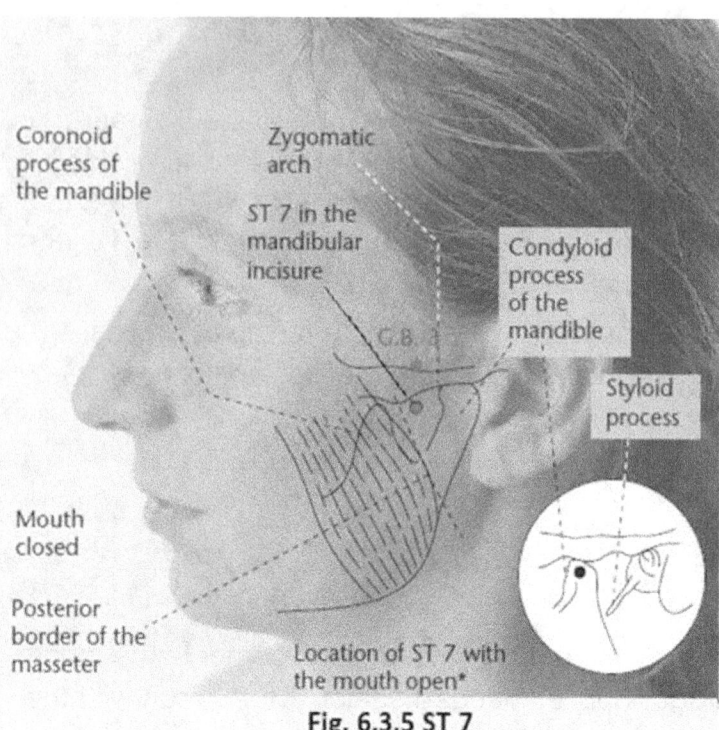

Coronoid process of the mandible

Zygomatic arch

ST 7 in the mandibular incisure

Condyloid process of the mandible

G.B.

Styloid process

Mouth closed

Posterior border of the masseter

Location of ST 7 with the mouth open*

Fig. 6.3.5 ST 7

mouth closed, it helps to ask the patient to open their mouth to locate the condyloid process more easily. If the finger rests on the condyloid process when the mouth is open, it will fall into ST 7 when the mouth is closed. See also Fig. 6.3.4.

Needling Technique: Perpendicular insertion 0.5 to 1 cun, followed by transverse insertion to connect with SI 19, ST 6, or SI 18.

Indications: Deafness, tinnitus, toothache, facial paralysis, facial pain, motor impairment of the jaw.

ST 8 "Head's Binding"

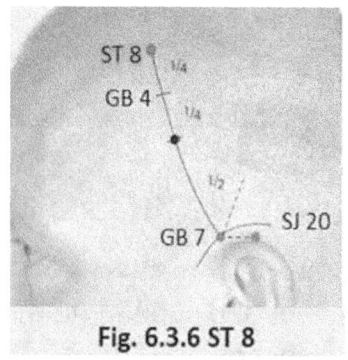

ST 8
GB 4
1/4
1/4
1/2
GB 7
SJ 20

Fig. 6.3.6 ST 8

Location: At the corner of the forehead, 0.5 cun within the anterior hairline and 4.5 cun lateral to DU 24.
Needling Technique: Transverse insertion 0.5 to 1 cun.
Indications: Headache, blurring of vision, eye pain, excessive lacrimation.

ST 16 "Breast Window"

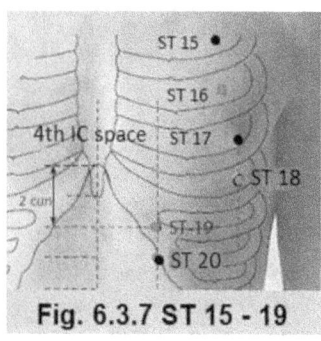

ST 15
ST 16
4th IC space   ST 17
ST 18
2 cun
ST 19
ST 20

Fig. 6.3.7 ST 15 - 19

Location: In the 3rd intercostal space, four cun lateral to the midline on the chest's mammillary line.
Needling Technique: Transverse insertion 0.5 to 0.8 cun along the intercostal space.

Indications: Lack of lactation, breast pain, chest fullness, hypochondriac pain, cough, asthma.

Caution: Avoid deep or perpendicular insertion due to the risk of pneumothorax.

ST 18 "Root of the Breast"

Location: In the 5th intercostal space, four cun lateral to the midline, below the root of the breast.
Needling Technique: Transverse-oblique insertion 0.5 to 1 cun.
Indications: Breast pain, insufficient lactation, chest pain, cough, asthma.
Caution: Risk of pneumothorax; avoid deep insertion.

ST 19 "Not Contained"

Location: 2 cun lateral to the midline and six cun superior to the umbilicus, level with REN 14.
Needling Technique: Perpendicular insertion 0.5 to 0.8 cun.
Indications: Abdominal distension, vomiting, gastric pain, anorexia.
Caution: Avoid deep insertion to prevent injury to the enlarged heart or liver.

ST 21 "Beam Gate"

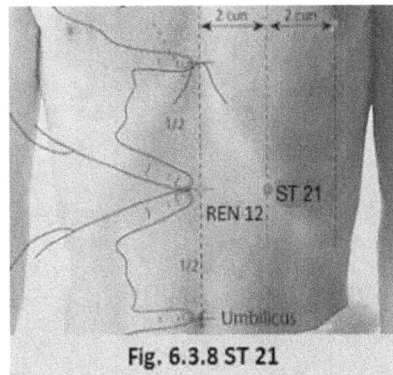

Fig. 6.3.8 ST 21

Location: 4 cun above the umbilicus, two cun lateral to REN 12.
Needling Technique: Perpendicular insertion 0.8 to 1.0 cun.
Indications: Gastric pain, vomiting, anorexia, abdominal distension, diarrhoea.

ST 24 "Slippery Flesh Gate"

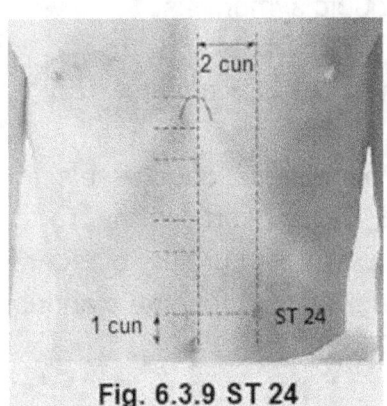

Fig. 6.3.9 ST 24

Location: 1 cun above the umbilicus, two cun lateral to REN 9.
Needling Technique: Perpendicular insertion 1 to 1.5 cun.
Indications: Epigastric pain, vomiting.
Caution: Deep needling in thin subjects may penetrate the peritoneal cavity.

ST 26 "Outer Mound"
Location: 1 cun below the umbilicus, two cun lateral to REN 7.
Needling Technique: Perpendicular insertion 1 to 1.5 cun.

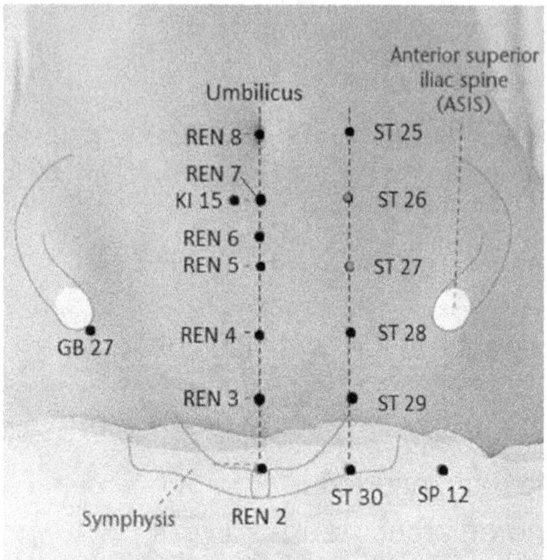

Indications: Abdominal pain, hernia, dysmenorrhoea.
Caution: Deep needling may penetrate the peritoneal cavity.

ST 27 (Daju, "Great Gigantic")
Location: 2 cun below the umbilicus, two cun lateral to REN 5.
Needling Technique: Perpendicular insertion 1 to 1.5 cun.
Indications: Lower abdominal distension, dysuria, hernia, and premature ejaculation.
Caution: Deep needling may penetrate the peritoneal cavity.

Fig. 6.3.10 ST 26, 27

ST 30 "Surging Qi"

Location: At the level of the superior border of the pubic symphysis, 2 cun lateral to the midline.
Needling Technique: Perpendicular insertion 1 to 1.5 cun.
Indications: Abdominal pain, borborygmus, hernia, genital pain or swelling, impotence, dysmenorrhoea, irregular menstruation.
Caution: Avoid deep upward insertion; ensure bladder is emptied before needling.

Stomach 30
Location: The two-cun line is halfway between the midline and the palpable lateral border of the rectus abdominis muscle. ST 30 lies on the lower abdomen and two cun lateral to the midline, at level with the superior border of the pubic symphysis.

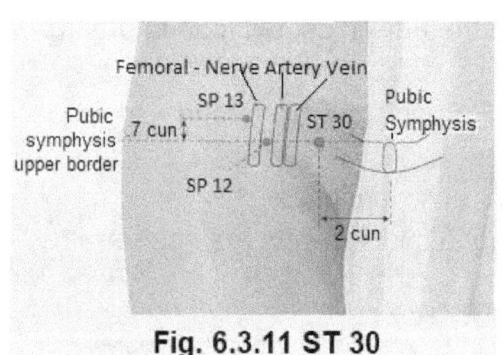

Fig. 6.3.11 ST 30

Needling Technique: ST 30 is needled with perpendicular insertion for 1 to 1.5 cun
Warning: In thin patients, deep insertion in a superior direction may penetrate blood vessels and the spermatic cord. Deep insertion may also damage the peritoneal cavity and urinary bladder. The patient should be asked to empty the bladder before needling.

Indications: Abdominal pain, borborygmus, hernia, swelling, pain of the external genitalia, impotence, dysmenorrhea, irregular menstruation.

ST 31 "Thigh Gate"

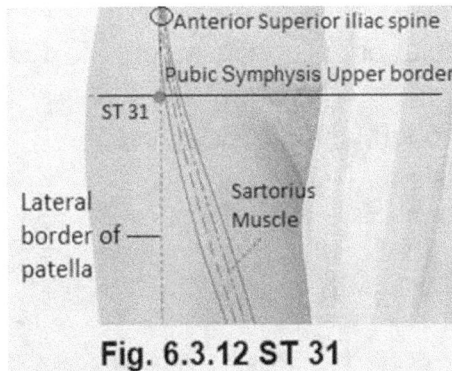

Fig. 6.3.12 ST 31

Location: On the upper thigh, lateral to the sartorius, at the intersection of vertical and horizontal lines from ASIS to pubic symphysis.
Needling Technique: Perpendicular or oblique insertion 1 to 2 cun.
Indications: Thigh pain, muscular atrophy, motor impairment, numbness, pain in lower limbs.

ST 34 "Ridge Mound"

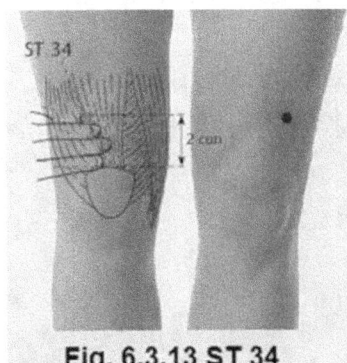

Fig. 6.3.13 ST 34

Location: 2 cun above the patella, on the line from ASIS to the lower lateral patella border.
Needling Technique: Perpendicular or oblique insertion 1 to 1.5 cun.
Indications: Knee pain and numbness, gastric pain, breast pain, and motor impairment of lower limbs.

ST 35 "Calf's Nose"

Location: Lateral to the patellar ligament in the hollow formed on knee flexion.

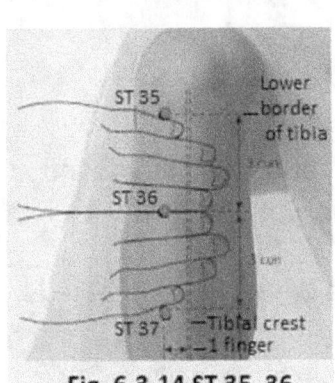

Fig. 6.3.14 ST 35, 36

Needling Technique: Perpendicular insertion 1 to 2 cun toward UB 40, or oblique insertion medial/superior.
Indications: Knee pain, numbness, motor impairment.

ST 36 "Leg Three Miles"
Location: 3 cun below ST 35, one fingerbreadth lateral to the tibia's anterior crest.
Needling Technique: Perpendicular insertion 1 to 1.5 cun.
Indications: Digestive disorders, diarrhoea, constipation, gastric pain, leg weakness, immune support, fatigue, insomnia.

ST 40 "Abundant Bulge"

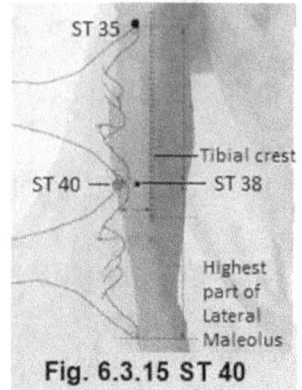

Fig. 6.3.15 ST 40

Location: Midway between knee and ankle, two fingerbreadths lateral to tibial crest.
Needling Technique: Perpendicular or oblique insertion 1 to 1.5 cun.
Indications: Phlegm disorders, cough, asthma, dizziness, headache, leg swelling, or paralysis.

ST 41 Jiexi, "Stream Divide"

Location: At the ankle, level with the lateral malleolus, between the extensor hallucis longus and extensor digitorum longus tendons.
Needling Technique: Perpendicular insertion 0.5 cun or oblique beneath tendons.
Indications: Ankle pain, leg weakness, dizziness, epilepsy, abdominal distension, constipation.
Caution: Avoid the anterior tibial artery and nerve.

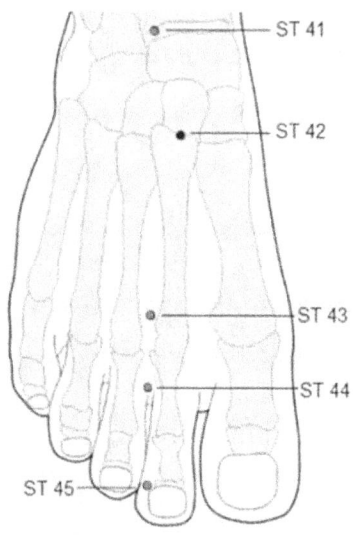

Fig. 6.3.16 ST 42 - 45

ST 43 Xiangu, "Sunken Valley"

Location: On the dorsum of the foot, between the second and third metatarsals, 1 cun proximal to ST 44.
Needling Technique: Perpendicular or oblique insertion 0.5 cun.
Indications: Foot pain/swelling, facial oedema, abdominal pain.

ST 44 "Inner Courtyard"

Location: On the dorsum of the foot, between the second and third toes, 0.5 cun proximal to the web margin.

Needling Technique: Perpendicular 0.5 cun or oblique insertion 0.5 to 1 cun directed proximally.
Indications: Facial pain, sore throat, gastric discomfort, diarrhoea, foot swelling, fever.

ST 45 "Strict Exchange"

Location: Lateral side of the second toe, 0.1 cun posterior to the nail corner.
Needling Technique: Subcutaneous insertion 0.1 cun.
Indications: Facial swelling, sore throat, hoarseness, abdominal distension, coldness of the leg and foot, fever, disturbed sleep.

Stomach Channel – Clinical Significance

The Stomach channel is one of the most essential and longest channels in the body. It treats various conditions related to digestion, metabolism, and disorders of the head, face, chest, abdomen, and lower limbs. It is frequently used for symptoms such as nausea, vomiting, acid reflux, abdominal pain, poor appetite, and constipation.

Because the channel passes through the face, it is also effective in treating facial paralysis, trigeminal neuralgia, toothache, and sinus disorders. Points around the eyes and jaw are often used in these cases.

-Modern Acupuncture-

6.4 Spleen Channel (SP)

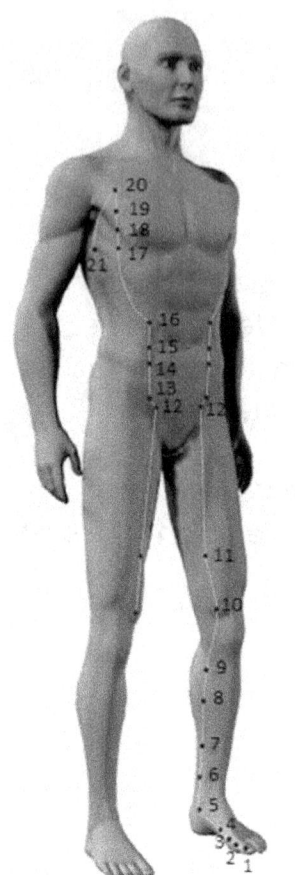

Fig. 6.4.1 Spleen Channel

The Spleen Channel, also called the Foot Tai Yin Channel, begins at SP 1 on the medial aspect of the big toe tip, after connecting with the Stomach channel. It travels along the medial foot at the red and white skin junction, ascends anterior to the medial malleolus, and continues upward along the medial leg. Passing through the anterior medial thigh, it reaches the inguinal region and travels along the anterior abdomen. The channel curves laterally from the midline, ascending through the intercostal spaces to the 2nd intercostal space. From there, it turns inferiorly midway between the axilla and the free end of the 11th rib to reach SP 21, then connects with the Heart channel.

Key points of the Spleen Channel 1, 2, 3, 4, 5, 6, 7, 8, 9, 10, 12, 15 are described below:

SP 1 "Hidden White"

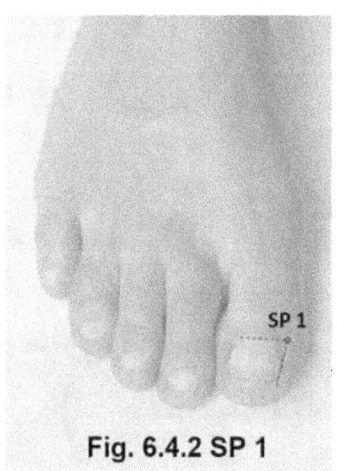

Fig. 6.4.2 SP 1

Location: On the dorsal aspect of the big toe, at the junction of lines along the medial nail border and nail base, about 0.1 cun from the nail corner.
Needling Technique: Perpendicular or oblique insertion directed proximally 0.1 to 0.2 cun, or prick to bleed.
Indications: Abdominal distension, uterine bleeding, mental disorders, insomnia, convulsions.

SP 2 "Great Metropolis"

Location: On the medial side of the big toe, in the depression distal and inferior to the first metatarsophalangeal joint.
Needling Technique: Oblique inferior insertion 0.3 to 0.5 cun.
Indications: Abdominal distension, gastric pain, constipation.

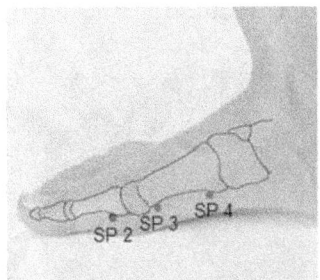

SP 3 "Supreme White"

Location: Proximal and inferior to the first metatarsophalangeal joint, in the depression at the red and white skin junction.
Needling Technique: Perpendicular insertion 0.5 to 1 cun.
Indications: Abdominal pain/distension, vomiting, diarrhoea,
constipation, dysentery, borborygmus.

Fig. 6.4.3 SP 2, 3 , 4

SP 4 "Grandfather Grandson"

Location: On the medial foot, in the depression distal and inferior to the base of the first metatarsal bone.
Needling Technique: Perpendicular insertion 0.5 to 1 cun.
Indications: Gastric pain, distention, diarrhoea, bloody stools, epigastric pain, poor appetite, chest congestion, irregular menstruation, postpartum faintness.

SP 5 "Shang Mound"

Location: On the medial ankle, in the depression formed by lines along the anterior and inferior borders of the medial malleolus.
Needling Technique: Perpendicular insertion 0.2 to 0.3 cun or transverse beneath tendons toward ST 41.
Indications: Abdominal issues, rigidity of the tongue, pain in the foot and ankle, haemorrhoids.

SP 6 (Sanyinjiao, "Three Yin Intersection")

Location: 3 cun directly above the tip of the medial malleolus, posterior to the medial tibial border.
Needling Technique: Perpendicular insertion 0.5 to 1 cun.
Indications: Commonly used for gynaecological, urological, gastrointestinal, neurological, and mental disorders.

SP 7 (Lougu, "Dripping Valley")

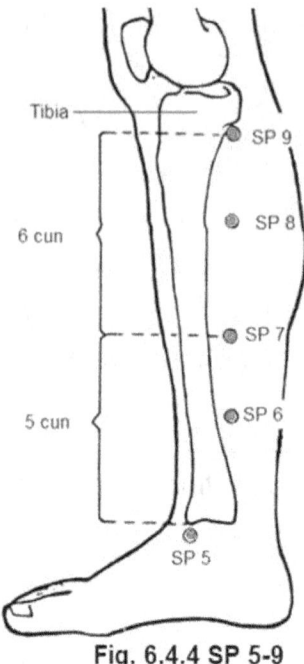

Fig. 6.4.4 SP 5-9

Location: 3 cun superior to SP 6, in a depression posterior to the medial tibial crest.
Needling Technique: Perpendicular or oblique insertion 1 to 1.5 cun.
Indications: Abdominal distension, borborygmus, cold/numbness/paralysis of the knee and leg.

SP 8 (Diji, "Earth Pivot")

Location: 3 cun inferior to SP 9, posterior to the medial crest of the tibia.
Needling Technique: Perpendicular or oblique insertion 1 to 1.5 cun.
Indications: Abdominal pain, diarrhoea, oedema, dysuria, irregular menstruation, dysmenorrhoea.

SP 9 (Yinlingquan, "Yin Mound Spring")

Location: In the depression below the medial condyle of the tibia, at the posterior border.
Needling Technique: Perpendicular insertion 1 to 1.5 cun.
Indications: Abdominal pain, diarrhoea, oedema, jaundice, dysuria, genital pain, dysmenorrhoea, knee pain.

SP 10 (Xuehai, "Sea of Blood")

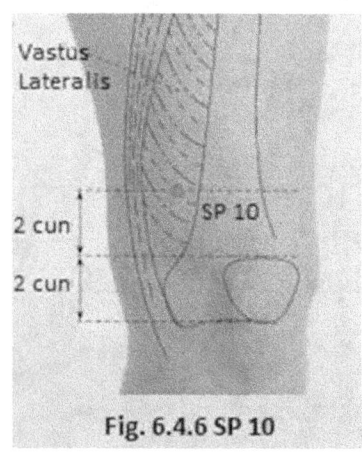

Fig. 6.4.6 SP 10

Location: 2 cun above the superior medial border of the patella, in the bulge of the medial portion of the quadriceps femoris.
Needling Technique: Perpendicular or oblique insertion 1 to 1.5 cun.
Indications: Irregular menstruation, dysmenorrhoea, uterine bleeding, urticaria, eczema, medial thigh pain.

SP 12 "Rushing Gate"

Location: Superior to the lateral end of the inguinal groove, lateral to the pulsating femoral artery, 3.5 cun lateral to REN 2.
Needling Technique: Perpendicular insertion 0.5 to 1 cun.
Caution: Avoid the artery, vein, and nerve.
Indications: Abdominal pain, hernia, dysuria.

SP 15 "Great Horizontal"

Location: In the depression at the lateral border of the rectus abdominis, four cun lateral to the umbilicus.
Needling Technique: Perpendicular insertion 0.5 to 1 cun.
Caution: Avoid puncturing an enlarged spleen or liver.
Indications: Abdominal pain/distension, diarrhoea, constipation, dysentery. Important for regulating the qi of the large intestine.

Spleen Channel, Clinical Significance

The Spleen channel plays a central role in digestion, energy production, and fluid metabolism. It is commonly used to treat poor appetite, bloating, loose stools, diarrhoea, and chronic fatigue. It supports the transformation and transportation of nutrients and fluids throughout the body.

Since it influences blood production and containment, this channel is valuable in managing bleeding disorders, varicose veins, prolapse, and uterine bleeding. Its role in holding things in place makes it key in treating organ prolapse and muscle weakness.

The Spleen also governs the muscles and limbs. Points on this channel help strengthen weak muscles and are used in muscle wasting or limb heaviness cases.

Emotionally, the Spleen is associated with overthinking and worry. The channel is involved in treating mental fatigue, lack of concentration, and emotional instability rooted in pensiveness or obsessive thought.

Additionally, because the channel passes through the genital region and connects with the Chong and Ren vessels, it helps treat gynecological disorders such as dysmenorrhea, irregular menstruation, and leukorrhea.

-Modern Acupuncture-

6.5 Heart Channel (HT)

The Heart Channel, also known as the Hand Shao Yin Channel, originates from its connection with the Spleen channel and begins at HT1, located in the center of the axilla. It descends along the posterior border of the medial aspect of the upper arm, passes through the cubital region at HT 3, and continues down to the pisiform area proximal to the palm at HT 7, where it enters the hand. It terminates at the medial aspect of the tip of the little finger at HT 9, where it connects to the Small Intestine channel.

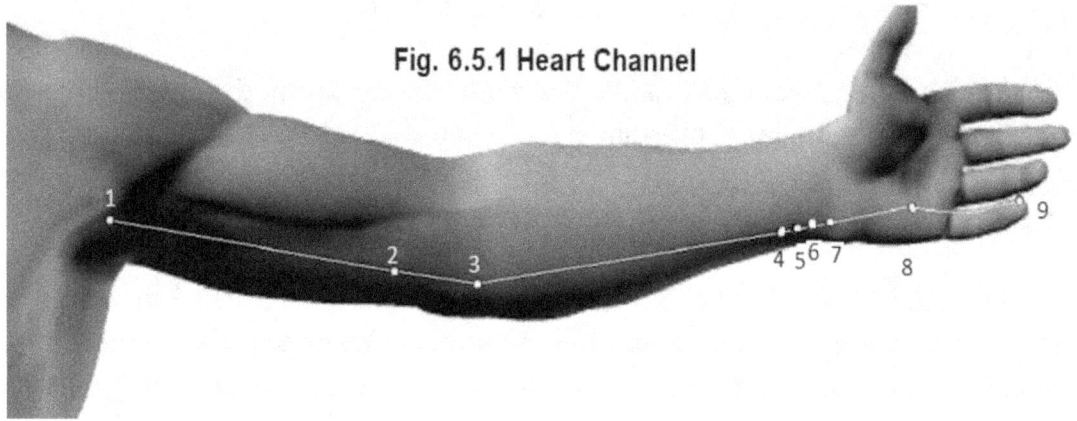

Fig. 6.5.1 Heart Channel

Key points HT 3, 4, and 7 along the Heart Channel are described below:

HT 3 "Lesser Sea"

Location: With the elbow flexed, this point lies at the midpoint of the line connecting the medial end of the cubital crease and the medial epicondyle of the humerus.
Needling Technique: Perpendicular insertion 0.5 to 1.0 cun.
Indications: Pain and numbness of the hand and arm, tremors of the hand, axillary pain, hypochondriac pain.

HT 4 "Spirit Path"

Location: On the radial side of the flexor carpi ulnaris tendon, 1.5 cun above the transverse crease of the wrist, with the palm facing upward.
Needling Technique: Perpendicular insertion 0.3 to 0.5 cun.
Indications: Spasmodic pain of the elbow and arm, sudden loss of voice. For cardiac-related chest pain (angina), acupuncture should not be used as first-line treatment unless emergency cardiac care is unavailable.

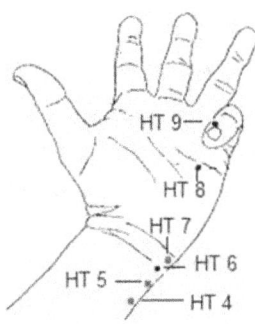

Fig. 6.5.3 HT 4-9

HT 5 "Penetrating the Interior"

Location: One cun above the transverse crease of the wrist, on the radial side of the flexor carpi ulnaris tendon, with the palm facing upward.
Needling Technique: Perpendicular insertion 0.3 to 0.5 cun.
Indications: Palpitations, dizziness, blurred vision, sore throat, sudden loss of voice, aphasia with tongue stiffness, pain in the wrist and elbow (only after excluding cardiovascular causes).

HT 7 "Spirit Gate"

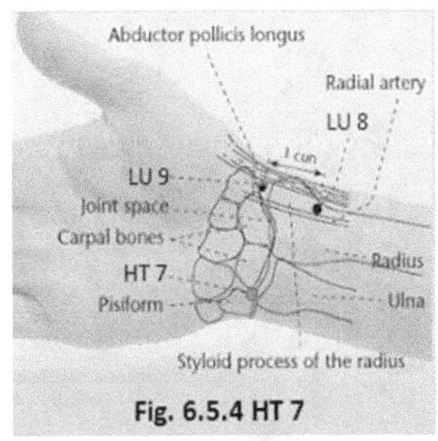

Fig. 6.5.4 HT 7

Location: At the ulnar end of the transverse wrist crease, in the depression on the radial side of the flexor carpi ulnaris tendon.
Needling Technique: Perpendicular insertion 0.3 to 0.5 cun.
Indications: Irritability, palpitations, hysteria, amnesia, insomnia, epilepsy, dementia, hypochondriac pain, feverish sensation in the palm.

Clinical Significance of Heart Channel

The Heart channel is closely linked to regulating blood circulation and stabilizing mental and emotional functions. It is commonly used to treat palpitations, chest pain, arrhythmias, and disorders affecting heart rhythm or blood flow.

Because the Heart is considered the seat of the mind (Shen) in traditional Chinese medicine, this channel plays a vital role in addressing emotional and psychological conditions. It is frequently used to manage insomnia, anxiety, restlessness, depression, poor memory, and excessive laughter or sadness.

The channel also runs along the inner arm and can help alleviate pain, numbness, or tingling in this area, including conditions such as medial epicondylitis (also known as golfer's elbow).

In some cases, Heart channel points are combined with Pericardium or Small Intestine points to harmonise emotional and cardiac symptoms, particularly when emotional stress and circulatory imbalance combine.

-Modern Acupuncture-

6.6 Small Intestine Channel (SI)

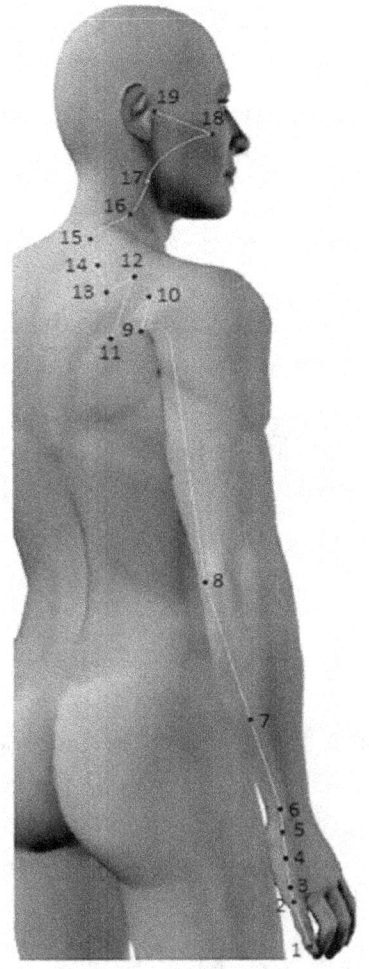

Fig. 6.6.1 Small Intestine Channel

The Small Intestine channel, also known as the Hand Tai Yang channel (Hand Greater Yang), originates from its connection with the Heart channel. It begins at the ulnar tip of the little finger at SI 1 and ascends along the ulnar aspect of the hand dorsum and posterior lateral arm, reaching the elbow at SI 8. From there, it travels around the scapular region, dips into the suprascapular fossa at SI 12, and ascends the neck to reach the cheek through the outer canthus of the eye at SI 18, before ending in front of the tragus at SI 19. It then links with the Urinary Bladder channel.

Important points of this channel, SI 1, 2, 3, 4, 5, 6, 8, 9, 10, 11, 18, and 19, are described below, along with their traditional names and meanings.

SI 1 – Shao Ze (Lesser Marsh)

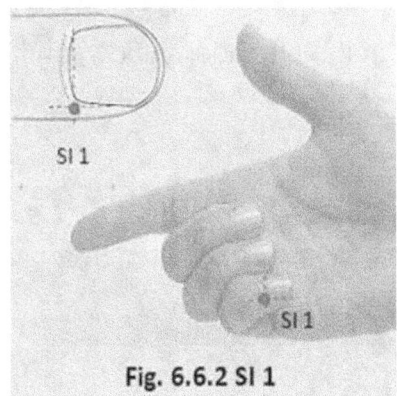

Fig. 6.6.2 SI 1

Location: On the ulnar side of the little finger, approximately 0.1 cun from the nail corner.
Needling Technique: Subcutaneous insertion of 0.1 cun or pricking to bleed.
Indications: Headache, fever, insufficient lactation, sore throat, redness of the eyes.

SI 2 – (Front Valley)

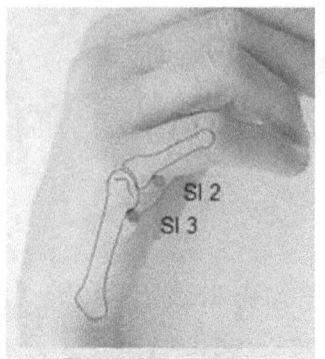

Location: On the ulnar end of the crease in front of the metacarpophalangeal joint of the little finger, at the junction of red and white skin, with a loose fist.
Needling Technique: Perpendicular insertion of 0.3 to 0.5 cun.
Indications: Finger numbness, fever, tinnitus, headache.

SI 3 – (Back Stream)

Fig. 6.6.3 SI 2, 3

Location: On the ulnar side of the hand, proximal to the fifth metacarpophalangeal joint, at the end of the transverse distal palmar crease, at the red-white skin junction with a loose fist.
Needling Technique: Perpendicular insertion in the depression between the base of the fifth metacarpal and the hamate bone.
Indications: Neck stiffness, tinnitus, deafness, sore throat, acute lumbar sprain, finger contracture/numbness, pain in the shoulder and elbow.

SI 4 – (Wrist Bone)

Location: On the ulnar side of the palm, in the depression between the base of the fifth metacarpal bone and the hamate bone.
Needling Technique: Perpendicular insertion of 0.3 to 0.5 cun.

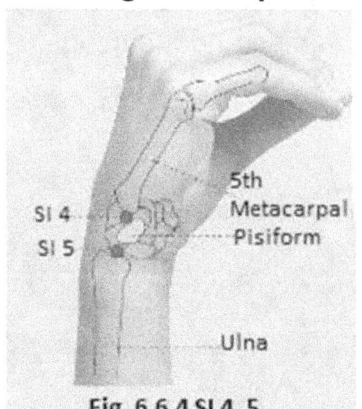

Indications: Headache, neck rigidity, finger contracture, wrist pain, jaundice.

SI 5 – (Yang Valley)

Location: In the bony cleft on the radial side of the styloid process of the ulna, with the palm facing the chest.
Needling Technique: Perpendicular insertion of 0.3 to 0.5 cun.
Indications: Blurred vision, pain in the shoulder, elbow, and arm.

Fig. 6.6.4 SI 4, 5

SI 6 – (Support for the Aged)

Location: In the bony cleft on the radial and dorsal side of the styloid process of the ulna.
Needling Technique: Perpendicular insertion of 0.3 to 0.5 cun.
Indications: Pain in the shoulder, elbow, and arm.

SI 8 – (Small Sea)

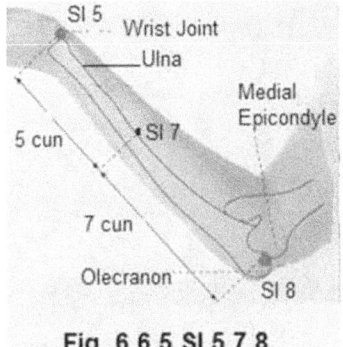

Fig. 6.6.5 SI 5,7,8

Location: In the depression between the olecranon and the medial epicondyle of the humerus, with the elbow flexed.
Needling Technique: Perpendicular insertion of 0.3 to 0.5 cun.
Indications: Headache, cheek swelling, pain in the nape, shoulder, arm, elbow, and epilepsy.

SI 9 – (True Shoulder)

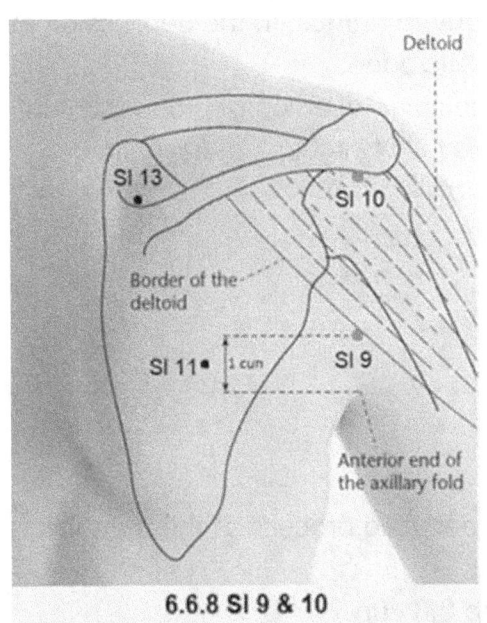

6.6.8 SI 9 & 10

Location: 1 cun above the posterior end of the axillary fold, posterior and inferior to the shoulder joint, with the arm adducted.
Needling Technique: Perpendicular insertion of 0.5 to 1.0 cun.
Indications: Scapular pain, motor impairment of the hand and arm.

SI 10 – (Upper Arm Transport Point)

Location: Directly above the posterior end of the axillary fold, in the depression inferior to the scapular spine when the arm is adducted.
Needling Technique: Perpendicular insertion of 0.5 to 1.0 cun.

Indications: Shoulder swelling, aching, and shoulder and arm weakness.

SI 11 – Tian Zong (Heavenly Gathering)

Location: On the scapula, in the centre of the subscapular fossa, level with the fourth thoracic vertebra.
Needling Technique: Perpendicular or oblique insertion of 0.5 to 1.0 cun. Caution: In thin individuals, avoid deep insertion to prevent lung injury.
Indications: Scapular pain, anterior/posterior arm pain, and asthma.

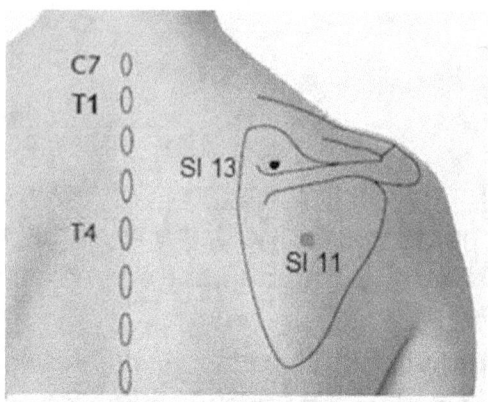

Fig. 6.6.9 SI 11

SI 18 – (Cheek Bone Hole)

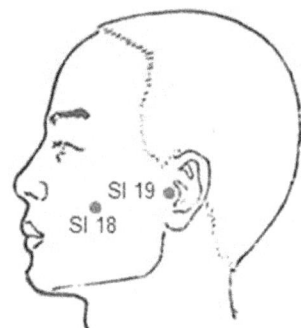

Fig. 6.6.10 SI 18, 19

Location: Directly below the outer canthus, in the depression at the lower border of the zygomatic bone.
Needling Technique: Perpendicular insertion of 0.5 to 0.8 cun.
Indications: Facial paralysis, eyelid twitching, facial pain, cheek swelling, toothache, yellow sclera.

SI 19 – (Palace of Hearing)

Location: Anterior to the tragus and posterior to the condyloid process of the mandible, in the depression formed when the mouth is open.
Needling Technique: Perpendicular insertion of 0.5 to 0.8 cun.
Indications: Facial paralysis, eyelid twitching, facial pain, toothache.

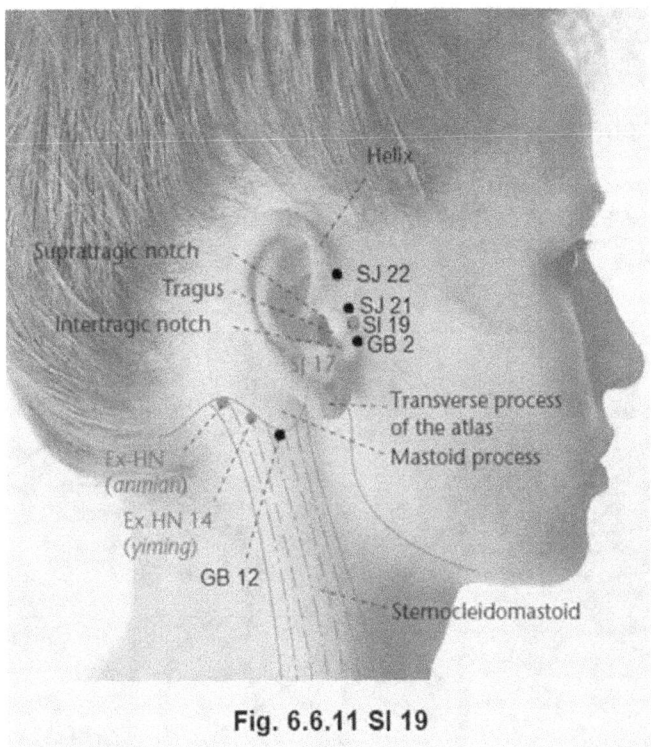

Fig. 6.6.11 SI 19

Small Intestine Channel – Clinical Significance

The Small Intestine channel, which runs along the posterior aspect of the arm and ascends to the face and ear, is often used to treat disorders of the head, neck, shoulder, and upper back. It is particularly helpful in neck stiffness, shoulder pain, scapular tension, and ear problems such as tinnitus, deafness, and otitis.

Though the Small Intestine is primarily known for its digestive function, in acupuncture, the channel is more involved in musculoskeletal and neurological conditions than direct gut issues. However, it can still assist with abdominal pain and digestive irregularities when used in conjunction with abdominal points.

This channel also clears internal heat and calms the mind. It is used for symptoms such as fever, restlessness, and mania. In traditional theory, it separates the pure from the impure, a metaphorical extension that is applied to mental clarity and discernment.

Emotionally, the Small Intestine channel helps individuals manage confusion, indecision, and the effects of prolonged emotional strain, particularly those affecting the heart-mind connection.

- Dr. Pardeshi Acupuncture -

6.7 Urinary Bladder Channel (UB)

The Urinary Bladder channel is also known as the Foot-Shaoyang channel. After receiving connection from the Small Intestine channel, it begins at UB 1, located at the inner canthus of the eye. It ascends through the forehead and connects to the DU channel at DU 3.

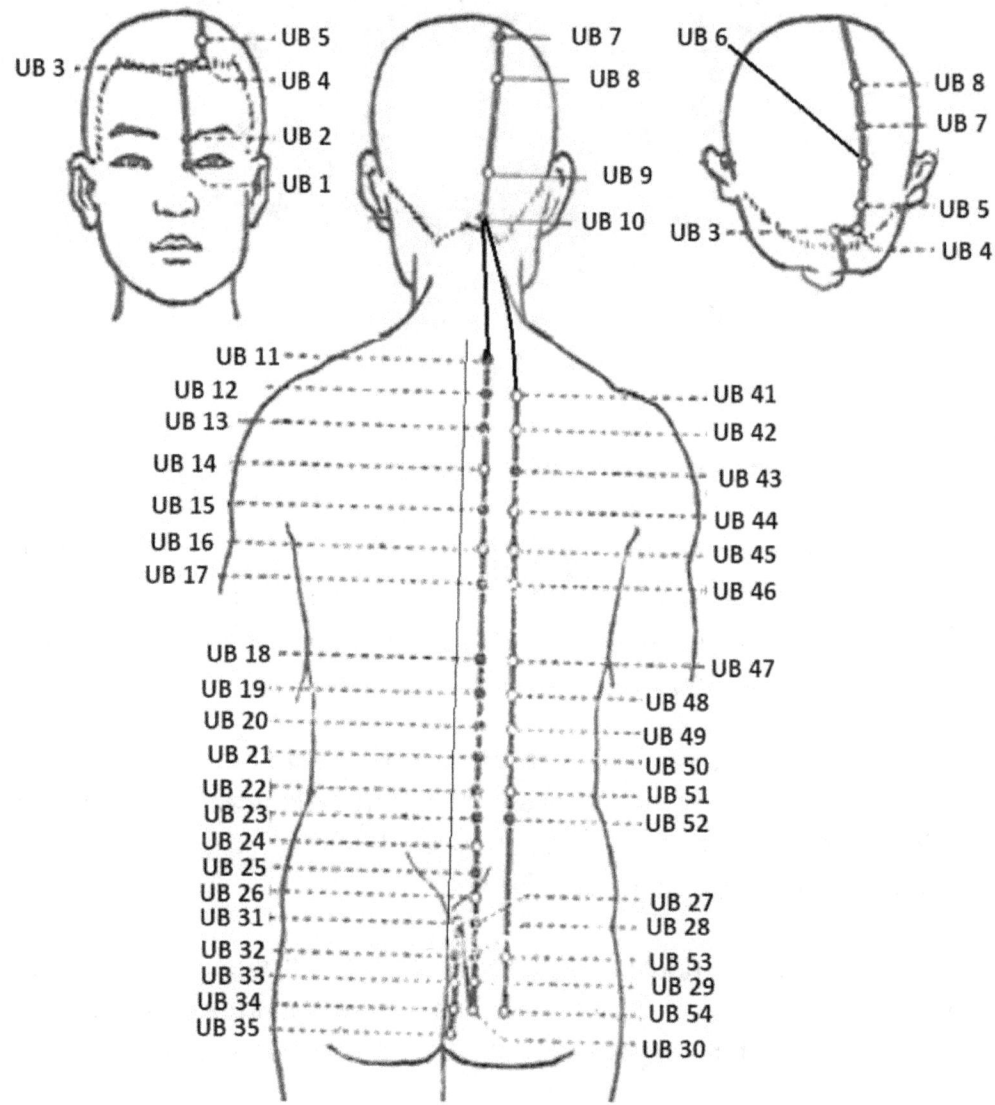

Fig. 6.7.1a Urinary Bladder Channel

A branch enters the brain, while the main channel continues over the vertex along the midline and reaches the posterior aspect of the neck at UB 10. From here, the pathway bifurcates and descends bilaterally along the back, running 1.5 cun lateral to the midline from UB 11 to UB 35.

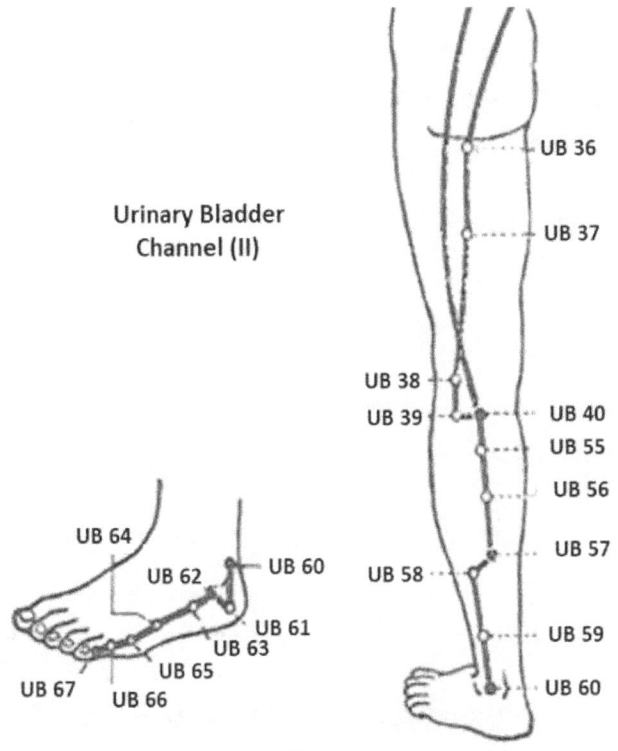

Urinary Bladder Channel (II)

Fig. 6.7.1b

Another branch descends from the gluteal region along the posterior thigh to the popliteal fossa UB 40, then travels downward along the gastrocnemius muscle. It courses along the posterior and inferior aspects of the lateral malleolus and terminates at UB 67, on the lateral side of the little toe. The channel subsequently connects with the Kidney channel.

The key points discussed below are: UB 2, 5, 7, 10, 11, 12, 13, 14, 17, 18, 19, 20, 21, 22, 23, 25, 27, 28, 31, 32, 33, 34, 40, 42, 43, 57, 60, 62, 65, and 67.

Urinary Bladder 2 (Gathered Bamboo)

Location: In the supraorbital notch, at the eyebrow's medial end.

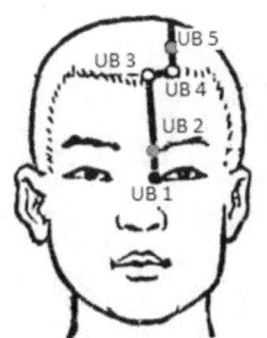

Fig. 6.7.2 UB 1 - 5

Needling Technique: Subcutaneous insertion of 0.3–0.5 cun or pricking to bleed.
Indications: Headache, supraorbital pain, lacrimation, eye redness/swelling, eyelid twitching, glaucoma.

Urinary Bladder 5 (Fifth Place)

Location: 1 cun above the anterior hairline and 1.5 cun lateral to the midline.
Needling Technique: Subcutaneous insertion of 0.3–0.5 cun.
Indications: Headache, epilepsy, convulsions.

Urinary Bladder 7 (Heavenly Connection)

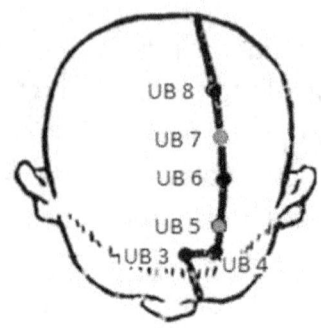

Fig. 6.7.3 UB 3 - 8

Location: 4 cun above the anterior hairline, 1.5 cun lateral to the midline.
Needling Technique: Subcutaneous insertion of 0.3–0.5 cun.
Indications: Headache, dizziness, nasal congestion, epistaxis, rhinorrhoea.

Urinary Bladder 10 (Celestial Pillar)

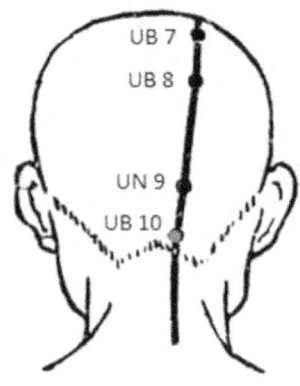

Fig. 6.7.4 UB 7 - 10

Location: 1.3 cun lateral to the posterior midline at the base of the skull.
Needling Technique: Perpendicular insertion of 0.5–0.8 cun.
Indications: Headache, shoulder/back pain, neck stiffness, sore throat.

Urinary Bladder 11 (Great Shuttle)

Location: 1.5 cun lateral to DU 13, level with the 1st thoracic vertebra.
Needling Technique: Oblique insertion of 0.5–0.7 cun.
Indications: Headache, neck/back pain, scapular pain, cough, fever.

Urinary Bladder 12 (Wind Gate)

Location: 1.5 cun lateral to the lower border of T2 spinous process.
Needling Technique: Oblique insertion of 0.5–0.7 cun.
Indications: Headache, neck rigidity, backache, cold, cough, fever.

Urinary Bladder 13 (Lung Shu)

Location: 1.5 cun lateral to DU 12, at T3 level.
Indications: Chest pain, cough, asthma.

Urinary Bladder 14 (Pericardium Shu)

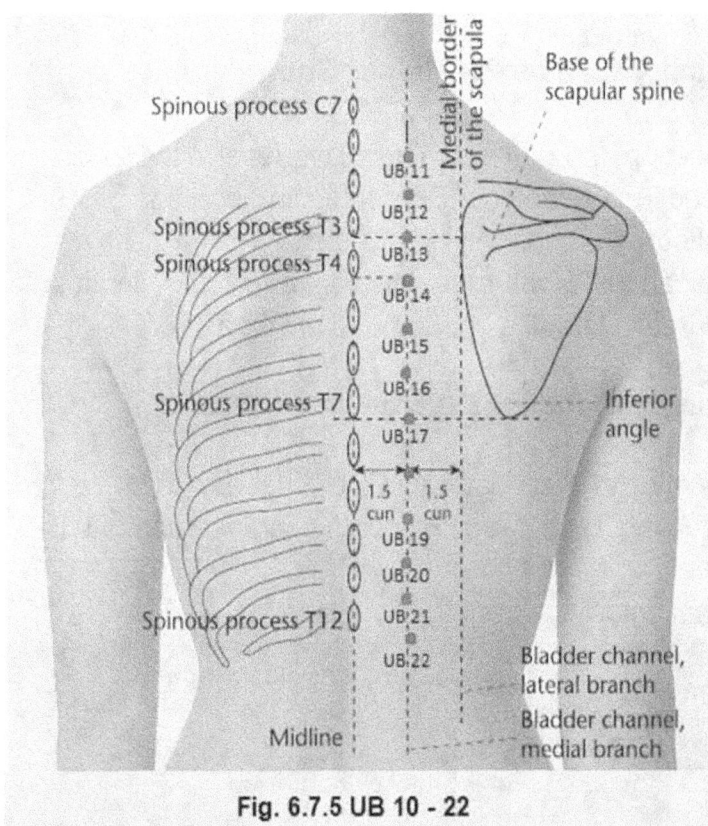

Fig. 6.7.5 UB 10 - 22

Location: 1.5 cun lateral to DU, level with T4.
Needling Technique: Oblique insertion of 0.5–0.7 cun.
Indications: Cough, palpitations, chest congestion, vomiting.

Urinary Bladder 17 (Diaphragm Shu)

Location: 1.5 cun lateral to DU 9, level with T7.
Needling Technique: Oblique insertion of 0.5–0.7 cun.
Indications: Vomiting, hiccups, belching, asthma, cough, measles.

Urinary Bladder 18 (Liver Shu)

Location: 1.5 cun lateral to DU 8, level with T9.
Needling Technique: Oblique insertion of 0.5–0.7 cun.
Indications: Hypochondriac pain, backache, epistaxis, jaundice, eye disorders, epilepsy.

Urinary Bladder 19 (Gallbladder Shu)

Location: 1.5 cun lateral to DU 7, level with T10.
Needling Technique: Oblique insertion of 0.5–0.8 cun.
Indications: Chest and hypochondriac pain, jaundice, bitter mouth taste.

Urinary Bladder 20 (Spleen Shu)

Location: 1.5 cun lateral to DU 6, level with T11.
Needling Technique: Oblique insertion of 0.5–0.7 cun.
Indications: Epigastric pain, distension, vomiting, diarrhoea, dysentery.

Urinary Bladder 21 (Stomach Shu)

Location: Same as UB 20; T12 level.
Needling Technique: Oblique insertion of 0.5–0.7 cun.
Indications: Digestive disorders, menorrhagia, oedema, backache.

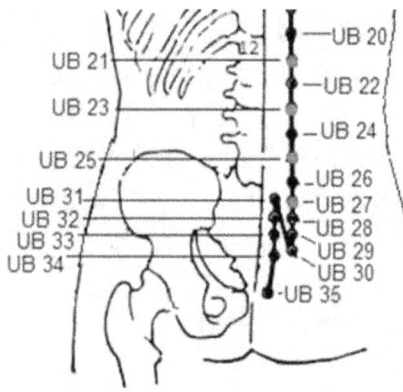

Fig. 6.7.6 UB 20 - 35

Urinary Bladder 23 (Kidney Shu)

Location: 1.5 cun lateral to DU 4, level with L2.
Needling Technique: Perpendicular insertion of 1.0–1.2 cun.
Indications: Nocturnal emission, backache, tinnitus, enuresis, infertility, oedema, diarrhoea.

Urinary Bladder 25 (Large Intestine Shu)

Location: 1.5 cun lateral to DU 3, level with L4.
Needling Technique: Perpendicular insertion of 0.8–1.2 cun.
Indications: Low back pain, abdominal disorders, constipation, sciatica.

Urinary Bladder 27 (Small Intestine Shu)

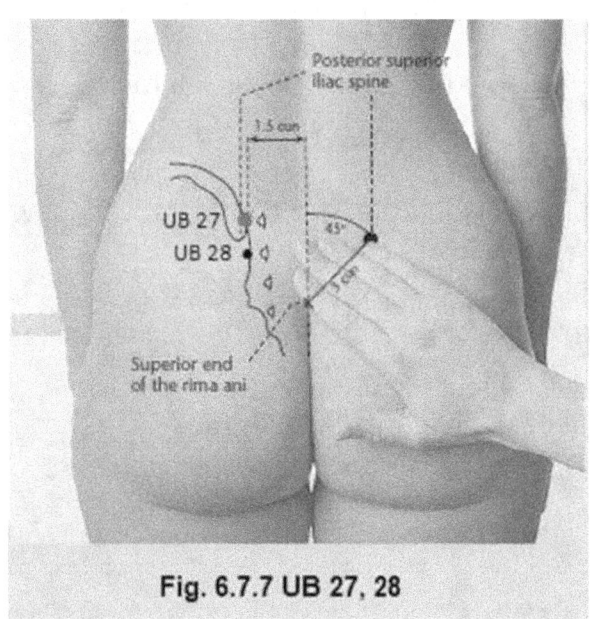

Location: 1.5 cun lateral to the 1st posterior sacral foramen.
Needling Technique: Perpendicular insertion of 0.8–1.2 cun.
Indications: Abdominal pain, dysentery, enuresis, leucorrhoea, sciatica.

Fig. 6.7.7 UB 27, 28

Urinary Bladder 31–34 (Upper, Second, Middle, Lower Crevice)

Location: At the first to fourth posterior sacral foramina.
Needling Technique: Perpendicular insertion of 0.8–1.2 cun.
Indications: Lumbosacral pain, menstrual disorders, leucorrhoea, urinary and bowel dysfunctions.

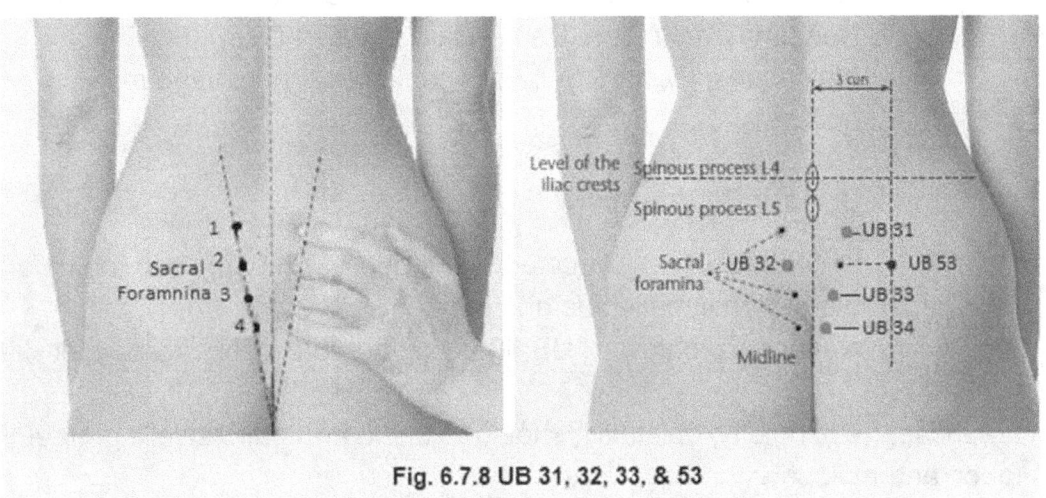

Fig. 6.7.8 UB 31, 32, 33, & 53

Urinary Bladder 40 (Middle of the Crook)

Location: Midpoint of the popliteal crease.
Needling Technique: Perpendicular 0.5–1.0 cun or pricking for bleeding.
Indications: Back pain, leg weakness, abdominal pain, hemiplegia, vomiting.

Urinary Bladder 42 (Door of the Corporeal Soul)

Location: 3 cun lateral to DU, level with T3.

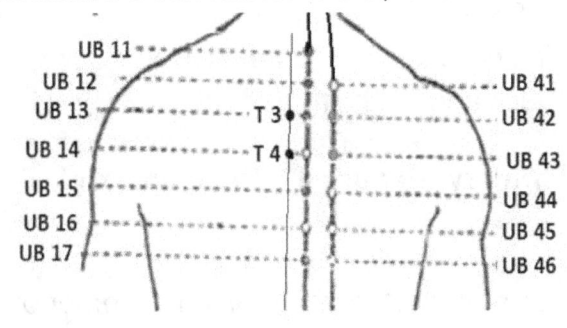

Fig. 6.7.10 UB 42, 43

Needling Technique: Oblique 0.3–0.5 cun.
Indications: Asthma, shoulder pain, neck rigidity.

Urinary Bladder 43 (Vital Region Shu)
Location: 3 cun lateral to DU, level with T4.
Needling Technique: Perpendicular 0.3–0.5 cun.
Indications: Weakness, asthma, memory loss, seminal emission.

Urinary Bladder 57 (Support the Mountain)

Location: Midline of the leg between UB 40 and UB 60, below the gastrocnemius belly.
Needling Technique: Perpendicular 0.8–1.2 cun.
Indications: Lumbago, calf cramps, haemorrhoids, constipation.

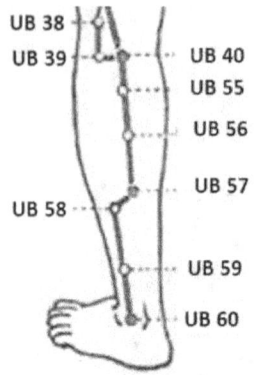

Fig. 6.7.11 UB 40, 57, 60

Urinary Bladder 60 (Kunlun Mountains)
Location: Between the lateral malleolus and Achilles tendon.
Needling Technique: Perpendicular 0.5–1.0 cun.
Indications: Pain of the head, neck, back, heel; labour pain; epilepsy.

Urinary Bladder 60

Location: UB 60 is located in the depression between the tip of the external malleolus and the Achilles tendon.
Needling Technique: UB 60 is punctured perpendicularly for 0.5 to 1.0 cun.
Indications: Headache, neck rigidity, epistaxis, shoulder, back, arm pain, swelling, heel pain, difficult labor, and epilepsy.

Urinary Bladder 62 (Extending Vessel)

Location: Depression directly below the lateral malleolus.
Needling Technique: Perpendicular 0.3 cun.
Indications: Epilepsy, insomnia, dizziness, back and leg pain.

Urinary Bladder 65 (Restraining Bone)
Location: Posterior to the fifth metatarsophalangeal joint.

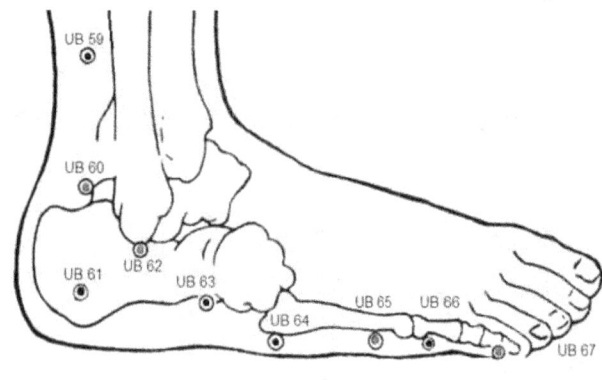

Fig 6.7.12 UB 50-67

Needling Technique: Perpendicular 0.3–0.5 cun.
Indications: Headache, blurred vision, neck and leg pain.

Urinary Bladder 67 (Reaching Yin)

Location: 0.1 cun lateral to the corner of the nail on the little toe.
Needling Technique: Superficial insertion of 0.1 cun.
Indications: Breech presentation, difficult labour, headache, nasal congestion, eye pain.

Clinical Significance: Urinary Bladder Channel

The Urinary Bladder channel is the longest in the body and significantly treats physical and mental conditions. It runs along the back and legs, making it highly effective for treating back pain, sciatica, neck stiffness, leg cramps, and tension in the paraspinal muscles.

It contains a special group of points, the Back-Shu points, located along the inner bladder line on the back. Each point corresponds to and influences a specific internal organ. These points are commonly used to regulate organ function and treat chronic internal disorders.

This channel also clears excesses such as heat, cold, and dampness from the body. It is valuable in treating urinary disorders such as painful urination, frequent urination, and urine retention, as well as gynaecological and reproductive problems.

Because the Urinary Bladder channel connects with the brain and governs the flow of Qi along the spine, it is essential in treating neurological conditions like epilepsy, paralysis, and anxiety. It also helps balance the autonomic nervous system, making it beneficial in stress-related disorders.

The outer line of the channel is used in emotional and psychological healing, addressing issues such as fear, grief, anger, and depression.

-Dr. Pardeshi Acupuncture-

6.8 Kidney Channel (KI)

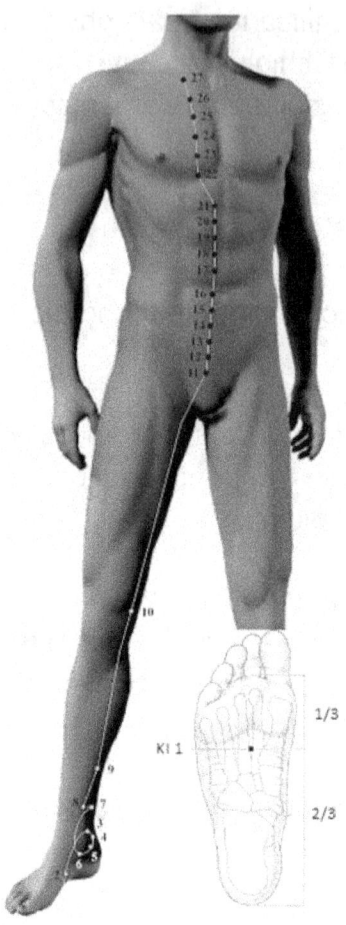

Fig. 6.8.1 KI Channel

The Kidney channel is also called the Foot Shao Yin channel, which, after getting a connection from the Urinary Bladder channel, starts with the point KI 1 in the sole in a depression of the foot in plantar flexion at the junction of the anterior one-third and posterior two-thirds of the line connecting the base of the 2nd and 3rd toes. It runs through a depression in the lower aspect of the tuberosity of the navicular bone (KI 2). It travels superiorly behind the medial malleolus and encircles it (KI 6). Ascending again along the medial side of the leg, it passes the medial side of the popliteal fossa (KI 10). It goes further upward along the posterior-medial aspect of the thigh. It forms a straight line 0.5 cun from the midline while traveling to the superior border of the pubic symphysis (KI 10). It ascends, diverging at the diaphragm, and ends in a depression on the lower border of the clavicle, two cun from the midline, at point KI 27. It connects further to the Pericardium channel.

Below are discussed the crucial points 1, 2, 3, 6, 7, 8, 10, 13, 14, 15, 17, 19, 21, and 27 of the Kidney channels.

Kidney 1 (Bubbling Spring)

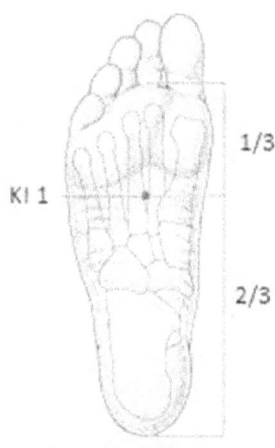

Fig. 6.8.2 KI 1

Location: KI 1 lies at the sole, in the depression when the foot is in plantar flexion, approximately at the junction of the anterior one-third and posterior two-thirds of the line connecting the base of the 2nd and 3rd toes and the heel.
Needling Technique: KI 1 is punctured perpendicularly for 0.3 to 0.5 cun.
Indications: Headache, blurred vision, dizziness, sore throat, dryness of the tongue, loss of voice, dysuria, burning sensation in the sole, loss of consciousness.

Kidney 2 (Blazing Valley)

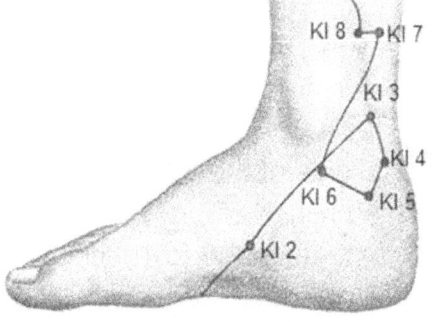

Fig. 6.8.3 KI 2 - 8

Location: KI 2 lies anterior and inferior to the medial malleolus in the depression on the lower navicular bone's tuberosity border.

Needling Technique: KI 2 is punctured perpendicularly for 0.3 to 0.5 cun.

Indications: Pruritus vulvae, prolapse of the uterus, irregular menstruation, nocturnal emission, thirst, diarrhoea, swelling, and pain of the foot's dorsum.

Kidney 3 (Supreme Stream)

Location: KI 3 lies at the depression between the tip of the medial malleolus and the Achilles tendon.

Needling Technique: KI 3 is punctured perpendicularly at a 0.3 to 0.5 cun depth.

Indications: Sore throat, toothache, deafness, tinnitus, dizziness, asthma, irregular menstruation, insomnia, nocturnal emission, impotence, frequency of micturition, pain in the lower back.

Kidney 6 (Shining Sea)

Location: KI 6 is situated in the depression below the medial malleolus.

Needling Technique: KI 6 is punctured perpendicularly at a depth of 0.3 to 0.5 cun.

Indications: Irregular menstruation, morbid leukorrhea, prolapse of the uterus, pruritus vulvae, frequency of micturition, retention of urine, constipation, epilepsy, insomnia, sore throat, and asthma.

Kidney 7 (Returning Current)

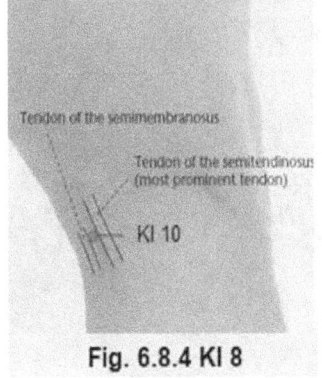

Fig. 6.8.4 KI 8

Location: KI 7 is directly above KI 3, located on the anterior border of the Achilles tendon.

Needling Technique: KI 7 is punctured perpendicularly at a depth of 0.5 to 0.7 cun.

Indications: Oedema, abdominal distension, diarrhoea, leg muscular atrophy, and spontaneous sweating.

Blood Supply: Deeper, anteriorly, the posterior tibial artery and vein.

Nerve Supply: The medial sural and medial crural cutaneous nerves; more profound, the tibial nerve.

Kidney 10 (Yin Valley)

Location: In the flexed knee position, KI 10 lies on the medial side of the popliteal fossa, level with UB 40, between the tendons of semitendinosus and semimembranosus.
Needling Technique: KI 10 is punctured perpendicularly to a depth of 0.8 to 1.0 cun.
Indications: Impotence, hernia, uterine bleeding, dysuria, pain in the knee and popliteal fossa, mental disorders.

Kidney 13 (Qi Cave)

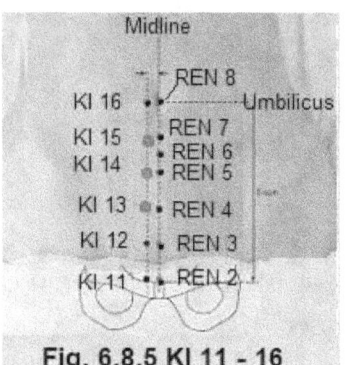
Fig. 6.8.5 KI 11 - 16

Location: KI 13 is three cun below the umbilicus and 0.5 cun lateral to REN 4.
Needling Technique: KI 13 is punctured perpendicularly for 0.5 to 1.0 cun.
Indications: Irregular menstruation, dysmenorrhea, dysuria, abdominal pain, diarrhoea.

Kidney 14 (Four Fullnesses)

Location: KI 14 lies two cun below the umbilicus, 0.5 cun lateral to REN 5.
Needling Technique: KI 14 is punctured perpendicularly for 0.5 to 1.0 cun.
Indications: Abdominal pain and distension, diarrhoea, nocturnal emission, irregular menstruation, dysmenorrhea, postpartum abdominal pain.

Kidney 15 (Middle Flow)

Location: KI 15 is one cun below the umbilicus, 0.5 cun lateral to REN 7.
Needling Technique: KI 15 is punctured perpendicularly for 0.5 to 1.0 cun.
Indications: Irregular menstruation, abdominal pain, constipation.

Kidney 17 (Shang Bend)

Location: KI 17 is two cun above the umbilicus, 0.5 cun lateral to REN 10.
Needling Technique: KI 17 is punctured perpendicularly for 0.5 to 1.0 cun.
Indications: Abdominal pain, diarrhoea, constipation.

Kidney 19 (Yin Metropolis)

Location: KI 19 is four cun above the umbilicus, 0.5 cun lateral to REN 12.
Needling Technique: KI 19 is punctured perpendicularly at a depth of 0.5 to 1.0 cun.
Indications: Abdominal pain, epigastric pain, constipation, vomiting.

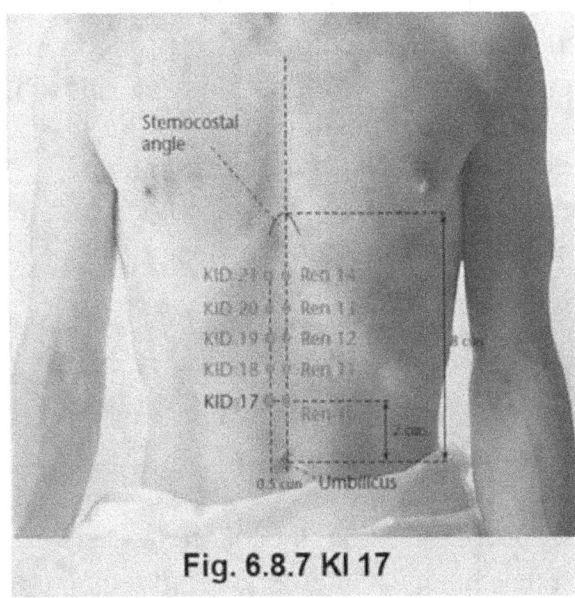

Fig. 6.8.7 KI 17

Kidney 21 (Dark Gate)

Location: KI 21 is six cun above the umbilicus, 0.5 cun lateral to REN 14.
Needling Technique: KI 21 is punctured perpendicularly at a depth of 0.3 to 0.7 cun. Deep insertion is not advisable to avoid injuring the liver.
Indications: Abdominal pain and distension, indigestion, vomiting, diarrhea, nausea, morning sickness.

Kidney 27 (Shu Mansion)

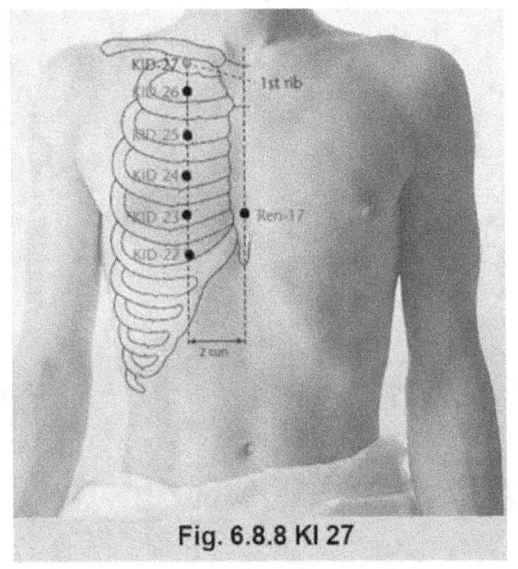

Fig. 6.8.8 KI 27

Location: KI 27 is located at the depression on the lower border of the clavicle, two cun lateral to the anterior midline.
Needling Technique: KI 27 is punctured obliquely for 0.3 to 0.5 cun to avoid lung injury.
Indications: Cough, asthma, chest pain.

Clinical Significance of Kidney Channel

The Kidney channel is fundamental in maintaining life essence, growth, development, and reproductive health. It is commonly used in conditions involving fatigue, infertility, irregular menstruation, sexual dysfunction, and menopausal symptoms. It supports the body's constitution and vitality, particularly in cases of chronic or degenerative illnesses.

This channel is also key in managing urinary disorders such as frequent urination, incontinence, and painful urination, as it governs the bladder and water metabolism. It is used for oedema, lower back pain, and weakness of the knees and ankles.

In traditional Chinese medicine, the kidneys are believed to store the essence (Jing), which is responsible for maintaining bone health, supporting brain function, and regulating developmental processes. Therefore, this channel treats osteoporosis, memory decline, hearing loss, and developmental delays.

Emotionally, the Kidney channel is related to willpower and fear. It is often used in cases of anxiety, insecurity, or trauma-induced psychological states. Strengthening the Kidney channel helps patients rebuild resilience and inner stability.

Additionally, the Kidney channel connects with the lungs and heart, supporting respiratory function and cardiac health in chronic asthma, shortness of breath, or palpitations due to deficient Qi or Yin.

-Modern Acupuncture-

6.9 Pericardium Channel (PC)

The Pericardium channel is also known as the Hand Jue Yin channel, which, after connecting to the Kidney channel, originates at point PC 1 in the chest, located laterally to the nipple. It then ascends to the axillary fossa and runs along the medial aspect of the upper arm, passing through the cubital fossa (PC 3). It continues downward to the forearm between the tendons of the palmaris longus and flexor carpi radialis muscles (PC 7). It enters the palm and travels along the middle finger to its tip at PC 9. The channel subsequently connects with the San Jiao channel.

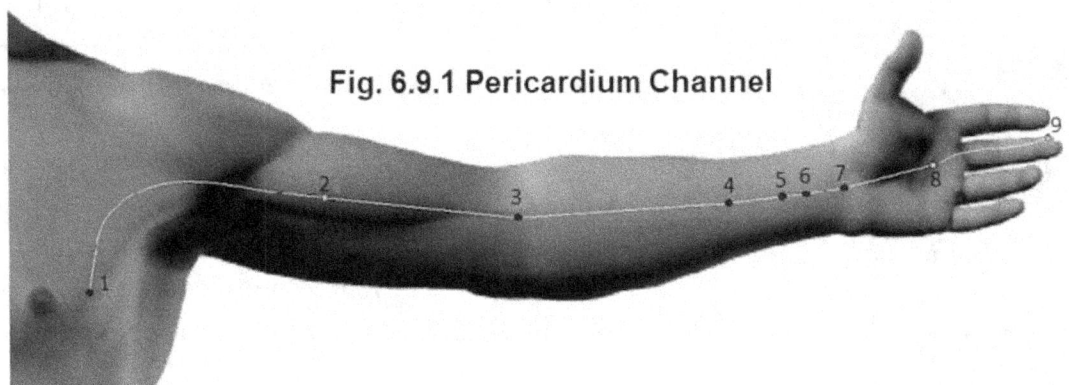

Fig. 6.9.1 Pericardium Channel

Below are discussed the critical points 3, 4, 5, 6, 7, and 9 of the Pericardium channels.

Pericardium 3 (Marsh at the Crook)

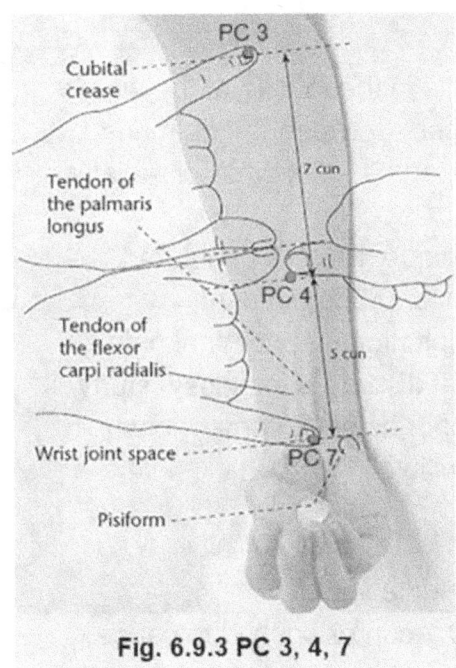

Fig. 6.9.3 PC 3, 4, 7

Location: PC 3 is situated at the transverse cubital crease, on the ulnar side of the biceps brachii muscle tendon.
Needling Technique: PC 3 is punctured perpendicularly for 0.5 to 0.7 cun or pricked with an injection needle to cause bleeding.
Indications: Palpitations, fever, irritability, abdominal pain, vomiting, pain in the elbow and arm, tremors of the hand and arm.

Pericardium 4 (Gate of Qi Reserve)

Location: PC 4 lies five cun above the transverse crease of the wrist, on the line connecting PC 3 and PC 7, between the tendons of the palmaris longus

and flexor carpi radialis muscles.
Needling Technique: PC 4 is punctured perpendicularly for 0.5 to 1.0 cun.
Indications: Palpitations, epistaxis, chest pain, furuncle, epilepsy.

Pericardium 5 (Intermediate Messenger)

Location: PC 5 is three cun above the wrist's transverse crease, between the palmaris longus tendons and the flexor carpi radialis muscles.

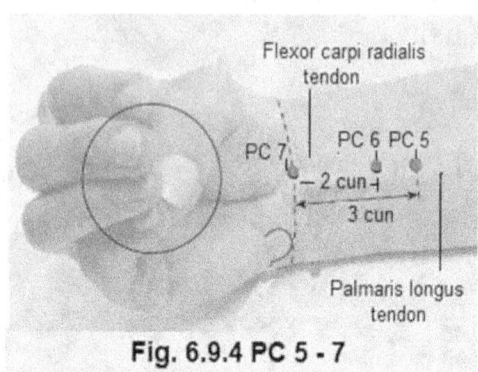

Fig. 6.9.4 PC 5 - 7

Needling Technique: PC 5 is punctured perpendicularly for 0.5 to 1.0 cun.
Indications: Palpitations, abdominal pain, vomiting, fever, irritability, malaria, mental disorders, epilepsy, swelling of the axilla, contracture of the elbow, and arm.

Pericardium 6 (Inner Pass)

Location: PC 6 is two cun above the wrist's transverse crease, between the palmaris longus tendons and the flexor carpi radialis muscles.
Needling Technique: PC 6 is punctured perpendicularly at 0.5 to 0.8 cun depth.
Indications: Palpitations, stuffy chest, hypochondriac pain, abdominal pain, nausea, vomiting, hiccups, mental disorders, epilepsy, insomnia, fever, irritability, contracture, and pain in the elbow and arm.

Pericardium 7 (Great Mound)

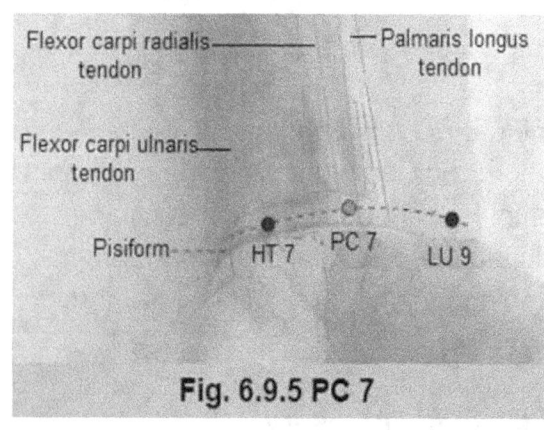

Fig. 6.9.5 PC 7

Location: PC 7 is in the middle of the wrist's transverse crease, between the palmaris longus tendons and the flexor carpi radialis muscles.
Needling Technique: PC 7 is punctured perpendicularly for 0.3 to 0.5 cun.
Indications: Palpitations, abdominal pain, vomiting, mental disorders, epilepsy, stuffy chest, hypochondriac pain, convulsions, insomnia, irritability.

Pericardium 9 (Middle Rushing)

Location: PC 9 is located at the centre of the tip of the middle finger.
Needling Technique: PC 9 is punctured superficially at 0.1 cun or pricked to cause bleeding.

Indications: Cardiac pain, palpitations, loss of consciousness, aphasia with stiffness of the tongue, heat stroke, feverish sensation in the palms.

Pericardium Channel – Clinical Significance

The Pericardium channel is associated with protecting the Heart, both physically and emotionally. It is commonly used to treat chest pain, palpitations, tightness in the chest, and irregular heartbeat. As a significant pathway for regulating the circulation of Qi and blood in the chest, it is also helpful in calming the chest in anxiety or panic attacks.

Due to its strong influence on mental and emotional states, this channel is frequently used in treating insomnia, irritability, restlessness, and depression. It helps stabilise the mind and is beneficial for emotional imbalances related to shock, trauma, or long-standing stress.

The channel also runs along the centre of the forearm, effectively managing wrist pain, carpal tunnel syndrome, and motor or sensory issues in the hand and forearm.

In addition, the Pericardium channel has applications in treating nausea, vomiting, and motion sickness, primarily through stimulation of the point PC 6 (Neiguan), which is also widely used in modern acupressure and medical devices for anti-nausea therapy.

-Modern Acupuncture-

6.10 San Jiao Channel (SJ)

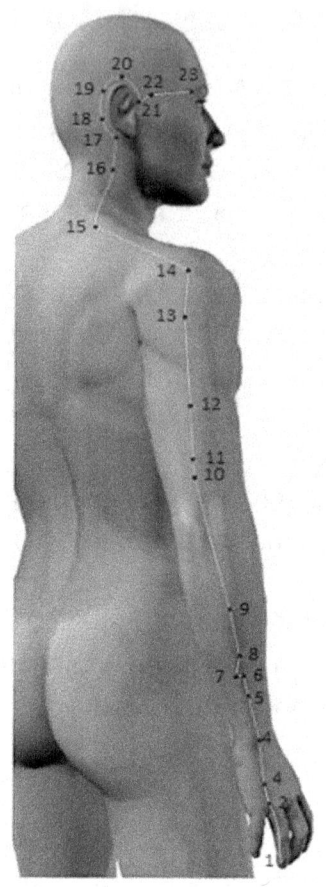

The San Jiao channel, also known as the *Hand Shao Yang* channel, originates from its connection with the Pericardium channel and begins at San Jiao 1 at the tip of the ring finger. It ascends between the fourth and fifth metacarpal bones, passes along the dorsum of the wrist (SJ 4) and the lateral side of the forearm between the radius and ulna, and courses through the olecranon (SJ 10). It continues along the lateral upper arm to the shoulder (SJ 14), then travels to the suprascapular fossa. Ascending to the neck, it follows the posterior border of the ear (SJ 19) and arcs to the forehead's corner. It then descends to the cheek and terminates in the depression at the lateral end of the eyebrow at SJ 23, connecting with the Gall Bladder channel.

Essential points discussed: **SJ 1, 2, 3, 4, 5, 6, 7, 8, 9, 10, 14, 15, 17, 20, 23**

Fig. 6.10.1 San Jiao Channel

San Jiao 1 (Rushing Pass)

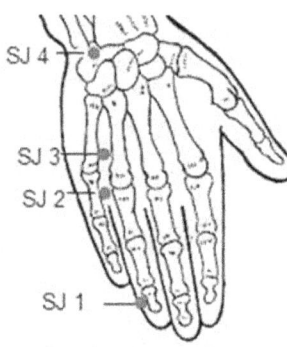

Fig. 6.10.2 SJ 1 - 4

Location: On the lateral side of the ring finger, approximately 0.1 cun from the nail corner.
Needling Technique: Superficial puncture for 0.1 cun or pricking with a needle to cause bleeding.
Indications: Headache, red eyes, sore throat, tongue stiffness, fever, irritability.

San Jiao 2 (Fluid Gate)

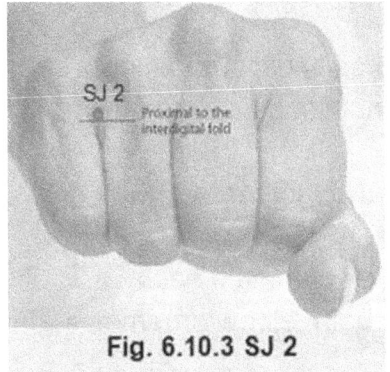

Fig. 6.10.3 SJ 2

Location: In the depression just proximal to the web margin between the ring and little fingers at the red and white skin junction when the fist is clenched.
Needling Technique: Oblique puncture for 0.3 to 0.5 cun directed between the metacarpal bones.
Indications: Headache, red eyes, sudden deafness, sore throat, arm pain.

San Jiao 3 (Middle Islet)

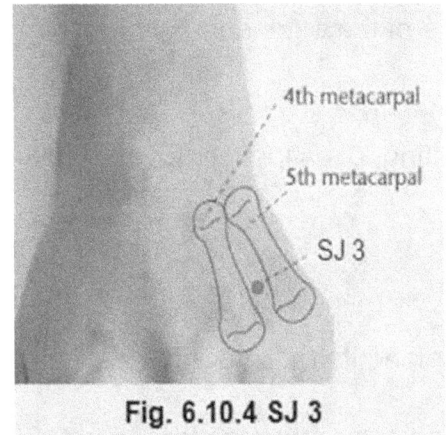

Fig. 6.10.4 SJ 3

Location: On the dorsum of the hand between the fourth and fifth metacarpal bones, in the depression proximal to the fourth metacarpophalangeal joint when the fist is clenched.
Needling Technique: Perpendicular puncture for 0.3 to 0.5 cun.
Indications: Headache, red eyes, deafness, tinnitus, sore throat, fever, elbow and arm pain, finger motor impairment.

San Jiao 4 (Yang Pool)

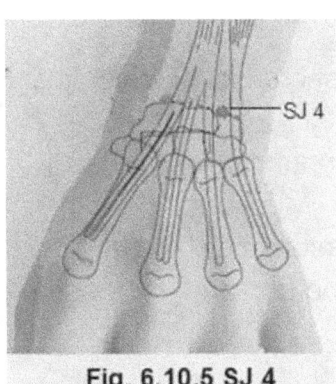

Fig. 6.10.5 SJ 4

Location: On the dorsum of the wrist, at the transverse crease, lateral to the extensor digitorum communis tendon.
Needling Technique: Perpendicular puncture for 0.3 to 0.5 cun.
Indications: Pain in the wrist, shoulder, arm, and deafness.

San Jiao 5 (Outer Pass)

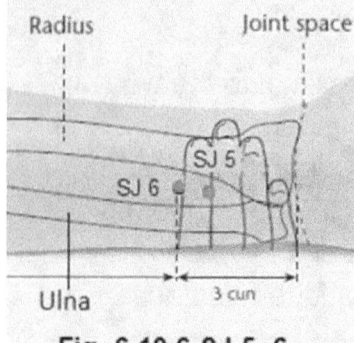

Fig. 6.10.6 SJ 5, 6

Location: 2 cun proximal to the dorsal wrist crease, between the radius and ulna on the line connecting SJ 4 and the olecranon.
Needling Technique: Perpendicular puncture for 0.5 to 1.0 cun.
Indications: Fever, headache, cheek pain, stiff neck, deafness, tinnitus, hypochondriac pain, elbow/arm motor issues, finger pain, hand tremor.

San Jiao 6 (Branch Ditch)

Location: 3 cun proximal to the wrist crease on the line between SJ 4 and the olecranon, between the radius and ulna, on the radial side of the extensor digitorum muscle.
Needling Technique: Perpendicular puncture for 0.8 to 1.2 cun.
Indications: Tinnitus, deafness, hypochondriac pain, vomiting, constipation, fever, heavy sensation in the shoulder/back, sudden hoarseness.

San Jiao 7 (Assembly of Ancestors)

Location: Level with SJ 6, on the ulnar side of the radius along its radial border.

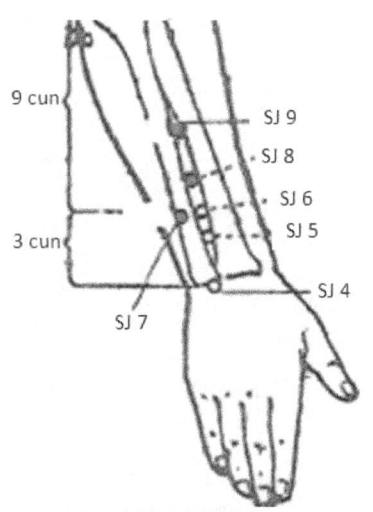

Fig. 6.10.7 SJ 7, 8

Needling Technique: Perpendicular puncture for 0.5 to 0.8 cun.
Indications: Deafness, ear pain, epilepsy, and arm pain.

San Jiao 8 (Three Yang Junction)

Location: 4 cun proximal to the wrist crease, between the radius and ulna.
Needling Technique: Perpendicular puncture for 0.5 to 1.0 cun.
Indications: Deafness, sudden hoarseness, chest and hypochondriac pain, pain in the hand and arm, toothache.

San Jiao 9 (Four Rivers)

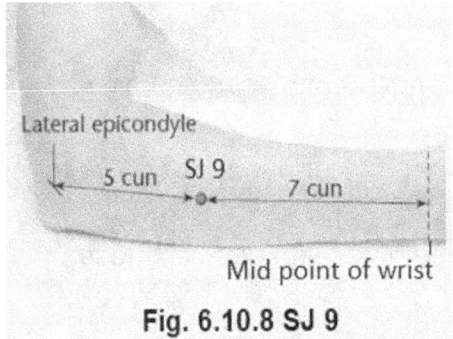

Fig. 6.10.8 SJ 9

Location: On the lateral forearm, five cun distal to the olecranon, between the radius and ulna.
Needling Technique: Perpendicular puncture for 0.5 to 1.0 cun.
Indications: Deafness, toothache, migraine, sudden hoarseness, and forearm pain.

San Jiao 10 (Celestial Well)

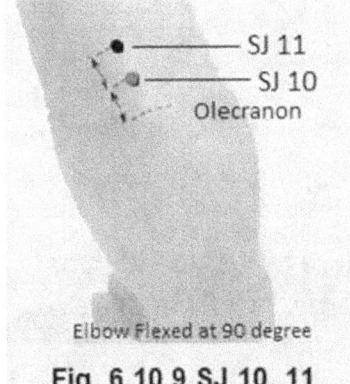

Fig. 6.10.9 SJ 10, 11

Location: In the depression, one cun superior to the olecranon when the elbow is flexed.
Needling Technique: Perpendicular puncture for 0.3 to 0.5 cun.
Indications: Pain in the neck, shoulder, and arm; epilepsy; goitre.

San Jiao 14 (Shoulder Crevice)

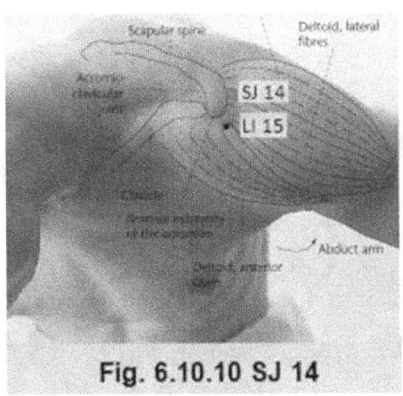

Fig. 6.10.10 SJ 14

Location: Posterior to LI 15, in the depression inferior and posterior to the acromion when the arm is abducted.
Needling Technique: Perpendicular puncture for 0.7 to 1.0 cun.
Indications: Shoulder and upper arm pain and motor impairment.

San Jiao 15 (Heavenly Crevice)

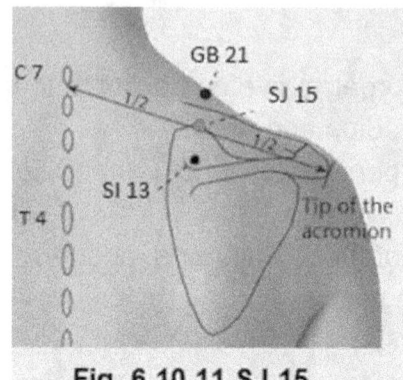

Fig. 6.10.11 SJ 15

Location: At the superior angle of the scapula, midway between GB 21 and SI 13.

Needling Technique: Perpendicular puncture for 0.3 to 0.5 cun.

Indications: Shoulder and elbow pain, neck stiffness.

San Jiao 17 (Wind Screen)

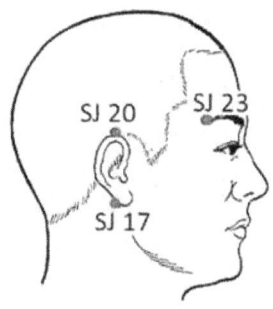

Fig. 6.10.12
SJ 17, 20, 23

Location: Posterior to the ear lobe, in the depression between the mandible and mastoid process.

Needling Technique: Perpendicular puncture for 0.5 to 1.0 cun.

Indications: Tinnitus, deafness, ear discharge, facial paralysis, cheek swelling, toothache.

San Jiao 20 (Minute Angle)

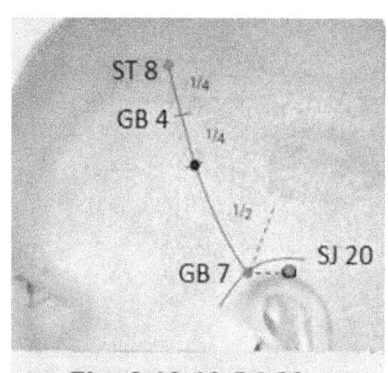

Fig. 6.10.13 SJ 20

Location: Within the hairline directly above the ear apex.

Needling Technique: Subcutaneous puncture for 0.3 to 0.5 cun.

Indications: Tinnitus, eye pain/redness/swelling, gum swelling, parotitis, toothache.

San Jiao 23 (Silken Bamboo Hollow)

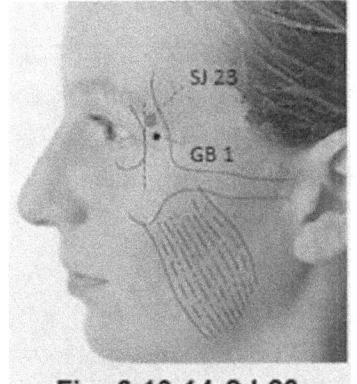

Fig. 6.10.14 SJ 23

Location: In the depression at the lateral end of the eyebrow.
Needling Technique: Subcutaneous puncture for 0.3 to 0.5 cun.
Indications: Headache, red and painful eyes, blurred vision, eyelid twitching, facial paralysis, toothache.

San Jiao Channel – Clinical Significance

The San Jiao channel is unique because it regulates the body's water pathways and the distribution of Qi among the upper, middle, and lower body regions, traditionally known as the triple burners. It treats fluid metabolism disorders, such as edema, urinary retention, and bloating.

The channel runs along the lateral arm, shoulder, neck, and ear, effectively treating pain or dysfunction in these areas, including frozen shoulder, lateral elbow pain (also known as tennis elbow), stiff neck, and tinnitus or deafness.

The channel passes around the ear and the sides of the head, making it helpful in treating migraines, temporal headaches, ear infections, and vertigo. It also clears heat and expels wind from the body, especially in febrile diseases or upper respiratory infections.

Emotionally, the San Jiao helps with stress-related tension, particularly those manifesting physically in the upper body. It also indirectly supports heart and pericardium functions through its connection and role in circulation and fluid transport.

Clinically, it is often combined with the Pericardium channel to balance internal and external aspects of heat, circulation, and emotional tension.

-Dr. Pardeshi Acupuncture-

6.11 Gall Bladder Channel (GB)

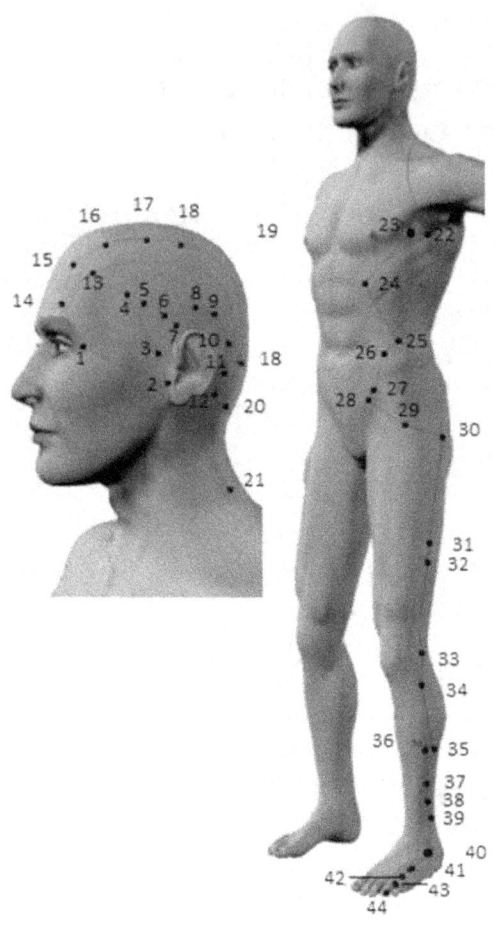

Fig. 6.11.1 Gall Bladder Channel

The Gall Bladder channel, known as the *Foot Shao Yang* channel, begins at Gall Bladder 1 near the outer canthus of the eye, after receiving input from the San Jiao channel. It descends to the front of the ear (GB 2), ascends to the corner of the forehead (GB 4), loops behind the ear, then moves forward again to the midpoint of the eyebrow (GB 14). It travels above the hairline to the side of the neck (GB 20), then descends to the top of the trapezius (GB 21) before entering the axilla and chest. Internally, it travels through the hypochondrium, emerging near the inguinal region (GB 28). It passes the pubic area, enters the hip (GB 30), and continues down the lateral thigh, knee (GB 33), and along the fibula to the lateral malleolus (GB 40). It ends on the lateral side of the fourth toe at GB 44, where it connects to the Liver channel.

Essential points discussed: GB 1, 2, 3, 4, 6, 8, 12, 14, 19, 20, 21, 30, 31, 32, 34, 38, 40, 41, 42, 43

Gall Bladder 1 (Pupil Crevice)

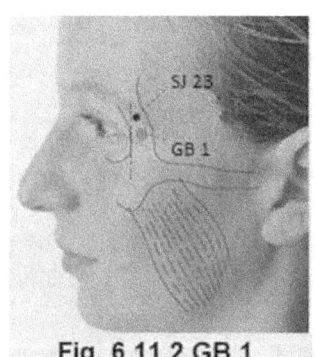

Fig. 6.11.2 GB 1

Location: Lateral to the outer canthus, on the orbit's lateral side.
Needling Technique: Horizontal puncture beneath the skin towards the affected side for 0.5 to 0.7 cun.
Indications: Tinnitus, deafness, toothache, TMJ pain, facial paralysis.

Gall Bladder 2 (Listening Meeting)

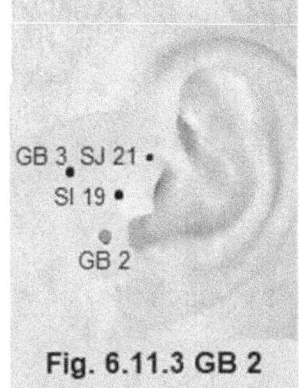

Fig. 6.11.3 GB 2

Location: Anterior to the inter-tragic notch, at the posterior border of the mandibular condyle, with the mouth open.
Needling Technique: Perpendicular puncture for 0.5 to 0.7 cun.
Indications: Tinnitus, deafness, toothache, TMJ dysfunction, deviation of eye/mouth.

Gall Bladder 3 (Above the Joint)

Location: Anterior to the ear, above ST 7, at the upper margin of the zygomatic arch.
Needling Technique: Perpendicular puncture for 0.3 to 0.5 cun. Deep needling is not advised.
Indications: Headache, tinnitus, deafness, facial deviation, toothache.

Fig. 6.11.4 GB 3

Gall Bladder 4 (Hanging Hair)

Location: Within the temporal hairline, at the junction of the upper 1/4th and lower 3/4th distance between ST 8 and GB 7.

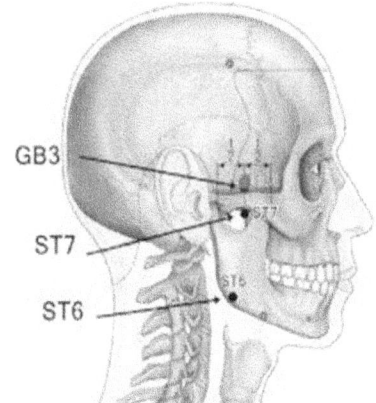

Needling Technique: Subcutaneous puncture for 0.3 to 0.5 cun.
Indications: Migraine, vertigo, tinnitus, outer canthus pain, epilepsy, convulsion.

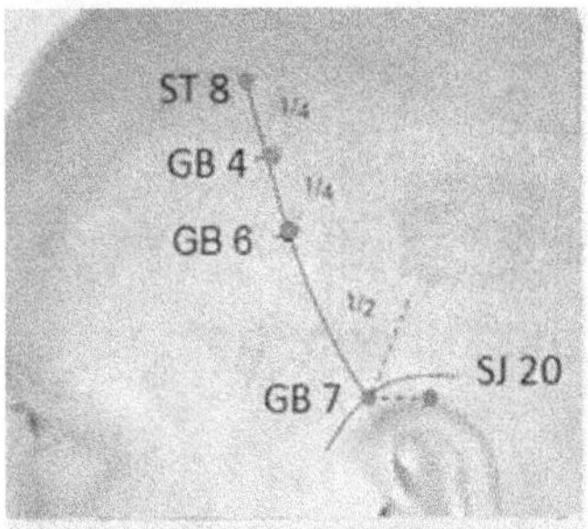

Gall Bladder 6 (Suspended Hair)

Fig. 6.11.5 GB 4, 6

Location: In the hairline at the junction of the lower 1/4th and upper 3/4th distance between ST 8 and GB 7.
Needling Technique: Subcutaneous puncture towards the treatment site for 0.3 to 0.5 cun.
Indications: Migraine, tinnitus, pain at the outer canthus, and frequent sneezing.

Gall Bladder 8 (Leading Valley)

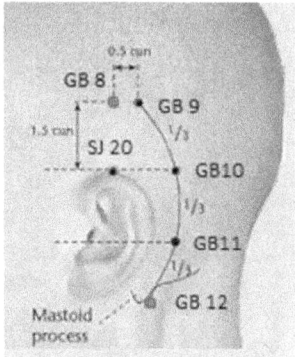

Fig. 6.11.6 GB 8, 9, 12

Location: 1.5 cun posterior to the auricular apex, within the hairline.
Needling Technique: Subcutaneous puncture for 0.3 to 0.5 cun.
Indications: Migraine, vertigo, vomiting.

Gall Bladder 12 (Completion Bone)

Location: In the depression posterior and inferior to the mastoid process.
Needling Technique: Oblique puncture for 0.3 to 0.5 cun.
Indications: Headache, insomnia, cheek swelling, retro-auricular pain, facial paralysis, toothache.

Gall Bladder 14 (Yang White)

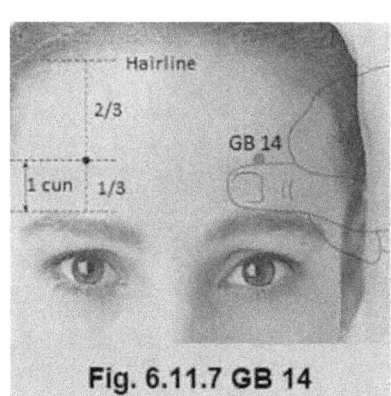

Fig. 6.11.7 GB 14

Location: 1 cun above the midpoint of the eyebrow, directly above the pupil.
Needling Technique: Subcutaneous puncture for 0.3 to 0.5 cun.
Indications: Frontal headache, eye pain, vertigo, eyelid twitching or ptosis, lacrimation.

Gall Bladder 19 (Brain Hollow)

Location: 2.25 cun lateral to the midline at the level of DU 17, on the superior border of the occiput.
Needling Technique: Subcutaneous puncture for 0.3 to 0.5 cun.
Indications: Headache, neck stiffness, tinnitus, vertigo, painful eyes, epilepsy.

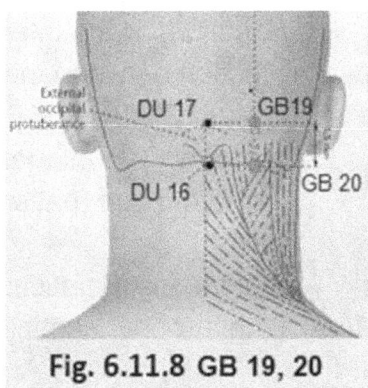

Fig. 6.11.8 GB 19, 20

Gall Bladder 20 (Wind Pool)

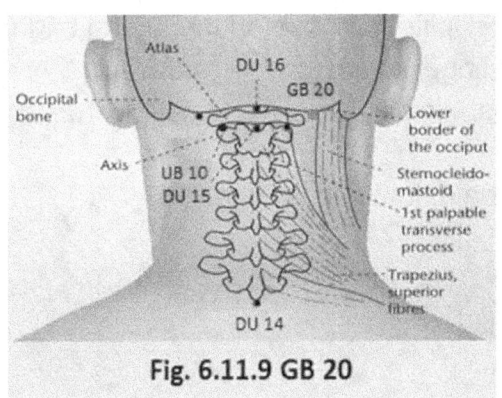

Fig. 6.11.9 GB 20

Location: In the depression between the upper SCM and trapezius, at the level of DU 16.

Needling Technique: Oblique puncture towards the nose for 0.3 to 0.5 cun.

Indications: Commonly used for headache, vertigo, insomnia, stiff neck, eye pain, glaucoma, convulsions, cold, and nasal obstruction.

Gall Bladder 21 (Shoulder Well)

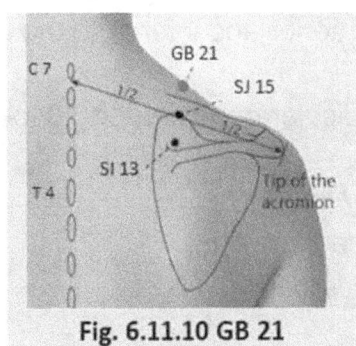

Fig. 6.11.10 GB 21

Location: Midpoint between DU 14 and the acromion, at the apex of the shoulder.

Needling Technique: Perpendicular puncture for 0.3 to 0.5 cun.

Indications: Neck rigidity, shoulder/back pain, arm dysfunction, lactation issues, mastitis, obstructed labour.

Gall Bladder 30 (Jumping Circle)

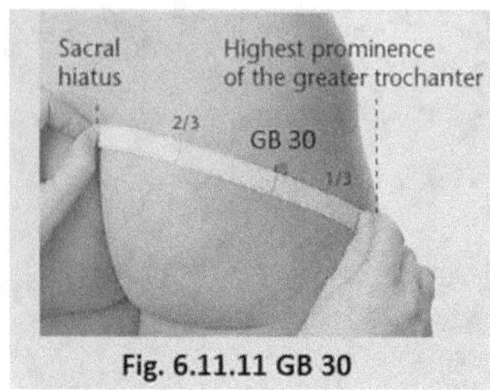

Fig. 6.11.11 GB 30

Location: At the lateral 1/3rd and medial 2/3rd junction between the greater trochanter and sacral hiatus (DU 2).
Needling Technique: Perpendicular puncture for 1.5 to 3.5 cun (patient in lateral position with thigh flexed).
Indications: Sciatica, lower back/thigh pain, lower limb atrophy, hemiplegia.

Gall Bladder 31 (Wind Market)

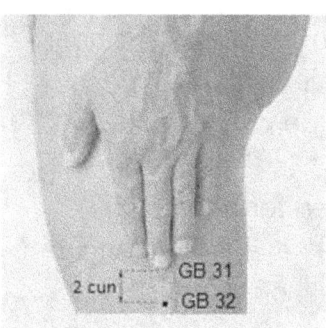

Fig. 6.11.12 GB 31, 32

Location: 7 cun above the popliteal crease on the lateral thigh midline (where the middle finger touches while standing).
Needling Technique: Perpendicular puncture for 0.7 to 1.2 cun.
Indications: Lumbar/thigh pain, lower limb paralysis, generalised itching.

Gall Bladder 34 (Yang Mound Spring)

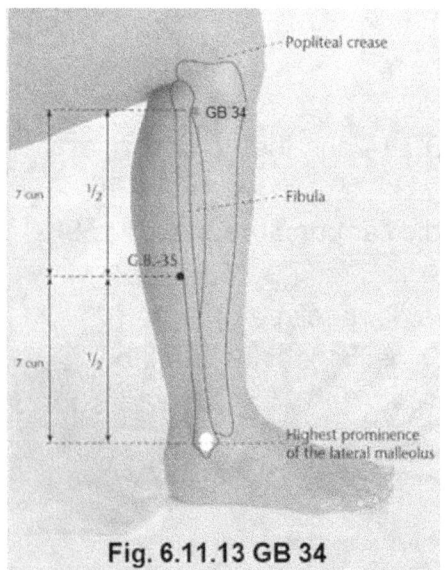

Fig. 6.11.13 GB 34

Location: In the depression anterior and inferior to the fibular head.
Needling Technique: Perpendicular puncture for 0.8 to 1.2 cun.
Indications: Hemiplegia, lower limb pain/weakness/numbness, knee swelling, hypochondriac pain, jaundice, vomiting.

Gall Bladder 38 (Yang Assistance)

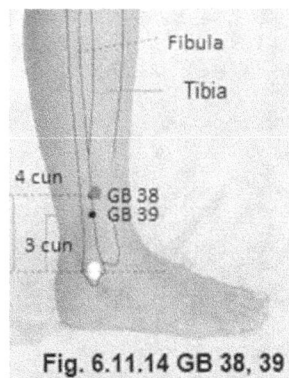

Fig. 6.11.14 GB 38, 39

Location: 4 cun above the tip of the lateral malleolus, slightly anterior to the fibula, between extensor digitorum longus and peroneus brevis.
Needling Technique: Perpendicular puncture for 0.5 to 0.7 cun.
Indications: Migraine, outer canthus pain, axillary pain, lumbar pain, chest and hypochondriac pain, lower limb pain.

Gall Bladder 40 (Mound of Ruins)

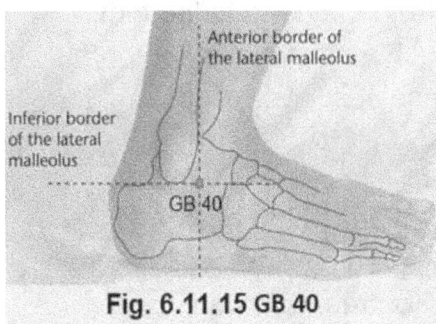

Fig. 6.11.15 GB 40

Location: Anterior and inferior to the lateral malleolus, lateral to the extensor digitorum longus tendon.
Needling Technique: Perpendicular puncture for 0.5 to 0.8 cun.
Indications: Neck pain, axillary swelling, hypochondriac pain, vomiting, acid regurgitation, leg atrophy, ankle pain/swelling.

Gall Bladder 41 (Foot Governor of Tears)

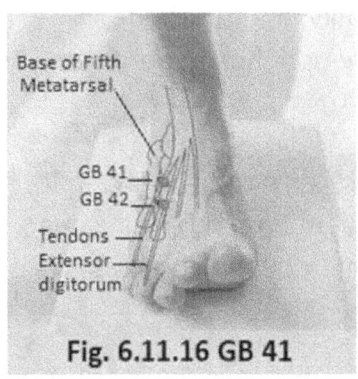

Fig. 6.11.16 GB 41

Location: Posterior to the 4th metatarsophalangeal joint, lateral to the extensor digiti minimi tendon.
Needling Technique: Perpendicular puncture for 0.3 to 0.5 cun.
Indications: Headache, vertigo, outer canthus pain, hypochondriac pain, breast pain, irregular menstruation, dorsum foot pain/swelling, toe spasm.

Gall Bladder 42 (Earth Five Meetings)

Location: Between the 4th and 5th metatarsals, medial to the extensor digiti minimi tendon.
Needling Technique: Perpendicular puncture for 0.3 to 0.5 cun.
Indications: Headache, canthus pain, tinnitus, breast distension, foot swelling/pain

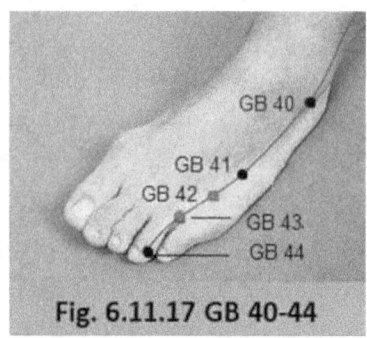

Fig. 6.11.17 GB 40-44

Clinical Significance - Gall Bladder Channel

The Gall Bladder channel traverses the side of the body from the head to the foot, making it highly effective in treating lateral body issues such as migraines, temporal headaches, jaw tension, neck and shoulder stiffness, hip pain, sciatica, and leg weakness.

It is one of the primary channels for addressing disorders affecting the head and sensory organs. It treats eye conditions, ear problems (like tinnitus and deafness), and facial paralysis. Points on this channel are often selected for treating sleep disturbances, especially difficulty falling asleep due to excessive thinking or emotional strain.

The Gall Bladder governs decision-making and courage. Emotionally, this channel treats indecision, timidity, irritability, and frustration. It is especially helpful when emotional stagnation leads to physical symptoms like tension headaches, digestive upset, or menstrual irregularities.

This channel also helps clear damp heat from the Liver-Gallbladder system, making it helpful in treating gallstones, a bitter taste in the mouth, nausea, and jaundice. It is also used in gynaecological and urogenital issues, particularly when emotional stress plays a role.

-Dr. Pardeshi Acupuncture-

6.12 Liver Channel (LV)

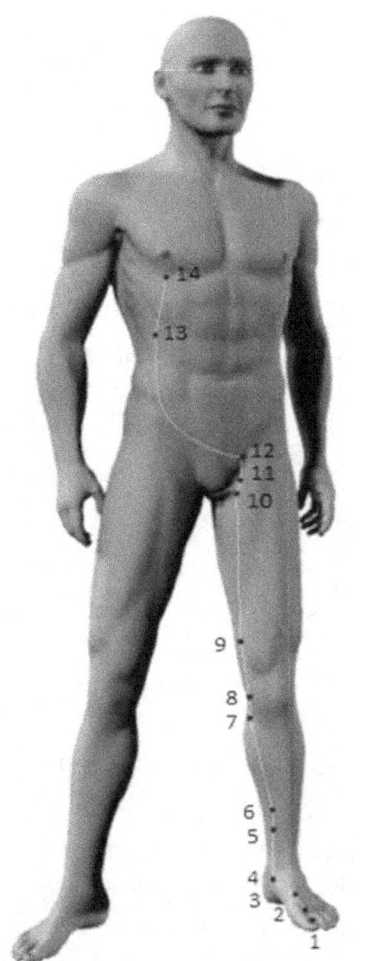

Fig. 6.12.1 LV Channel

The Liver channel is also called the *Foot Jue Yin* channel. After establishing a connection from the Gall Bladder channel, it begins at LV 1 on the lateral side of the great toe. It ascends along the dorsum of the foot and passes anterior to the medial malleolus (LV 4). It travels upward along the medial aspect of the lower leg and thigh, reaching the pubic region at the level of the iliac crest (LV 11). It then encircles the external genitalia, crosses to the opposite side of the lower abdomen, and terminates directly below the nipple at LV 14, where it links to the Lung channel.

The crucial points of the Liver channel discussed below include: 1, 2, 3, 5, 7, 8, and 9.

Liver 1 (LV 1) *(Big Mound)*

Location: On the lateral side of the terminal phalanx of the great toe, approximately 0.1 cun from the nail's corner.
Needling Technique: Subcutaneous insertion 0.1 to 0.2 cun.
Indications: Hernia, enuresis, uterine bleeding, uterine prolapse, epilepsy.

Liver 2 (LV 2) *(Moving Between)*

Location: On the dorsum of the foot between the first and second toes, just proximal to the margin of the web at the junction of the red and white skin.
Needling Technique: Oblique insertion 0.3 to 0.5 cun.
Indications: Hypochondriac pain, abdominal distension, headache, dizziness, eye pain

and swelling, deviation of the mouth, hernia, painful urination, urinary retention, irregular menstruation, epilepsy, insomnia, convulsions.

Liver 3 (LV 3) *(Great Rushing)*

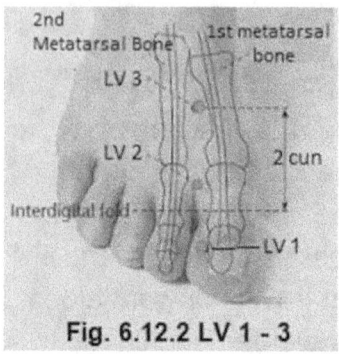

Fig. 6.12.2 LV 1 - 3

Location: On the dorsum of the foot, in the depression distal to the junction of the first and second metatarsal bones.
Needling Technique: Perpendicular insertion 0.3 to 0.5 cun.
Indications: Headache, dizziness, insomnia, depression, eye disorders, mouth deviation, hypochondriac pain, abnormal uterine bleeding, hernia, enuresis, urinary retention, epilepsy, pain at the medial malleolus.

Liver 5 (LV 5) *(Woodworm Canal)*

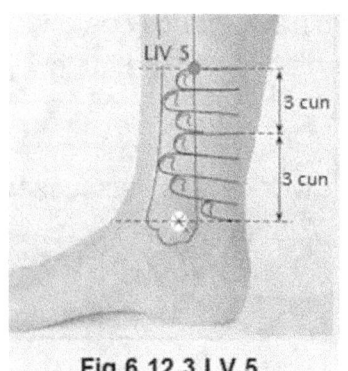

Fig 6.12.3 LV 5

Location: Five cun above the tip of the medial malleolus, on the medial surface of the tibia.
Needling Technique: Subcutaneous insertion 0.3 to 0.5 cun.
Indications: Urinary retention, enuresis, hernia, irregular menstruation, leucorrhoea, pruritus vulvae, weakness, and leg atrophy.

Liver 7 (LV 7) *(Knee Joint)*

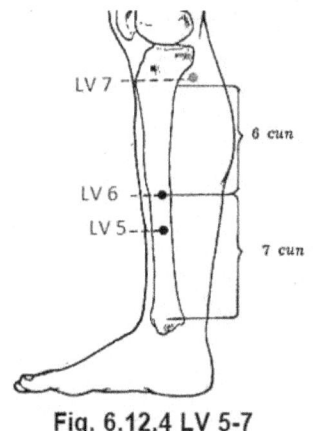

Fig. 6.12.4 LV 5-7

Location: Posterior and inferior to the medial condyle of the tibia, in the upper part of the medial head of the gastrocnemius muscle, one cun posterior to SP 9.
Needling Technique: Perpendicular insertion 0.5 to 1.0 cun.
Indications: Knee pain.

Liver 8 (LV 8) *(Spring at the Crook)*

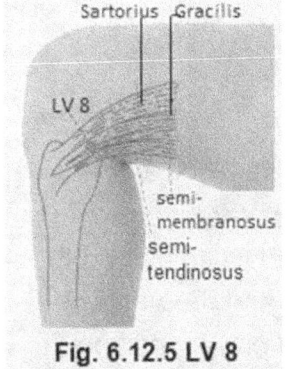

Fig. 6.12.5 LV 8

Location: At the medial end of the popliteal crease, posterior to the medial epicondyle of the tibia, in the depression between the insertions of the semimembranosus and semitendinosus muscles. Locate with the knee flexed.
Needling Technique: Perpendicular insertion 0.5 to 0.8 cun.
Indications: Uterine prolapse, lower abdominal pain, urinary retention, external genital pain, pruritus vulvae, medial knee and thigh pain.

Liver 9 (LV 9) *(Yin Bladder)*

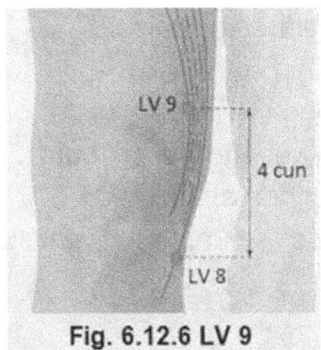

Fig. 6.12.6 LV 9

Location: Four cun above the medial epicondyle of the femur, between the vastus medialis and sartorius muscles.
Needling Technique: Perpendicular insertion 0.5 to 0.7 cun.
Indications: Lumbosacral pain, lower abdominal pain, enuresis, urinary retention, irregular menstruation.

Liver Channel – Clinical Significance

The Liver channel plays a key role in regulating the smooth flow of Qi, blood, and emotions throughout the body. It is frequently used in the treatment of gynaecological disorders such as irregular menstruation, dysmenorrhoea, PMS, and infertility. Due to its path along the lower abdomen and genitals, it also treats hernia, genital pain or swelling, and urinary problems.

This channel is essential in managing emotional imbalances, especially anger, irritability, frustration, and mood swings. It is often selected in stress-related conditions where emotional constraint leads to physical symptoms such as tension headaches, digestive upset, or insomnia.

The Liver channel influences the tendons and is vital in treating muscle spasms, cramps, tremors, and restricted joint movement, especially in the legs and lower body. It also nourishes the eyes and is used in blurry vision, dry eyes, and red or painful eyes.

-Modern Acupuncture-

6.13 DU Channel (GV)

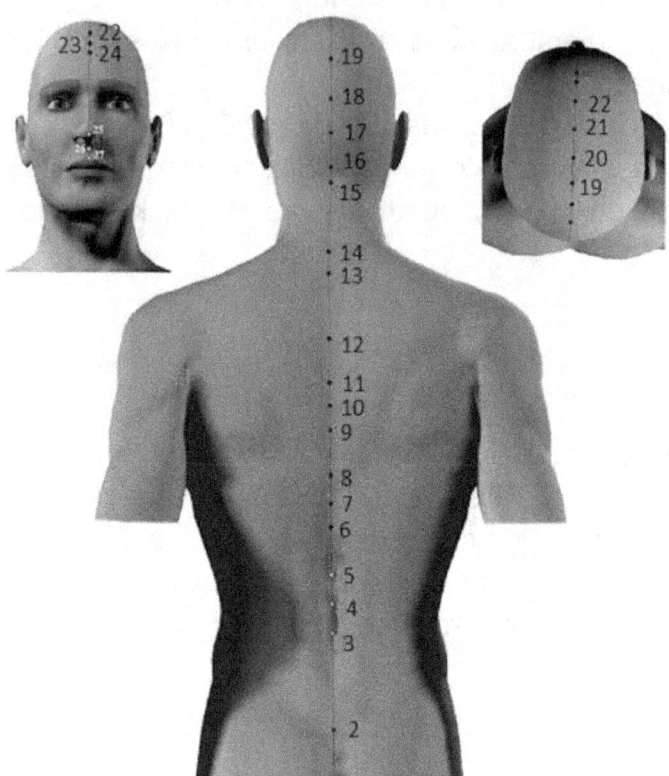

Fig. 6.13.1 DU Channel

The DU channel is also referred to as the *Governing Vessel*. It begins at DU 1, located midway between the tip of the coccyx and the anus, with the patient in the prone position. It ascends along the midline of the back, travelling through the spinal column to the nape of the neck (DU 14), then continues upward to the vertex (DU 20). From there, it descends along the midline of the forehead and nose to the philtrum (DU 26), and ends at the labial frenulum inside the upper lip with DU 28.

The critical points of the DU channel discussed below include: 3, 4, 9, 11, 14, 15, 17, 20, 24, 26, and 28.

DU 3 (Lumbar Yang Gate)

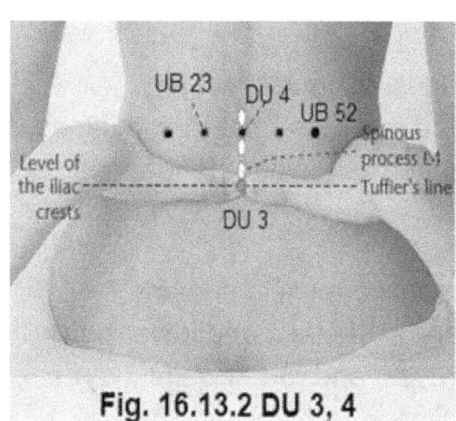

Fig. 16.13.2 DU 3, 4

Location: Below the spinous process of the fourth lumbar vertebra, at the level of the iliac crest.
Needling Technique: Perpendicular insertion 0.5 to 1.0 cun.
Indications: Irregular menstruation, nocturnal emission, impotence, lumbosacral pain, muscular atrophy, motor impairment, numbness, and lower limb pain.

DU 4 (Gate of Life)

Location: Below the spinous process of the second lumbar vertebra.
Needling Technique: Perpendicular insertion 0.5 to 1.0 cun.
Indications: Impotence, spermatorrhoea, lumbago, back stiffness, diarrhoea, indigestion, fatigue.

DU 9 (Reaching Yang)

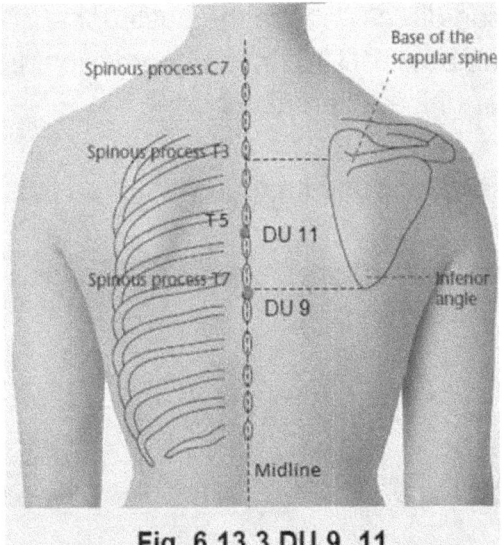

Fig. 6.13.3 DU 9, 11

Location: Below the spinous process of the seventh thoracic vertebra, approximately level with the inferior angle of the scapula.
Needling Technique: Oblique upward insertion 0.5 to 1.0 cun.
Indications: Jaundice, cough, asthma, back stiffness, chest and upper back pain.

DU 11 (Spirit Pathway)
Location: Below the spinous process of the fifth thoracic vertebra.
Needling Technique: Oblique upward insertion 0.5 to 1.0 cun.
Indications: Poor memory, anxiety, palpitations, back pain and stiffness, and cough.

DU 14 (Great Vertebra)

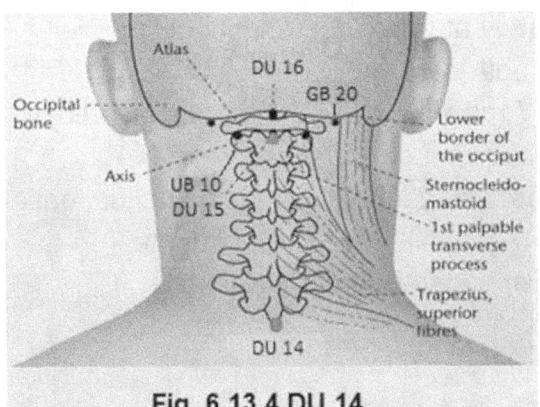

Fig. 6.13.4 DU 14

Location: Below the spinous process of the seventh cervical vertebra, approximately at shoulder level.
Needling Technique: Oblique upward insertion 0.5 to 1.0 cun.
Indications: Neck stiffness and pain, fever, epilepsy, cough, asthma, common cold, and rigidity of the back.

DU 15 (Gate of Muteness)
Location: 0.5 cun above the midpoint of the posterior hairline, in the depression below the spinous process of the first cervical vertebra.
Needling Technique: Perpendicular insertion 0.5 to 0.8 cun.
Warning: Deep or oblique upward needling is contraindicated due to proximity to the

medulla oblongata.

Indications: Mental disorders, epilepsy, sudden loss of voice, deafness, stroke, tongue stiffness, aphasia, occipital headache, neck rigidity.

DU 17 (Brain's Door)

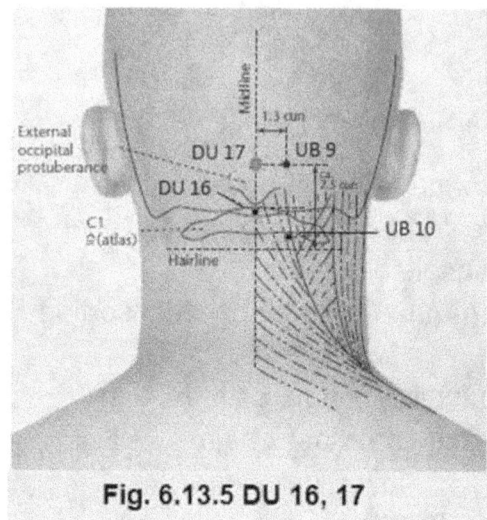

Fig. 6.13.5 DU 16, 17

Location: 2.5 cun directly above the posterior hairline, 1.5 cun above DU 16, in the depression at the upper border of the external occipital protuberance.

Needling Technique: Subcutaneous insertion 0.3 to 0.5 cun.

Indications: Epilepsy, dizziness, neck pain, and stiffness.

DU 20 (Hundred Meetings)

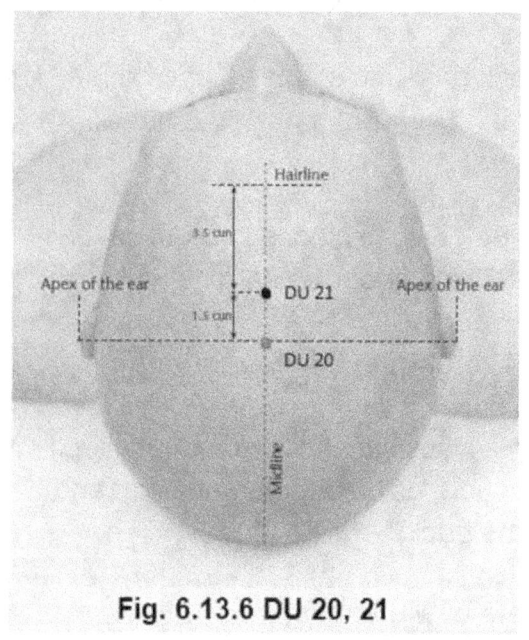

Fig. 6.13.6 DU 20, 21

Location: On the midline of the head, five cun above the midpoint of the anterior hairline, approximately at the midpoint connecting the apexes of both ears.

Needling Technique: Subcutaneous insertion 0.3 to 0.5 cun.

Indications: Headache, dizziness, tinnitus, nasal obstruction, aphasia after stroke, mental disorders, prolapse of rectum or uterus.

DU 24 (Spirit Court)

Location: 0.5 cun above the midpoint of the anterior hairline.
Needling Technique: Subcutaneous insertion 0.3 to 0.5 cun or pricking to cause bleeding.
Indications: Epilepsy, anxiety, palpitations, insomnia, headache, vertigo, and nasal discharge.

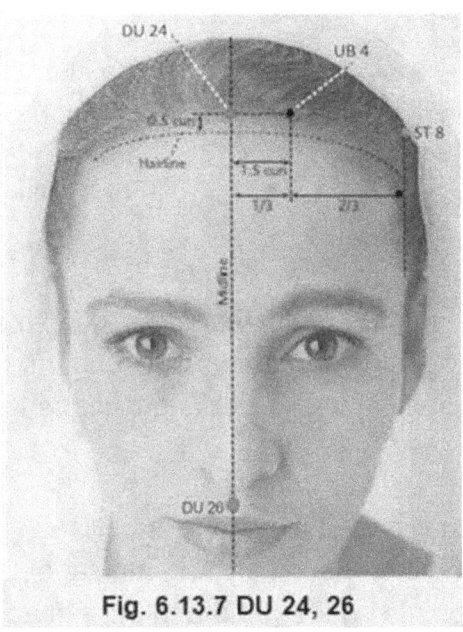

Fig. 6.13.7 DU 24, 26

DU 26 (Water Trough)
Location: At the philtrum's upper third and middle third junction.
Needling Technique: Oblique upward insertion 0.3 to 0.5 cun.
Indications: Mental disorders, epilepsy, hysteria, coma, deviation of the mouth and eyes, facial swelling, and acute lumbar pain.

DU 28 (Gum Intersection)

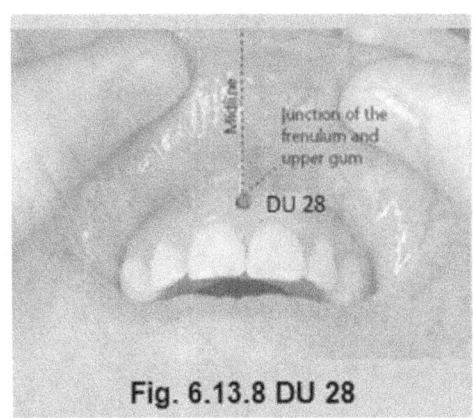

Location: At the junction of the frenulum and gum of the upper lip.
Needling Technique: Oblique upward insertion 0.1 to 0.2 cun or pricked to bleed.
Indications: Mental disorders, gum pain and swelling, and nasal discharge.

Fig. 6.13.8 DU 28

DU Channel – Clinical Significance

The Du channel, also known as the Governing Vessel, runs along the midline of the posterior body from the perineum to the head. It is closely linked to the brain, spinal cord, and central nervous system. This channel is especially significant in neurological, musculoskeletal, and mental health conditions.

Clinically, it is used to treat spinal disorders, including stiffness, pain, scoliosis, and vertebral injuries. It is also indicated in conditions involving paralysis, tremors, seizures, and post-stroke recovery, particularly in cases of hemiplegia. Due to its pathway through the brain, it plays a crucial role in managing conditions such as epilepsy, vertigo, headaches, and poor memory.

The Du channel regulates Yang energy in the body and is often selected for symptoms of Yang deficiency or collapse, such as fatigue, incontinence, organ prolapse, or chronic cold sensations. It is also helpful in cases of Yang rising, such as hypertension or anxiety with heat signs.

Emotionally and psychologically, the Du channel stabilises the Shen (mind-spirit), and is commonly used in psychiatric disorders including mania, depression, obsessive thinking, and insomnia. Its points on the head and upper back are particularly calming and regulating for the brain and mind.

Many of its points are used in emergency and revival situations, including those related to shock, coma, and collapse.

-Modern Acupuncture-

Dr. C Pardeshi MD

6.14 REN Channel (REN)

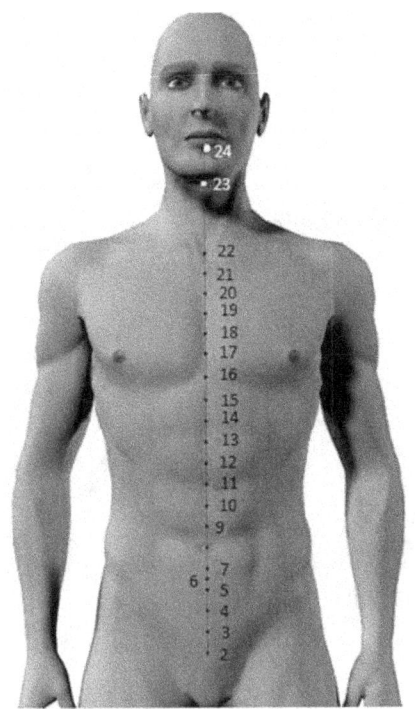

Fig. 6.14.1 REN Channel

The REN channel is also called the *Conception Vessel*. It begins at REN 1, located at the midpoint between the anus and the scrotum in males, and between the anus and the posterior labial commissure in females. It ascends anteriorly through the pubic region (REN 2), runs along the anterior midline of the abdomen (REN 15), passes through the chest and throat, and ends at REN 24, located in the depression of the mento-labial groove.

The crucial points of the REN channel discussed below include: 2, 3, 4, 5, 6, 8, 9, 10, 15, and 24.

REN 2 (Curved Bone)

Location: At the midpoint of the upper border of the symphysis pubis.
Needling Technique: Perpendicular insertion 0.5 to 0.8 cun.
Caution: During pregnancy, points from REN 2 to REN 13 should be needled with extreme care.

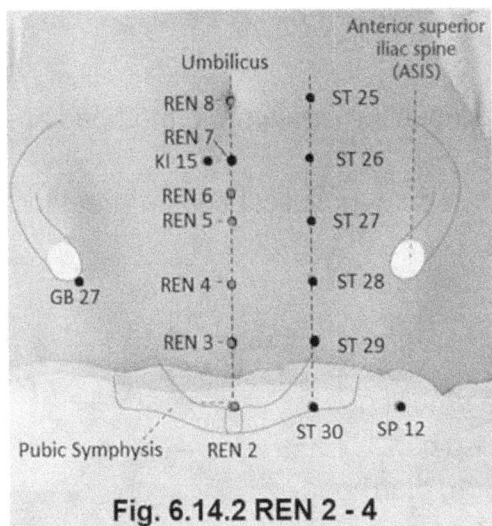

Fig. 6.14.2 REN 2 - 4

Indications: Urinary retention and dribbling, enuresis, nocturnal emission, impotence, chronic leucorrhoea, irregular menstruation, dysmenorrhoea, and hernia.

REN 3 (Middle Pole)

Location: On the anterior midline, four cun below the umbilicus.
Needling Technique: Perpendicular insertion 0.5 to 1.0 cun.
Indications: Enuresis, nocturnal emission, impotence, hernia, uterine bleeding, irregular

menstruation, dysmenorrhoea, leucorrhoea, frequent or retained urination, lower abdominal pain, uterine prolapse, vaginitis.

REN 4 (Gate of Origin)

Location: On the anterior midline, three cun below the umbilicus.
Needling Technique: Perpendicular insertion 0.8 to 1.2 cun.
Indications: Urinary disturbances, hernia, menstrual irregularities, leucorrhoea, dysmenorrhoea, uterine bleeding, postpartum haemorrhage, lower abdominal pain, indigestion, diarrhoea, rectal prolapse.

REN 5 (Stone Gate)

Location: On the anterior midline, two cun below the umbilicus.
Needling Technique: Perpendicular insertion 0.5 to 1.0 cun.
Indications: Abdominal pain, diarrhoea, oedema, hernia, anuria, enuresis, amenorrhoea, chronic leucorrhoea, uterine bleeding, postpartum haemorrhage.

REN 6 (Sea of Qi)

Location: On the anterior midline, 1.5 cun below the umbilicus.
Needling Technique: Perpendicular insertion 0.8 to 1.2 cun.
Note: REN 6 is a significant point for tonification.
Indications: Abdominal pain, enuresis, nocturnal emission, impotence, hernia, oedema, diarrhoea, dysentery, uterine bleeding, irregular menstruation, amenorrhoea, leucorrhoea, postpartum haemorrhage, constipation, asthma.

REN 8 (Spirit Gate)

Location: In the centre of the umbilicus.
Needling Technique: **Needling contraindicated.** Moxibustion or warming methods are used instead.
Indications: Collapse, diarrhoea due to cold, abdominal cold, umbilical spasm (treated with moxibustion).

REN 9 (Water Separation)

Location: On the anterior midline, one cun above the umbilicus.
Needling Technique: Perpendicular insertion 0.5 to 1.0 cun.
Indications: Abdominal pain, oedema, urinary retention, diarrhoea.

REN 10 (Lower Cavity)

Location: On the anterior midline, two cun above the umbilicus.
Needling Technique: Perpendicular insertion 0.5 to 1.2 cun.
Indications: Epigastric pain, abdominal distension, indigestion, vomiting, diarrhoea.

REN 15 (Turtledove Tail)

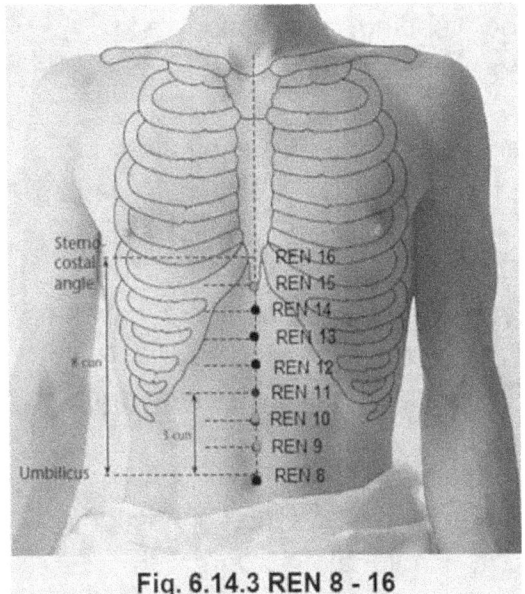

Fig. 6.14.3 REN 8 - 16

Location: On the anterior midline, one cun below the xiphisternal synchondrosis. Locate the patient in a supine position with arms raised.
Needling Technique: Oblique downward insertion 0.4 to 0.6 cun.
Caution: Avoid deep needling to prevent cardiac injury.
Indications: Chest and cardiac pain, nausea, mental disorders, epilepsy.

REN 24 (Container of Fluids)

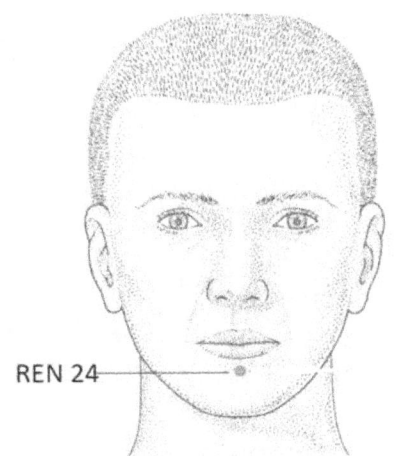

Fig. 6.14.4 REN 24

Location: In the depression at the centre of the mento-labial groove.
Needling Technique: Oblique upward insertion 0.2 to 0.3 cun.
Indications: Facial puffiness, gum swelling, toothache, drooling, mental disorders, deviation of the mouth and eyes.

Clinical Significance - Ren Channel

The Ren channel, also known as the Conception Vessel, runs along the midline of the anterior body from the perineum to the chin. It is considered the Sea of Yin and governs all the Yin channels in the body. This channel is deeply involved in reproductive, urogenital, respiratory, and digestive functions.

It is especially important in treating gynaecological and reproductive issues such as irregular menstruation, infertility, leucorrhoea, uterine bleeding, and menopausal symptoms. In men, it is used for conditions like impotence, prostatitis, and hernia.

The Ren channel regulates the uterus and the lower abdomen and is also commonly used for abdominal pain, bloating, constipation, diarrhoea, and urinary difficulties such as retention or incontinence.

It plays a key role in supporting prenatal and postnatal Qi and is often used in cases of chronic fatigue, poor development, or recovery from long-term illness. It also strengthens the body's Yin aspect and nourishes the fluids, effectively treating dryness, night sweats, and Yin deficiency heat.

Emotionally, the Ren channel helps stabilize the mind and supports the connection between the heart and kidneys. It is frequently used in emotional disorders with underlying hormonal or reproductive links.

-Modern Acupuncture-

Summary of Clinical Significance of Channels

Channel	Clinical Significance
Lung	Regulates respiration, Qi, and body fluids; treats cough, asthma, skin issues, and emotional grief.
Large Intestine	Treats facial/head disorders, toothache, fever, digestive irregularities, and emotional rigidity.
Stomach	Addresses digestive problems, facial paralysis, fluid retention, and emotional overthinking.
Spleen	It supports digestion, muscle tone, and blood production and treats gynecological and emotional worry.
Heart	Manages cardiac symptoms, insomnia, anxiety, and emotional disorders; stabilizes the mind.
Small Intestine	It treats pain in the neck/shoulder, ear issues, and neurological tension and supports mental clarity.
Bladder	Key for spinal pain, urinary issues, neurological disorders, and emotional distress.
Kidney	It supports the essence, reproduction, bones, and hearing, and treats chronic fatigue, fear, and lower back pain.
Pericardium	It protects the heart and treats chest and emotional disorders, nausea, and wrist/forearm issues.
San Jiao	Regulates water pathways, treats lateral arm/neck/ear pain, febrile illness, and stress tension.
Gall Bladder	Treats migraines, side-body pain, eye/ear issues, emotional frustration, and damp-heat in the liver.
Liver	Regulates Qi flow, menstruation, emotions, and treats tendon problems, eye disorders, and hypertension.
DU (Governing Vessel)	Controls Yang treats spinal and neurological disorders, mental imbalance, and collapse.
REN (Conception Vessel)	Governs Yin, supports reproductive health, digestion, urination, Yin deficiency, and emotional balance.

6.15 Extra Acupuncture Points

Extra acupuncture points are those not located on the traditional fourteen meridians. Although not formally integrated into the classical meridian system of Traditional Chinese Medicine (TCM), these points have demonstrated distinct therapeutic benefits and are widely used in clinical acupuncture. Many were initially derived from frequently stimulated *Ashi points* (tender or reactive points) and thus do not necessarily conform to traditional Chinese medicine (TCM) principles, such as the Yin-Yang or Five Elements theory.

Despite this, specific extra points anatomically align with conventional meridians. For example, Yintang lies on the Governing Vessel, Erbai on the Pericardium meridian, and Taiyang on the San Jiao meridian. As new extra points are identified and clinically validated, their utility in modern acupuncture continues to expand.

Some important extra acupuncture points are described below:

Sishencong (Ex HN 1) *(Four Alert Spirit Points)*

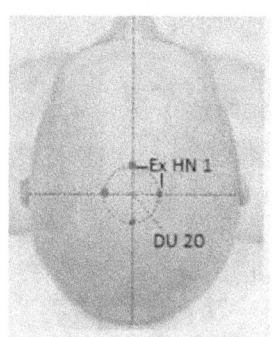

Fig. 6.15.1 Ex HN 1 Sisbencong

Location: Four points, each one cun anterior, posterior, and lateral to **DU 20**, located on the vertex.
Needling Technique: Subcutaneous insertion 0.5 to 1.0 cun toward the treatment direction.
Indications: Headache, vertigo, insomnia, poor memory, epilepsy.

Yintang (Ex HN 3) *(Hall of Impression)*
Location: Midpoint between the medial ends of the eyebrows.
Needling Technique: Subcutaneous insertion 0.3 to 0.5 cun.
Indications: Frontal headache, heaviness of the head, epistaxis, rhinorrhoea, insomnia, infantile convulsions.

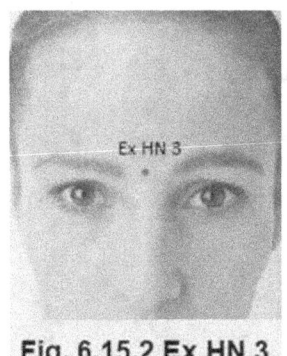

Fig. 6.15.2 Ex HN 3
Yintang

Taiyang (Ex HN 5) *(Supreme Yang)*

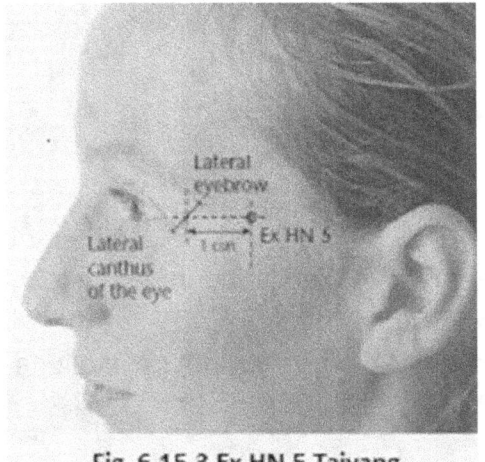

Fig. 6.15.3 Ex HN 5 Taiyang

Location: In the depression, approximately one fingerbreadth is posterior to the midpoint between the lateral eyebrow and the outer canthus.
Needling Technique: Perpendicular insertion 0.3 to 0.5 cun or prick to bleed.
Indications: Headache, eye disorders, deviation of the eyes and mouth.

Yuyao (Ex HN 6) *(Fish Waist)*

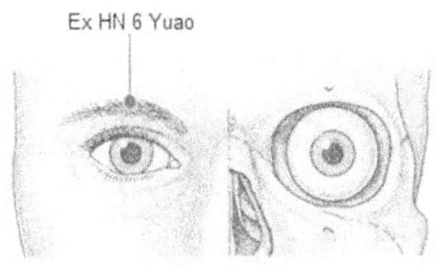

Fig. 6.15.4 Ex HN 6 Yuao

Location: At the midpoint of the eyebrow, directly above the pupil.
Needling Technique: Subcutaneous insertion 0.3 to 0.5 cun.
Indications: Supraorbital pain, eyelid twitching, ptosis, corneal clouding, eye redness, and swelling.

Jinjin & Yuye *(Golden Liquid & Jade Fluid)*

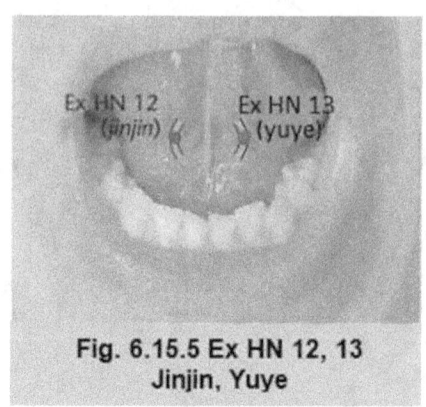

Location: On the veins of the tongue's frenulum **Jinjin** on the left, **Yuye** on the right.
Needling Technique: Prick to cause bleeding.
Indications: Tongue swelling, vomiting, aphasia due to tongue stiffness.

Fig. 6.15.5 Ex HN 12, 13 Jinjin, Yuye

Anmian (Ex HN 54) *(Peaceful Sleep)*

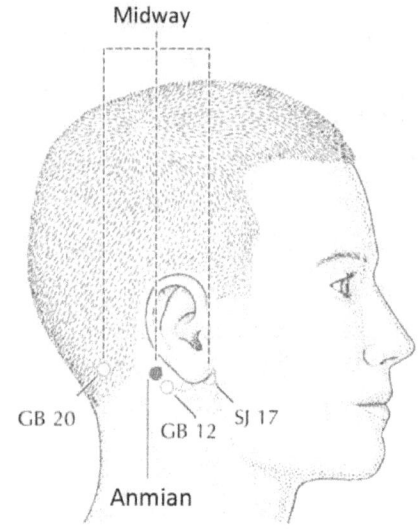

Location: Midpoint between SJ 17 and GB 20.
Needling Technique: Perpendicular insertion 0.5 to 0.8 cun.
Indications: Insomnia, headache, vertigo, palpitations, mental disorders.

Fig. 6.15.6 Anmian

Huatuojiaji *(Hua Tuo's Paraspinal Points)*

Location: 34 points, 0.5 cun lateral to the lower border of each spinous process from T1 to L5, bilaterally.
Needling Technique: Perpendicular insertion: 0.5 to 1.0 cun (cervical/thoracic), 1.0 to 1.5 cun (lumbar).
Indications: Disorders corresponding to segmental innervations (see Fig. 6.15.7).

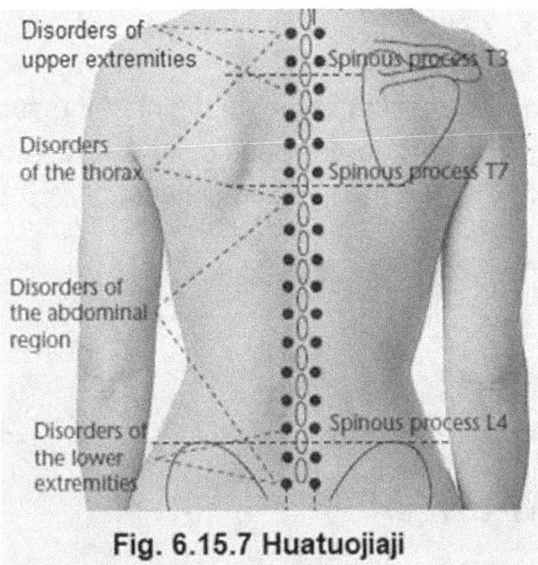

Fig. 6.15.7 Huatuojiaji

Jianqian (Jianneiling) *(Front of the Shoulder)*

Location: Midway between the end of the anterior axillary fold and **LI 15**.
Needling Technique: Perpendicular insertion 0.8 to 1.2 cun.
Indications: Shoulder and arm pain, upper limb paralysis.

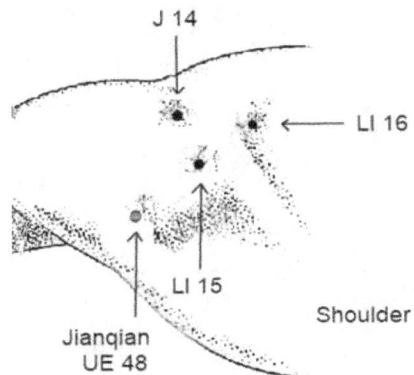

Fig. 6.15.8 Jianqian

Shanglianquan *(Upper Ridge Spring)*

Location: One cun below the jaw's midpoint, between the hyoid and the mandible.
Needling Technique: Oblique insertion 0.8 to 1.2 cun toward the root of the tongue.
Indications: Excessive salivation, tongue stiffness, sore throat, dysphagia, aphonia.

Heding (Ex LE 2) *(Crane's Summit)*

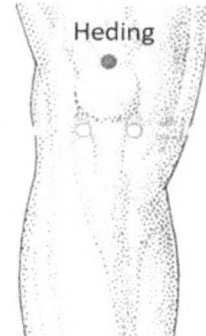

Location: Depression at the midpoint of the superior patellar border.
Needling Technique: Perpendicular insertion 0.3 to 0.5 cun.
Indications: Knee pain, leg weakness, paralysis.

Fig. 6.15.10
Heding

Xiyan (Ex LE 5) *(Eyes of the Knee)*

Location: Pair points in the medial and lateral depressions to the patellar ligament (knee flexed). Lateral Xiyan overlaps with **ST 35**.
Needling Technique: Perpendicular insertion 0.5 to 1.0 cun.
Indications: Knee pain, lower limb weakness.

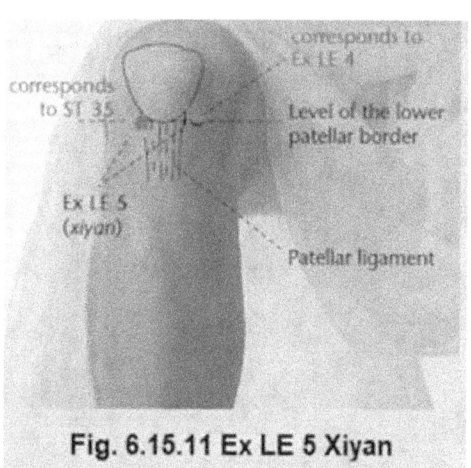

Fig. 6.15.11 Ex LE 5 Xiyan

Lanweixue (Ex LE 7) *(Appendix Point)*

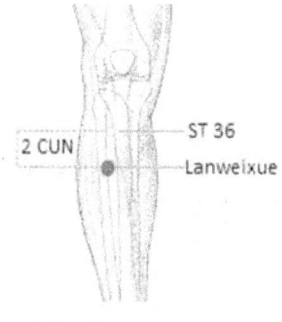

Location: On the anterior lateral lower leg, two cun below **ST 36**, one fingerbreadth lateral to the tibial crest.
Needling Technique: Perpendicular insertion 1.5 to 2.0 cun.
Indications: Acute/chronic appendicitis, dyspepsia, leg pain, paralysis.

6.15.12 Lanweixue

Erjian *(Tip of the Ear)*

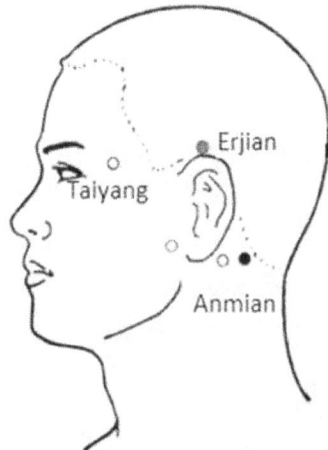

Fig. 6.15.13 Ex HN 6 Erjian

Location: Apex of the auricle (folded).
Needling Technique: Perpendicular insertion 0.1 to 0.2 cun or prick to bleed.
Indications: Eye redness and swelling, fever, febrile disease.

Dingchuan *(Calm Dyspnoea)*

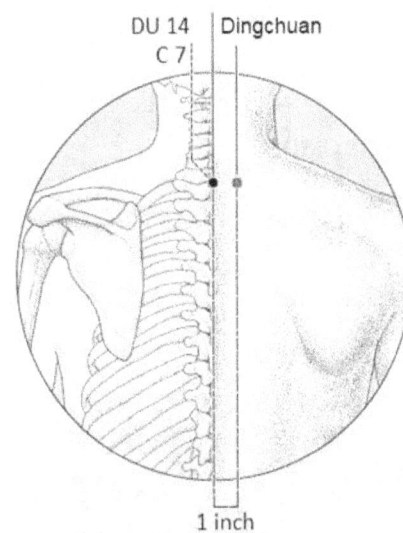

Fig. 6.15.14 Dingchuan

Location: 0.5 cun lateral to **DU 14**.
Needling Technique: Perpendicular insertion 0.5 to 0.8 cun.
Indications: Asthma, cough, neck stiffness, upper back pain.

Baxie (Ex UE 9) *(Eight Pathogens)*

Location: At the dorsum of the hand, in the web margins at the junction of red and white skin (loose fist).
Needling Technique: Oblique insertion 0.3 to 0.5 cun or prick to bleed.
Indications: Finger numbness, contracture, hand swelling, and pain.

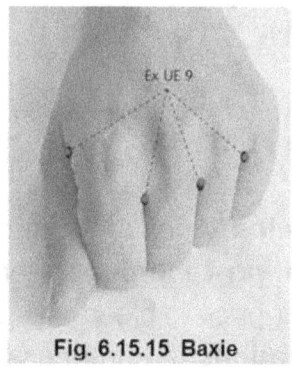

Fig. 6.15.15 Baxie

Qiduan (Ex LE 12) *(Ten Ends)*

Location: On the tip of each toe, 0.1 cun lateral to the nail corners.
Needling Technique: Perpendicular insertion 0.1 cun; retention for 20 minutes advised.
Indications: Toe numbness, pain, swelling, and emergency treatment for stroke.

Erbai (Ex UE 29) *(Two Whites)*

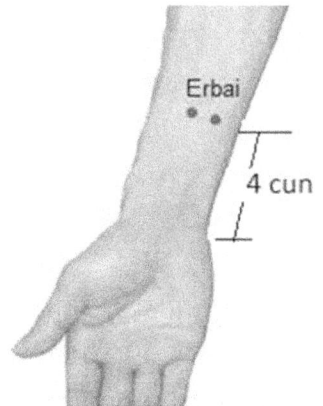

Location: Palmar forearm, four cun above the transverse wrist crease, on either side of the **flexor carpi radialis** tendon.

Needling Technique: Perpendicular insertion 0.5 to 1.0 cun.
Indications: Haemorrhoids, rectal prolapse.

Fig. 6.15.16 Erbai

Bafeng (Ex LE 10) *(Eight Winds)*

Location: In the depressions of the toe webs, proximal to web margins, at red-white skin junctions.
Needling Technique: Oblique insertion 0.5 to 0.8 cun.
Indications: Toe pain, swelling, and redness of the dorsum of the foot.

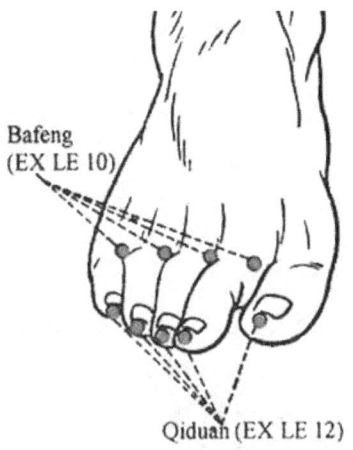

Fig. 6.15.17
Ex LE 10 Bafeng, Ex LE 12 Qiduan

Mu Guan and Gu Guan *(Wood Pass & Bone Pass)*

Location: **Mu Guan**: 0.5 cun distal to the pisiform bone at the palm base.

Gu Guan: 0.5 cun distal to the scaphoid bone at the palm base.
Needling Technique: Perpendicular insertion until bone contact; tapping against bone is preferred.
Indications: Arthritis, plantar fasciitis, viral fever, common cold.

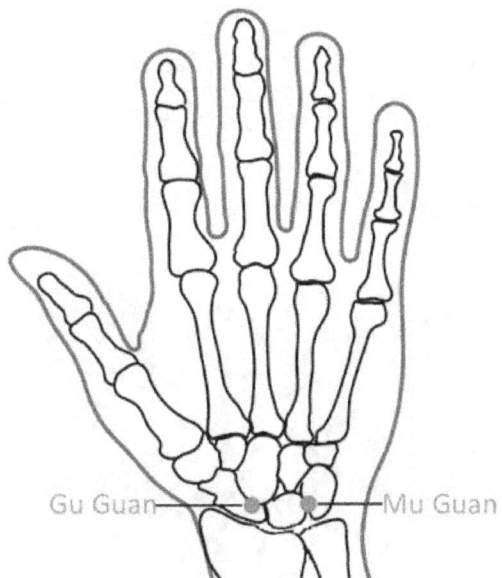

Fig. 6.15.18 Mu Guan, Gu Guan

Clinical Significance of Extra Acupuncture Points

Extra acupuncture points are specific locations on the body that lie outside the fourteen regular meridians but have proven therapeutic value through clinical use. Though not integrated into the classical meridian system, they have unique functions, indications, and local effects.

Clinically, extra points are often used for pain management, neurological disorders, musculoskeletal conditions, and certain systemic or organ-specific diseases. For example, Yintang is widely used for calming the mind and relieving anxiety, while Sishencong aids in improving memory and treating insomnia. Extra points, such as Baichongwo, are applied in dermatological conditions, while points like Jinjin–Yuye are valid in tongue or speech disorders.

These points often arise from empirical practice and are chosen based on their effectiveness rather than theoretical placement. Many extra points coincide with muscle motor points or neurovascular junctions, making them powerful in musculoskeletal and neurological therapies.

They are especially valuable in modern acupuncture for their focused actions, ease of location, and compatibility with various treatment protocols, including scalp acupuncture, electroacupuncture, and microsystems therapy.

-Modern Acupuncture-

7. Tung Acupuncture

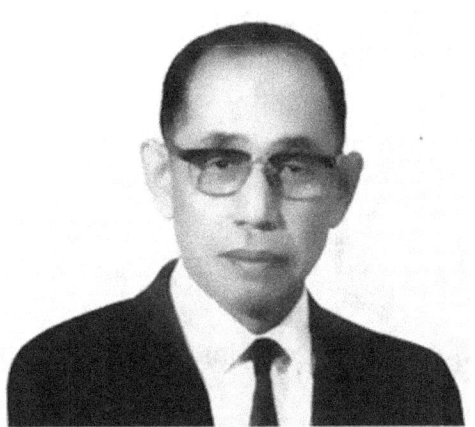

Master Tung Ching Chang
(1916–1975)

Tung was born in 1916 into an acupuncture family in Ping Du County, Shandong Province, China, and began his career as an acupuncturist at 18. During World War II, he served in the Kuo Min Tang (KMT) army and applied his acupuncture skills to help his fellow soldiers. In 1949, following the Communist Party of China's victory, the Nationalists (KMT) retreated to Taiwan, where Chiang Kai-shek established a permanent base. In the 1960s, he established a private acupuncture clinic in Taiwan. However, in the 1970s, Taiwan began formal licensing for TCM practitioners. Tung was denied a license due to his lack of formal schooling and was consequently forced to cease practice. He passed away in 1975, shortly after this setback.

Tung Ching Chang was the first acupuncturist to teach the Tung acupuncture system outside his family. He accepted his first disciple, Lin Ju Chu, in 1962 Taipei, Taiwan. Previously, the Tung method remained a secret family tradition, but Tung Ching Chang chose to share it with the public. This decision led to the Tung method gaining widespread recognition and becoming an essential branch of acupuncture globally.

Tung acupuncture is a unique system recognized for its effectiveness in treating pain, musculoskeletal disorders, internal medicine conditions, etc. The system is particularly appreciated for its rapid and powerful therapeutic effects, which are attributed to specific acupuncture points that directly influence corresponding body areas.

Tung points are primarily on the extremities, especially the hands and feet. A hallmark of this system is "mirroring" or "contralateral needling," where points on one side of the body are needled to treat issues on the opposite side. For instance, pain in the right knee might be treated by needling points on the left foot or hand.

Basic Premise – Human Microcosm

The foundational concept of Tung acupuncture is that humans are microcosms of the universe. This idea is rooted in Chinese philosophical thought, including the teachings of Confucian scholars, who believed that the same laws and forces that govern the

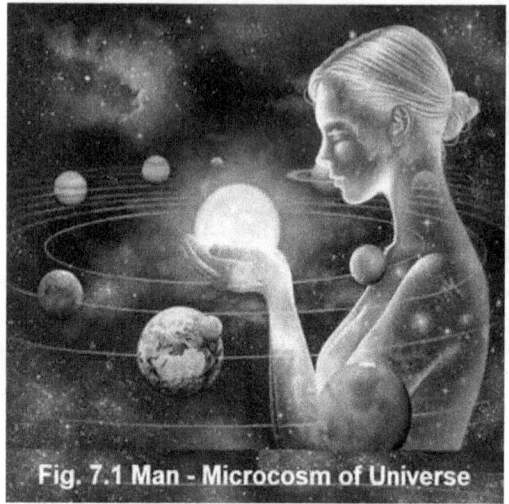

Fig. 7.1 Man - Microcosm of Universe

universe also govern human beings. The holographic acupuncture technique derives from the principle that the local reflects the general. Just as a hologram contains the complete image in every part, each area of the human body contains a representation of the whole.

According to this view, one part of the body can affect or be affected by another part that is distant in space. Tung acupuncture distinguishes itself by not relying on traditional Chinese medicine (TCM) diagnostic theories, allowing for more streamlined clinical applications.

Correspondence

Tung acupuncture identifies three main types of correspondences:

A. Image Correspondence B. Channel Correspondence C. Tissue Correspondence.

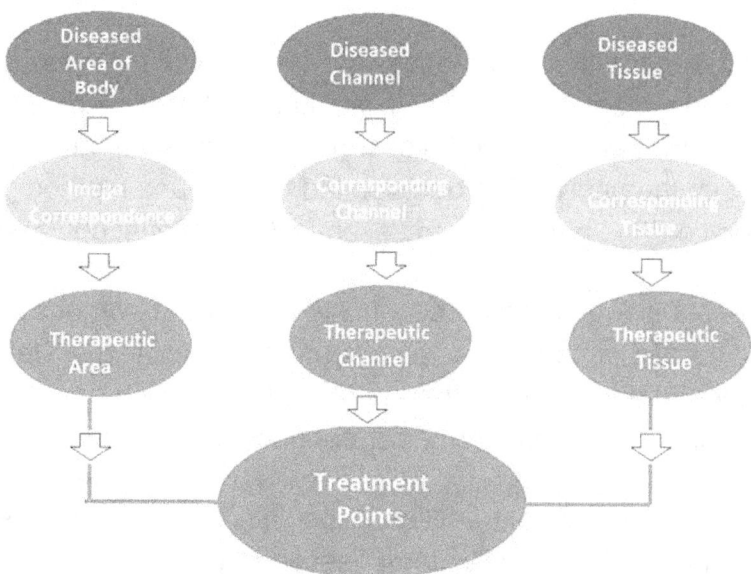

Fig. 7.2 Identifying Treatment Points for a Diseased Area

A. Image Correspondence

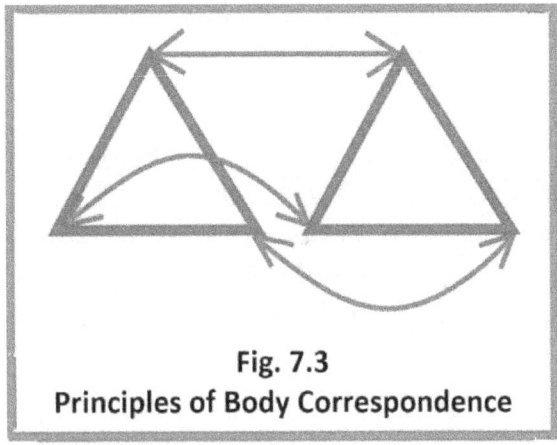

Fig. 7.3
Principles of Body Correspondence

This principle posits that various body parts mirror each other. Pain or disease in one area can often be treated by addressing a corresponding area elsewhere. The following examples explain this concept:

Upper Limb to Upper Limb in the Same Direction

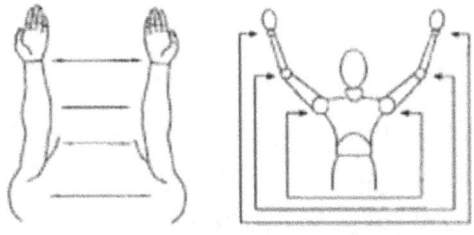

Fig. 7.4 Upper Limb to Opposite Upper Limb in Same Direction

Place both arms side by side. The right shoulder corresponds to the left shoulder, and the right elbow to the left elbow. Thus, a left tennis elbow can be treated by right LI 11.

Lower Limb to Lower Limb in the Same Direction

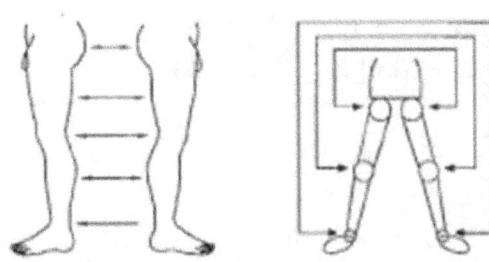

Fig. 7.5 Lower Limb to Opposite Lower Limb in Same Direction

Position both legs side by side. The right knee corresponds to the left knee. For example, right knee pain can be treated by left ST 35.

Upper Limb to Lower Limb in the Same Direction

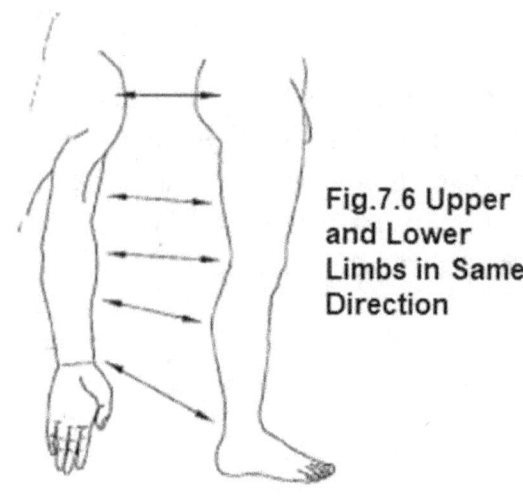

Fig.7.6 Upper and Lower Limbs in Same Direction

Imagine the elbow at the level of the knee. The wrist corresponds to the ankle, and the shoulder to the hip. For example, PC 6 can treat ankle pain. LI 5 and ST 41, SJ 3 and GB 41, and SJ 5 and GB 39 are reciprocal pairs.

Lower Limb to Upper Limb in the Opposite Direction

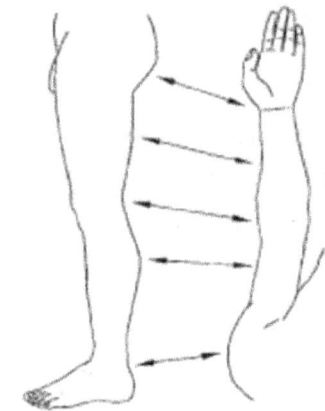

Fig. 7.7 Upper Limb and Lower Limbs in Opposite Directions

Imagine the elbow and knee aligned but facing in opposite directions. The ankle corresponds to the shoulder, and the hip to the wrist. Hence, 44.06 can treat ankle pain; ST 41 can treat shoulder pain.

Upper Limb and Trunk in the Same Direction, Fig. 7.8

Wrist and fingers correspond to the external genitalia and the lower lumbar region. The shoulder corresponds to the chest and upper back. For example, 33.06 treats backache; 11.01 treats inguinal hernia.

Upper Limb to Trunk in the Opposite Direction, Fig. 7.8

Wrist and fingers correspond to the head and neck. The shoulder corresponds to the pelvic region. The elbow corresponds to the waist. SI 3 treats neck pain; finger points are used to treat headaches. PC 6, 33.04, and 33.05 treat chest symptoms. SI 11 and 44.11 treat vaginal discharge.

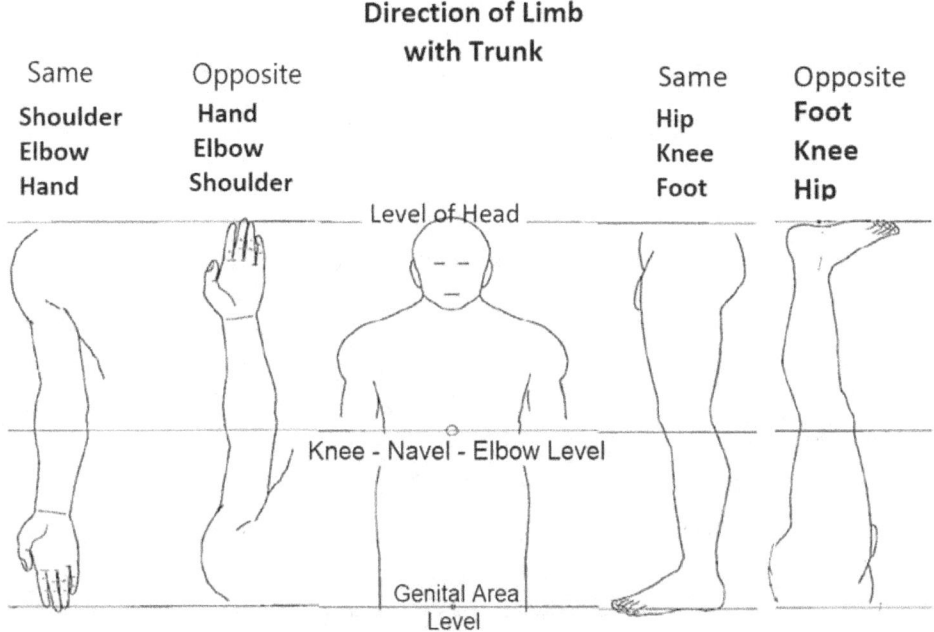

Fig. 7.8 Limbs to Trunk Correspondence

Lower Limb to Trunk in the Same Direction, Fig. 7.8

The thigh corresponds to the abdomen and back. Hip corresponds to chest. The foot corresponds to the genital organs. 88.01–03 treat lung and heart issues. 66.06 treats dysmenorrhea. The knee corresponds to the umbilicus.

Lower Limb to Trunk in the Opposite Direction, Fig. 7.8

The ankle corresponds to the neck. Knee to umbilicus. Foot to head. GB 41 and ST 43 are used to treat migraines. UB 65 treats occipital headaches. LV 1 and LU 11 (ghost points) treat depressive psychosis.

Top to Bottom and Bottom to Top

The entire body, in a head-to-toe orientation, can be treated on the opposite level. As heel pain can effectively be treated by DU 20, neck pain can also be treated by 77.01 at the Tendo Achilles tendon. Similarly, 55.xx at the sole treats the eye, and Jaw at ST 6 can treat pain at the dorsum of the foot.

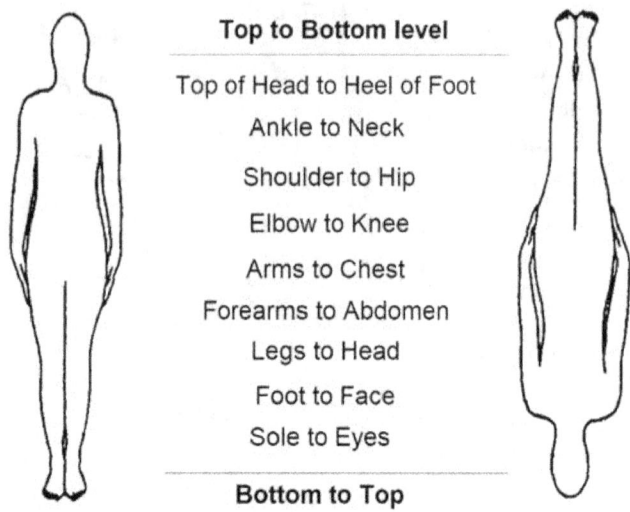

Top to Bottom level

Top of Head to Heel of Foot

Ankle to Neck

Shoulder to Hip

Elbow to Knee

Arms to Chest

Forearms to Abdomen

Legs to Head

Foot to Face

Sole to Eyes

Bottom to Top

Fig. 7.9 Whole Body Top to Bottom Correspondence

Inter-Related Mirror Image Treatment Areas of Limbs and Trunk

Inter-Related Mirror Image Treatment Areas of Limbs and Trunk		
Area Treated of limbs.	Target Area	Target Reverse Area
Fingers/Toes	Testicles and Anus	Top of Head
Hand/ Foot	Sacrum, Coccyx, Genitals	Head
Wrist/ Ankle	Lumbo-sacral area, Bladder	Neck
Forearm/ Legs	Lower Abdomen, Lower Back	Upper Abdomen, Lower Thorax, Chest, Mid-Back,
Elbow/ Knee	Umbilicus	Umbilicus
Upper Arm/ Thigh	Upper Abdomen, Lower Thorax, Chest, Mid-Back,	Lower Abdomen, Lower Back

Shoulder/ Hip Joint	Neck, Jaw, the base of the Skull	Genitals
Top of Shoulder/ Hip	Top of Head	Testicles, Anus

All Directions to the Centre

Correspondence also exists from all limbs and the face toward the body centre. DU 20 treats prolapsed rectum; DT 17 treats headaches.

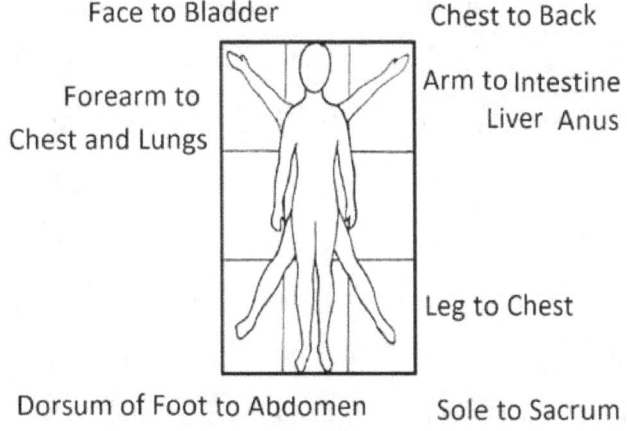

Face to Bladder   Chest to Back

Forearm to Chest and Lungs   Arm to Intestine Liver Anus

Leg to Chest

Dorsum of Foot to Abdomen   Sole to Sacrum

Fig. 7.10 Centre to Periphery to Centre

B. Channel Correspondence

The following table outlines the **corresponding relations of acupuncture channels** that can be utilized for therapeutic targeting when a specific meridian is affected by disease. It provides three alternate approaches to select a treatment channel: (1) the *same-name channel on the contralateral side*, (2) the *opposite paired channel on the foot or hand*, and (3) the *interior–exterior paired channel on the contralateral side*. This system is especially useful in balance method acupuncture, contralateral needling, and distal point therapy. Understanding these relationships enhances point selection, allowing for effective treatment without the need to directly needle the affected channel, thereby increasing safety and systemic balance.

Same Channel: Pain on a point, such as UB 2, can be treated at UB 67.

Same Name Channel on Upper/Lower Limb: For example, Hand Tai Yang (SI) can be treated by Foot Tai Yang (UB). Pain in the ST channel (leg) can be treated by the LI channel (arm).

Exterior–Interior Coupling: Yang channels, such as SJ, can be treated through their Yin counterparts, like PC, either on the same or opposite side.

Same Name External–Internal Channel (Upper/Lower): SJ pain can be treated through the Liver channel on the opposite limb. *See the following table.*

If Diseased Channel is -		Target Channel can be - Same Name Channel on Contralateral		Target Channel - Opposite Channel on Foot/ Hand		Target Channel - Interior - Exterior on Contralateral side	
Hand Tai Yin	LU	Foot Tai Yin	SP	Foot Tai Yang	UB	Hand Yang Ming	LI
Hand Yang Ming	LI	Foot Yang Ming	ST	Foot Jue Yin	LV	Hand Tai Yin	LU
Foot Yang Ming	ST	Hand Yang Ming	LI	Hand Jue Yin	PC	Foot Tai Yin	SP
Foot Tai Yin	SP	Hand Tai Yin	LU	Hand Tai Yang	SI	Foot Yang Ming	ST
Hand Shao Yin	HT	Foot Shao Yin	KI	Foot Shao Yang	GB	Hand Tai Yang	SI
Hand Tai Yang	SI	Foot Tai Yang	UB	Foot Tai Yin	SP	Hand Shao Yin	HT
Foot Tai Yang	UB	Hand Tai Yang	SI	Hand Tai Yin	LU	Foot Shao Yin	KI
Foot Shao Yin	KI	Hand Shao Yin	HT	Hand Shao Yang	SJ	Foot Tai Yang	UB
Hand Jue Yin	PC	Foot Jue Yin	LV	Foot Yang Ming	ST	Hand Shao Yang	SJ
Hand Shao Yang	SJ	Foot Shao Yang	GB	Foot Shao Yin	KI	Hand Jue Yin	PC
Foot Shao Yang	GB	Hand Shao Yang	SJ	Hand Shao Yin	HT	Foot Jue Yin	LV
Foot Jue Yin	LV	Hand Jue Yin	PC	Hand Yang Ming	LI	Foot Shao Yang	GB

Corresponding Relations of Channels Useful in Treatments

C. Tissue Correspondence

Tung acupuncture also incorporates correspondence between similar tissue types:

Bone Treats Bone: Sciatica treated by needling near the bone (e.g., 22.05, 22.04).

Tendon Treats Tendon: Tendon issues like gastrocnemius strain or neck stiffness treated by 77.01, 77.02, and LU 5.

Muscle Treats Muscle: General muscle pain and atrophy treated at 88.17–19.

Blood Vessel Treats Blood Vessel: 44.08 and 44.09 near large arm vessels treat vascular conditions.

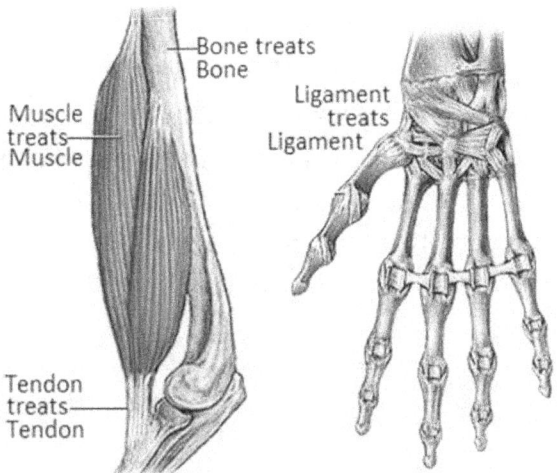

Fig. 7.11 Tissue Correspondence

D. Venous Congestion Correspondence

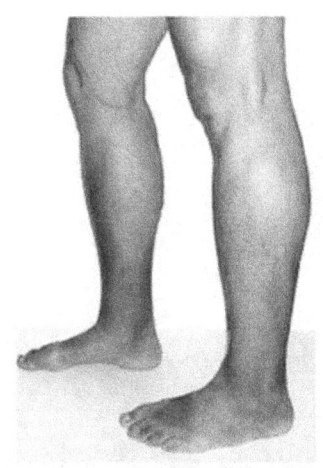

Fig. 7.12 Correspondence of Venous Congestion

Internal diseases often manifest as venous congestion in the corresponding external areas.

Examples:

Lung disease reflected at 1010.19 and 1010.20 (mouth)
Cervical spondylitis and shoulder disease reflected at 22.01 and 22.02
Hand and foot issues reflected in the fingers (11.27)
Cardiac/lung pathology in children may show signs on the middle finger
Anoxic conditions reflected at LU 5 and UB 40—bleeding relieves symptoms in 5–7 days

– Modern Acupuncture –

8. Tung Acupuncture Zones and Points

Tung acupuncture points are grouped according to their specified location on the body or zones. The groups are as follows - those on fingers are series - 11.xx, hand - 22.xx, lower arm - 33.xx, upper arm - 44.xx, sole - 55.xx, dorsum of foot - 66.xx, leg - 77.xx, thigh - 88.xx, ear - 99.xx, head and face - 1010.xx, ventral part (front) of the trunk - VT.xx, and dorsal part (back) of the trunk DT.xx. They are referred to in terms of numbers in that order. The advantage of Tung acupuncture points' peripheral distal distribution is that they are conveniently located away from the disease site, making them ideal for treatment. It also allows patients to move while the needle is still in place.

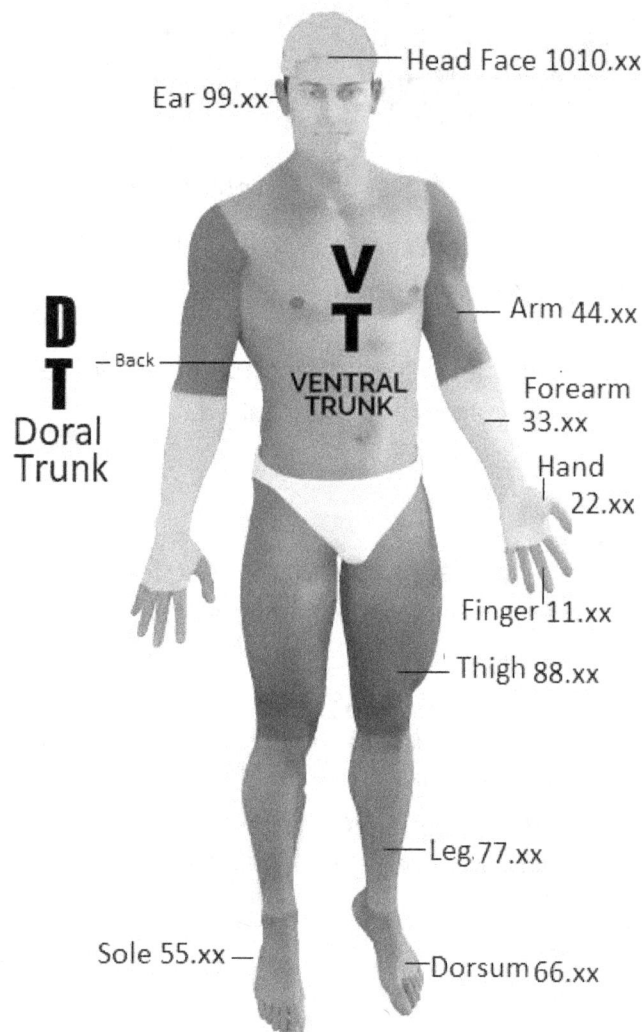

Fig. 8 Tung Acupuncture Zones

8.1 Tung Points on Fingers – 11.xx

The Tung acupuncture points on the fingers are classified under the 11.xx series. A clear anatomical understanding of the fingers is crucial for accurately locating these points and administering effective treatment. For instructional purposes, the tip of the left-hand finger demonstrates the imaginary lines. These lines should be well-visualised before attempting point location. For the right-hand fingers, a mirror image approach must be applied.

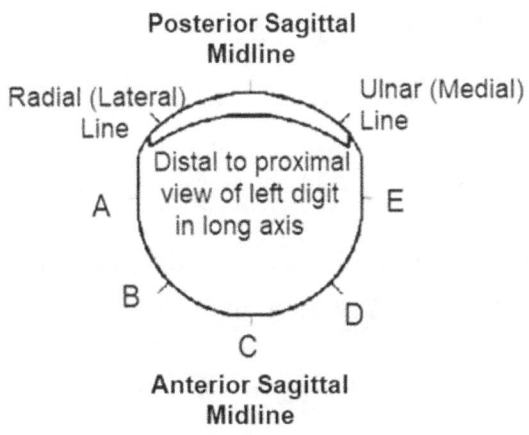

Fig. 8.11.1 Reference Lines on Fingers

There are 27 points located on the fingers. Through image correspondence, these points influence the opposite fingers, toes, pelvis, lower abdomen, head, and face. Additionally, they can affect the knees and chest. Thus, needling finger points is clinically effective for treating conditions associated with these regions.

11.01

Location: 0.33 cun radial to the centre of the proximal phalanx of the index finger, on Line B, level with point 11.05.
Needling Technique: Insert 0.2–0.3 cun deep.

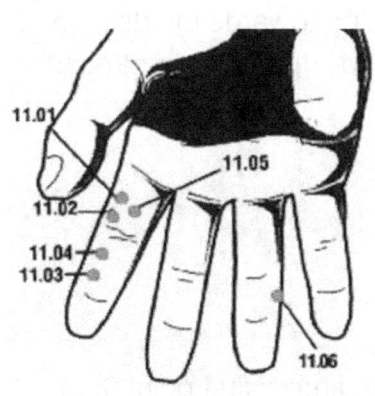

Fig. 8.11.2

Indications: Knee pain, inguinal hernia, pain at the outer eye corner, bearing-down testicular pain.

11.02

Location: On the upper part of the proximal phalanx of the index finger, 0.2 cun distal to 11.01, also on Line B.
Needling Technique: Insert 0.2–0.25 cun deep.
Indications: Bronchitis, chest tightness, palpitations, knee pain, inguinal hernia, outer eye pain, enteritis.

11.03

Location: 0.2 cun radial to the midline of the middle phalanx of the index finger.
Needling Technique: Insert 0.2–0.25 cun deep.
Indications: Inguinal hernia, urethritis, toothache, abdominal pain.

11.04

Location: 0.2 cun radial to the midline of the middle phalanx of the index finger, at its distal third; 0.66 cun from the distal crease.
Needling Technique: Insert 0.2–0.25 cun deep.
Indications: Inguinal hernia, urethritis, toothache, abdominal pain.

11.05

Location: Centre of the proximal phalanx of the index finger, on Line C.
Needling Technique: Insert 0.1–0.2 cun deep.
Indications: Palpitations, chest oppression, knee pain, dizziness, hernia. Commonly used for inguinal hernia, often combined with bleeding at the medial malleolus.

11.06

Location: On the middle phalanx of the ring finger, ulnar side of Line E.
Needling Technique: Insert 0.2–0.3 cun deep.
Indications: Dysmenorrhoea, fibroids, endometritis, irregular menstruation, leucorrhoea, tubal block, frequent urination, vaginal swelling, recurrent miscarriage.

11.10

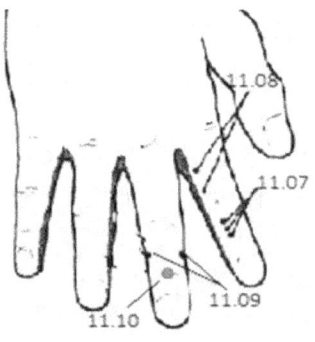

Location: Centre of the middle phalanx of the middle finger, dorsal side.
Needling Technique: Oblique needling towards the distal end, just touching but not striking bone. Allow the hand to hang to support needle retention.
Indications: Hemiplegia.

Fig. 8.11.3

11.12

Location: Dorsal midline of the proximal phalanx of the middle finger; first point 0.33 cun from the second finger crease, second point 0.66 cun from the same crease.
Needling Technique: Oblique insertion distally with a fine needle; touch the bone.
Indications: Lumbar sprain, supraorbital bone pain, and nasal bone pain.

11.13

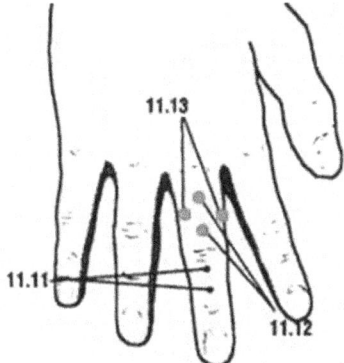

Fig. 8.11.4

Location: Two points on the dorsal side of the proximal phalanx of the middle finger at the radial and ulnar midline.
Needling Technique: Insert 0.1–0.2 cun deep by the bone's side.
Indications: Knee pain, palpitations, infantile irritability.

11.14

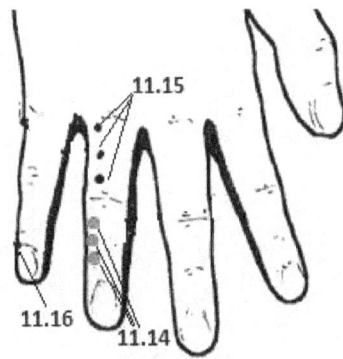

Fig. 8.11.5

Location: Three points on the dorsal-ulnar aspect of the proximal phalanx of the ring finger—one at midline, the others 0.3 cun above and below it.
Needling Technique: Insert 0.1–0.2 cun deep alongside the bone.
Indications: Facial paralysis, breast swelling, muscle atrophy, irritability.

11.17

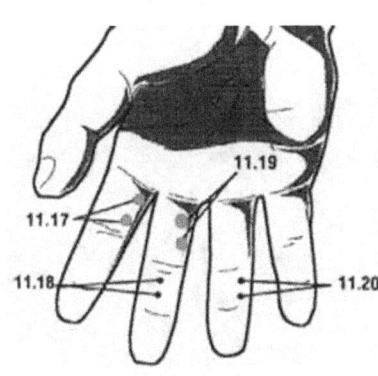

Fig. 8.11.6

Location: Two points on the palmar-medial side of the first phalanx of the index finger, 0.2 cun from the midline, on Line D.
Needling Technique: Insert 0.2–0.3 cun deep.
Indications: Irritability.

11.19

Location: Two points on the palmar-ulnar side of the proximal phalanx of the middle finger; 0.33 cun and 0.66 cun from the second digital crease.
Needling Technique: Insert 0.1–0.2 cun deep.
Indications: Palpitations, rheumatism.

11.23

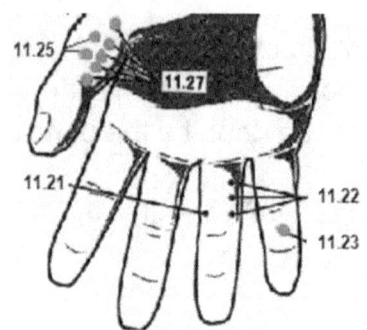

Fig. 8.11.7

Location: Palmar side of the middle phalanx of the little finger on Line C.
Needling Technique: Insert 0.1–0.2 cun deep.
Indications: Jaundice.

11.24

Location: Two points on the ulnar-dorsal side of the proximal phalanx of the thumb; one 0.3 cun from midline, the other 0.5 cun from the second crease.
Needling Technique: Insert 0.2–0.3 cun deep close to the phalanx.
Indications: Female infertility, endometritis, PID, fibroids, lower abdominal distension, irregular menstruation, dysmenorrhoea, menorrhagia, scanty menstruation.

11.27 Fig. 8.11.7

Location: Five points along the radial-palmar aspect of the proximal phalanx of the thumb, 0.2 cun apart on the Line A.
Needling Technique: Insert 0.2–0.4 cun deep depending on the nearby or distal problem focus.
Indications: Pain and soreness in the fingers, ankle, heel, dorsum of foot, toes, headache, arthritis, tenosynovitis, joint swelling, pneumonia, cough, tonsillitis.

8.2 Tung Points on Hand – 22.xx

The Tung acupuncture points on both the dorsal and palmar sides of the hand are classified under the 22.xx series. This group has eleven points (eight primary and three additional), most of which are located on the dorsal surface. Points on the palmar side are more sensitive and require precise needling to minimise patient discomfort.

According to the principle of image correspondence, hand points influence and treat conditions of the lower back, abdomen, head, face, shoulders, the opposite hand, and both feet. Additionally, chest-related diseases often respond effectively to points in the 22.xx series.

22.01

Location: Situated on the thenar eminence, approximately one cun below the skin fold between the first and second metacarpals and two cun from the skin fold. It has cross-communication with point 22.05 on the dorsal aspect of the hand.

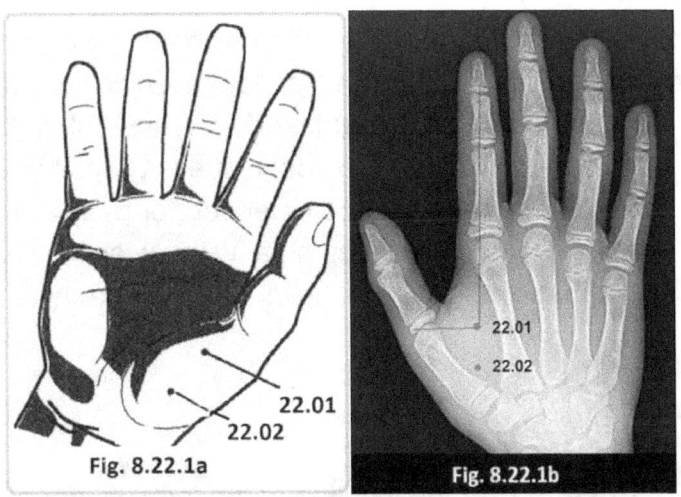

Fig. 8.22.1a   Fig. 8.22.1b

Needling Technique: Insert one cun deep. Typically used in conjunction with 22.02.
Indications: Back pain, pneumonia (particularly effective), common cold, cough, and childhood asthma.

22.02

Location: Located between the first and second metacarpal bones, two cun from the skin fold. With the fingers closed together, extend the C-line of the index finger to the palmar surface and draw a horizontal line from the thumb's proximal knuckle. Point 22.01 is at the intersection; 22.02 is located one cun obliquely below 22.01 on the C-

line.
Needling Technique: Insert one cun deep. Used with 22.01.
Indications: Back, shoulder, neck, and chest pain; fever, palpitations, knee pain, hemiplegia, and respiratory disorders, including pneumonia.

22.03

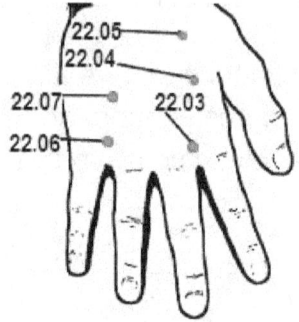

Fig. 8.22.2 03, 06, 07

Location: On the dorsum of the hand, 0.5 cun proximal to the metacarpophalangeal joint of the index and middle fingers.
Needling Technique: Insert 0.3–0.5 cun deep.
Indications: Sciatica; lumbar, back, shoulder, and neck pain; wrist sprain (radial side); red eyes (combine with 11.17), conjunctivitis, and eye itching.

22.04

Location: On the dorsum of the hand, in the depression 0.5 cun from the index-thumb joint or between the first and second metacarpal bones. Lock fingers in a grip to locate.

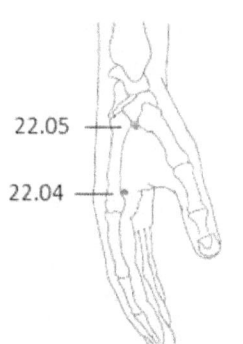

Needling Technique: Insert 0.5–1 cun along the second metacarpal bone. This technique is typically used with 22.05. An injection needle is recommended for paediatric asthma, high fever, and acute pneumonia, with excellent results.
Indications: Sciatica, childhood asthma, high fever (very effective).

22.05

Fig. 8.22.3 04, 05

Location: At the junction of the index finger and thumb, between the 1st and 2nd metacarpal bones, 1.2 cun proximal to 22.04 and directly opposite 22.02. Close to LI 4. Lock fingers in a grip to locate.
Needling Technique: Insert two cun deep.
Indications: Effective for sciatica, lower back pain, chest trauma, knee and foot disorders, shoulder and groin pain, dysuria, hemiparesis, irregular menstruation, amenorrhoea, difficult labour, tinnitus, migraine, and chronic cough. Combine with 22.04, GB 31, 11.18, or DT.04 for hemiplegia.

22.06

Location: Between the metacarpals of the ring and little fingers, 0.5 cun proximal to the metacarpophalangeal joint. Lock fingers in a grip to locate.

Needling Technique: Insert 0.3–0.5 cun deep.

Indications: Pain in the lower back, spine, shoulder, neck, lateral malleolus, and generalised body aches; hypertension, tinnitus, dizziness, and astigmatism. Commonly paired with 22.07 in cases of fatigue.

22.07

Location: Between the 4th and 5th metacarpals on the dorsum, 1.5 cun proximal to the metacarpophalangeal joint and one cun posterior to 22.04. Lock fingers in a grip to locate.

Needling Technique: Insert 0.3–0.5 cun deep.

Indications: Often used with 22.06 for acute lumbar sprain, waist pain, biliary colic, renal colic, and toothache.

22.08

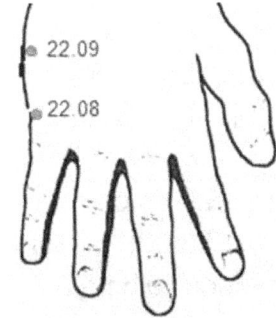

22.09

22.08

Fig. 8.22.4 08, 09

Location: Lateral side of the 5th metacarpal bone on the dorsum, 2.5 cun distal to the wrist crease and 0.5 cun posterior to SI 3.

Needling Technique: Insert 0.5 cun deep.

Indications: Headache, sciatica, bilateral lumbar heaviness and pain, and discomfort in the popliteal fossa.

22.09

Location: Dorsal aspect of the lateral 5th metacarpal bone, 1.5 cun distal to the wrist crease and one cun posterior to 22.08.

Needling Technique: Insert 0.5 cun deep.

Indications: Epistaxis, dental and ocular pain, tinnitus, lumbar pain.

-Modern Acupuncture-

8.3 Tung Points on Lower Arm – 33.xx

Tung acupuncture points on the forearm are grouped under the 33.xx series. According to the mirror image theory in Tung acupuncture, the forearm corresponds to the opposite forearm, the lower leg, the lower abdomen (especially the pelvic organs), the lower back, and the lower chest. Therefore, points on the forearm help treat disorders in these regions. The forearm contains 16 Tung points.

33.01

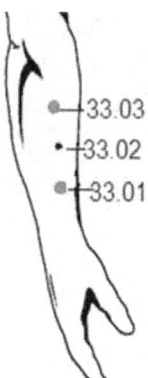

Fig. 8.33.1

Location: Two cuns are proximal to the wrist crease on the radial side of the forearm, along the line between LI 5 and LI 11.
Needling Technique: Insert the needle obliquely distally toward LI 5 to a depth of 0.2–0.5 cun.
Indications: Irregular menstruation, leukorrhea, prolapsed rectum, and haemorrhoidal pain.

33.03

Location: Situated on the radial side of the forearm, halfway between LI 5 and LI 11 (6 cun from the wrist crease), two cun posterior to 33.02 and four cun posterior to 33.01.
Needling Technique: Insert obliquely distally toward LI 5 to a depth of 0.2–0.5 cun, with the patient supine. This technique is commonly used with 33.01 and 33.02.
Indications: Irregular menstruation, leukorrhea, prolapsed rectum, haemorrhoid pain, and abdominal bloating.

33.04

Location: Three cun proximal to the wrist crease on the dorsal midline of the forearm, in the depression between the radius and ulna. It corresponds anatomically with SJ 6.
Needling Technique: Insert 0.3–0.5 cun deep.
Indications: Acute lumbar sprain.

33.05

Location: Two cun proximal to 33.04, with the palm placed on the chest.
Needling Technique: Insert 0.5–1 cun deep.
Indications: Chest pain, stuffiness, distension, and hand cramps.

33.06

Location: One and a half cun proximal to 33.05 (i.e., two cun from 33.05), with the palm on the chest.
Needling Technique: Insert 0.5–1 cun deep.
Indications: Chest distension, pain or cramps in the forearm and hand, and sciatica radiating along the lateral thigh.

33.07

Location: Two cun proximal to 33.06, on the muscle prominence with the palm placed on the chest.
Needling Technique: Insert 0.5–1 cun deep.
Indications: Cough, asthma, common cold, rhinitis, sciatica, leg pain, and lower back pain.

33.08

Location: On the lateral side of the ulna, 6.5 cun proximal to the lateral side of the pisiform bone, 0.5 cun lateral to 33.06.
Needling Technique: Insert 0.3–0.5 cun deep.
Indications: Sciatica, abdominal pain, distension of the leg, numbness, and pain in the feet.

33.09

Location: One and a half cun proximal to 33.08 (eight cun from the pisiform bone), on the lateral side of the ulna.
Needling Technique: Insert 0.5–0.8 cun deep.
Indications: Sciatica, calf pain, abdominal pain, leg distension, and foot numbness or pain.

33.11

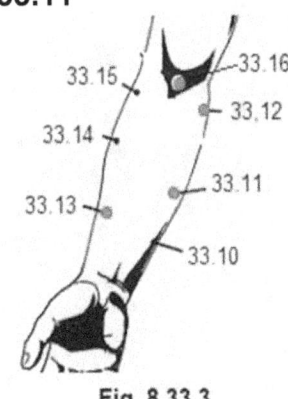

Fig. 8.33.3

Location: On the ulnar side, six cun proximal to the pisiform bone, with the palm on the chest.
Needling Technique: When used in Dao Ma style for hepatitis, insert 0.3–0.5 cun deep on the left side.
Indications: Hepatitis (used with points 88.12, 88.13, 88.14, and 33.10).

33.12

Location: In the depression on the medial side of the inferior ulna, five cun distal to the elbow, near SI 8, with the palm on the chest.

Needling Technique: Insert 0.3–0.5 cun deep on the left side for hepatitis in Dao Ma technique.

Indications: Sciatica involving the medial thigh or groin, pain of the sacrum and tailbone, knee pain, palpitations, chest tightness, and vomiting.

33.13

Location: On the medial side of the radius, four cun proximal to the wrist crease on the ventral forearm, near the styloid process.

Needling Technique: Insert 0.5 cun deep for asthma and pain syndromes; insert one cun deep for palpitations.

Indications: Asthma, pain of the palm, fingers, shoulder, arm, and back; palpitations.

33.16

Location: In the cubital crease, the biceps brachii tendon's radial side corresponds to LU 5.

Needling Technique: Insert 0.3–0.5 cun deep.

Indications: Elbow inflammation, frozen shoulder, chest pain, congestion, asthma, tonsillitis, pneumonia, laryngitis, and palpitations.

-Dr. Pardeshi Acupuncture-

8.4 Tung Points on Upper Arm – 44.xx

Tung acupuncture points on the upper arm are grouped under the 44.xx series. According to holographic principles, these points treat conditions of the opposite arm, upper abdomen, chest, shoulder, upper back, and knee. The upper arm contains **17 (10)** points.

44.06

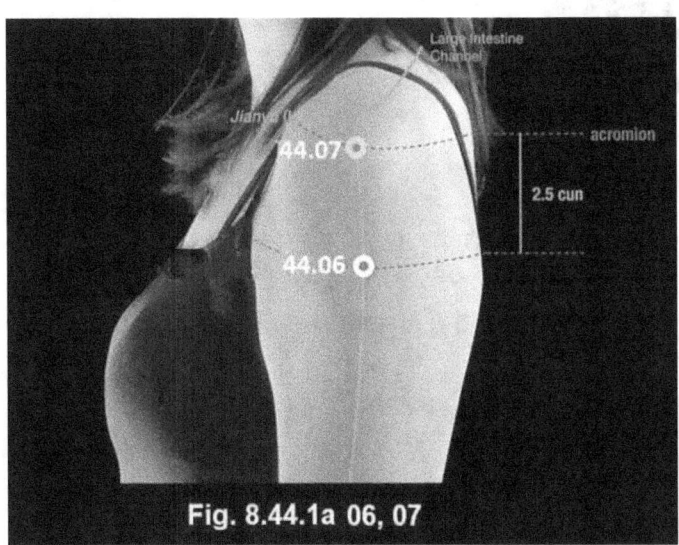

Fig. 8.44.1a 06, 07

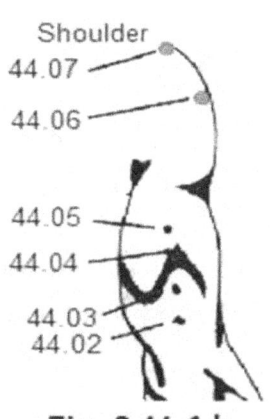

Fig. 8.44. 1 b

Location: Located on the lateral side of the humerus, 2.5 cun inferior to the acromion joint.
Needling Technique: Insert 0.5–1 cun deep.
Indications: Knee pain (most effective), dermatosis (especially in the neck region), shoulder pain, polio, hemiplegia, palpitations, arteriosclerosis, and nosebleeds.

44.11

Location: Located one cun anterior and superior to point 44.06.
Needling Technique: Insert 0.3–0.5 cun deep.
Indications: Vaginitis, vaginal pain, leukorrhea, and polio. Particularly effective for gynaecological conditions. Combined with 44.06, it also addresses weakness and distending calf pain.

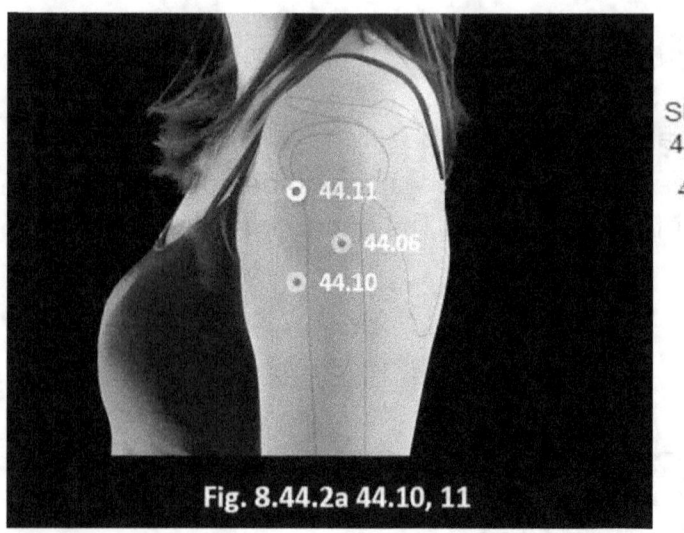

Fig. 8.44.2a 44.10, 11

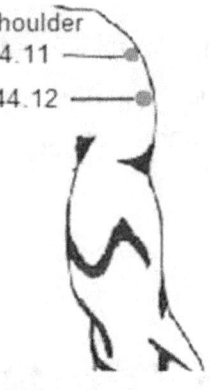

Fig. 8.44.2 b

44.16

Location: Located on the posterior upper arm, one cun posterior to 44.06.
Needling Technique: Insert 0.6–1.5 cun deep.
Indications: Polio, sciatica, arm pain, hypertension, and distended calf pain. Bloodletting is used for cirrhosis and hepatitis. This point is primary in treating polio and lower extremity weakness, often combined with 44.15, 44.11, and 44.12.

44.17

Location: Located on the posterior upper arm, two cun obliquely posterior and inferior to 44.07.
Needling Technique: Insert 0.3–0.5 cun deep.
Indications: Nephritis, kidney stones, lower back pain, leg aches, general debility, and pain of the arm, wrist, and hand dorsum.

8.5 Tung Points on Sole – 55.xx

The Tung acupuncture points of the 55.xx series are located on the sole. Holographically, the sole corresponds to the opposite sole, palm, head, face, lower abdomen, and pelvis. Needling these points can treat disorders in these regions. The plantar surface of the foot has six points that tend to be relatively painful when needled.

55.01

Location: At the centre of the distal crease on the plantar side of the second toe.
Needling Technique: Insert 0.3–0.5 cun deep. Bleeding is performed using an injection needle.
Indications: Liver disease, difficult labour, retained placenta, hernia, irregular menstruation, and emergency bloodletting for angina pectoris.

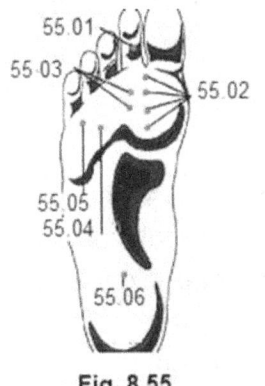

Fig. 8.55

55.02

Location: Comprises a group of four points situated between the first and second metatarsal bones on the plantar surface. The first point is 0.5 cun posterior to the joint of the big toe and second toe; the following three points are located successively 0.5 cun and then 0.8 cun posterior to each other.
Needling Technique: Insert 0.5–1 cun deep.
Indications: Eye pain, eyelid inflammation, aching of the nasal bone. These points lie opposite LV 2 and LV 3 and are primarily used for diseases of the eyes and eyebrows.

55.03

Location: Composed of two points located between the second and third metatarsal bones on the plantar surface. The first is one cun posterior to the second toe joint, and the second is 0.5 cun behind the first.
Needling Technique: Insert 0.5–1 cun deep.
Indications: Weakness of the fingers and pain in the arms.

55.06

Location: Located at the centre of the anterior edge of the heel.
Needling Technique: Insert up to a maximum of 0.5 cun. Deeper needling is contraindicated as it may cause irritability.
Indications: Plantar fasciitis, headache, nasal congestion, and nosebleeds.

8.6 Tung Points on Dorsum of Foot – 66.xx

Tung acupuncture points on the dorsum of the foot are grouped under the 66.xx series. This area is significant in treating a wide range of disorders. According to holographic mapping, the foot corresponds to the opposite foot, hand, fingers, head, face, neck, pelvic organs, and lower abdomen. The dorsal surface of the foot has 15 Tung points.

66.01

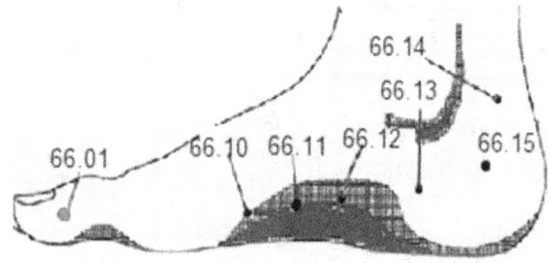

Fig. 8.66.1

Location: Located at the centre of the medial side of the big toe, in the red and white skin area near the base of the toenail.
Needling Technique: Insert 0.1–0.3 cun deep.
Indications: Conjunctivitis, hernia, thumb and index finger pain, and vaginitis.

66.02

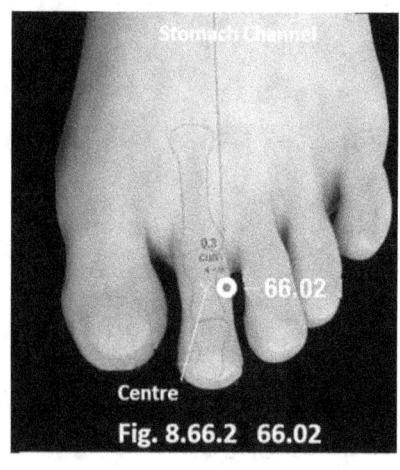

Fig. 8.66.2 66.02

Location: Located 0.3 cun lateral to the centre of the middle segment of the second toe on the dorsal side.
Needling Technique: Insert 0.2–0.4 cun deep, closely along the phalanx to reduce pain.
Indications: Leukorrhea, irregular menstruation, dysmenorrhoea, endometritis, and tubal obstruction.

66.03

Location: Located on the dorsal surface between the first and second metatarsal bones, 0.5 cun from the metatarsophalangeal joints.
Needling Technique: Insert 0.5–1 cun deep.
Indications: Palpitations, dizziness, retained placenta, chin pain, difficulty in opening the mouth, coma, endometritis, and uterine fibroids.

66.04

Location: Located in the depression one cun posterior to 66.03, between the first and second metatarsal bones. Fig. 8.66.3
Needling Technique: Insert 0.5–1.5 cun deep.
Indications: Difficult labour, liver and stomach diseases, pain in hands and feet,

endometritis, uterine fibroids, headache, dizziness, sore throat, deviation of mouth and eye, vaginal pain, and hernia.

66.06

Location: Located in the depression anterior to the junction of the third and fourth metatarsal bones, 1.5 cun from the metatarsophalangeal joints and one cun proximal to 66.07.
Needling Technique: Insert 1–1.5 cun deep.

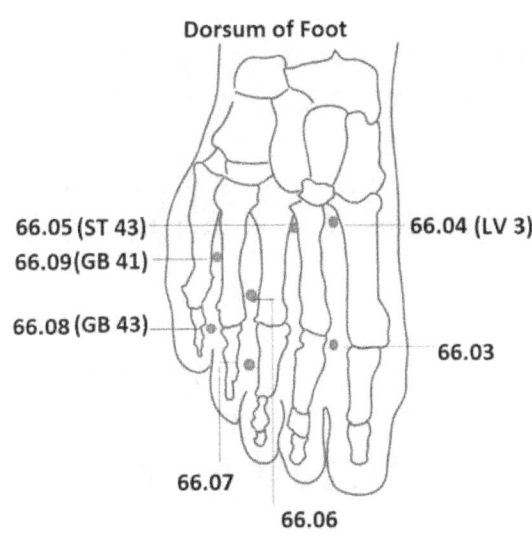

Dorsum of Foot

66.05 (ST 43)
66.09 (GB 41)

66.08 (GB 43)

66.04 (LV 3)

66.03

66.07

66.06

Fig. 8.66.3 03 - 09

Indications: Joint stiffness or pain in the middle and ring fingers, stiff neck, shoulder pain, trigeminal neuralgia, earache, spleen enlargement, indigestion, liver disease, fatigue, and gall bladder disease. Often used in conjunction with 66.07 in the Dao Ma technique.

66.07

Location: Located between the third and fourth metatarsal bones, 0.5 cun proximal to the metatarsophalangeal joint and one cun distal to 66.06.
Needling Technique: Insert 0.5–1 cun deep.
Indications: Splenomegaly, indigestion, liver disease, fatigue, gallbladder disease, and polio.

66.09

Location: Located one cun proximal to 66.08 between the fourth and fifth metatarsal bones.
Needling Technique: Insert 0.5–1 cun deep.
Indications: Neuralgia of the neck and arm, lower back pain, calf tightness, limb oedema, abdominal distension, uterine disorders, tinnitus, and itchy eyes.

8.7 Tung Points on Leg – 77.xx

Tung acupuncture points on the leg are grouped under the 77.xx series. There are **28 points** on the lower leg. According to holographic principles, the legs, forearms, lower abdomen, chest, neck, and head correspond to each other. Therefore, points on the leg help treat conditions involving the head, face, neck, shoulder, lower abdomen, lower back, and other areas.

77.01

Location: Located in the centre of the Achilles tendon, 3.5 cun superior to the heel.
Needling Technique: Insert 0.5–0.8 cun deep into the tendon, enough to touch the bone.

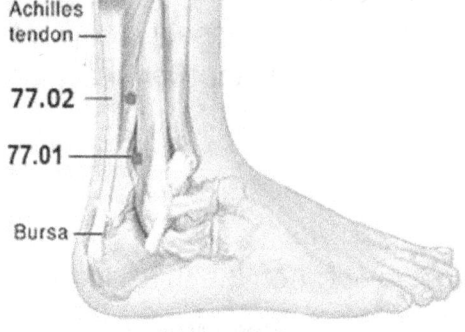

Fig. 8.77.1

Indications: Spinal, lumbar, and neck pain from sprain, stomach spasms, and leg cramps.

77.02

Location: Located two cun superior to 77.01 in the centre of the tendon.
Needling Technique: Insert two cun deep into the tendon.
Indications: Spinal, lumbar, and neck pain, abdominal spasms, and leg cramps. Used with 77.01.

77.03

Location: Located two cun above 77.02 in the centre of the tendon.
Needling Technique: Insert 0.5–1 cun deep.

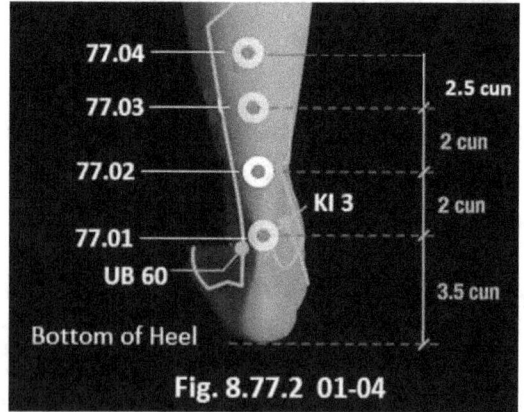

Fig. 8.77.2 01-04

Indications: Shoulder and back pain, lower back pain, sciatica, and leg muscle spasms.

77.04

Location: Located 2.5 cun superior to 77.03.
Needling Technique: Insert 1–2 cun deep.
Indications: Backache, nosebleed, and haemorrhoids due to bleeding the vessels around the point.

77.05

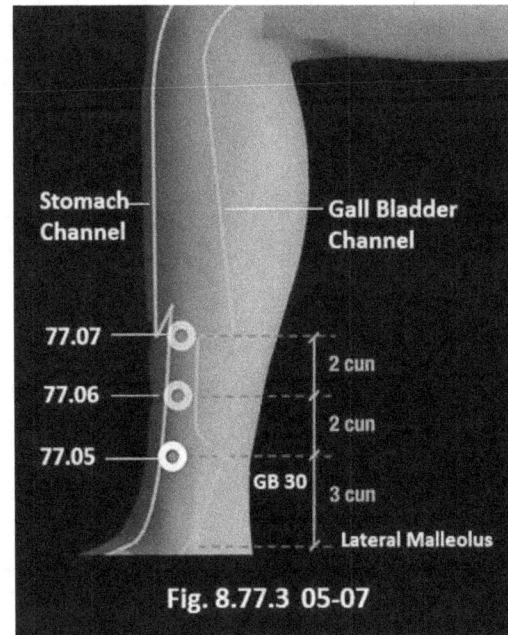

Stomach Channel
Gall Bladder Channel
77.07
77.06
77.05
2 cun
2 cun
GB 30
3 cun
Lateral Malleolus

Fig. 8.77.3 05-07

Location: Located three cun superior to the lateral malleolus and one cun anterior to the fibula.
Needling Technique: Insert 1–2 cun deep.
Indications: Hyperthyroidism, exophthalmos, tonsillitis, facial deviation, migraine, lumps, and liver disease.

77.06

Location: Located two cun superior to 77.05.
Needling Technique: Insert 1–2 cun deep.
Indications: Hyperthyroidism, exophthalmos, tonsillitis, facial deviation, migraine, and liver disease.

77.07
Location: Located two cun directly superior to 77.06.
Needling Technique: Insert 1–2 cun deep.
Indications: Trigeminal neuralgia, pain in the shoulder, arm, and wrist, migraine, hyperthyroidism, exophthalmos, tonsillitis, facial deviation, and liver disease.

77.08

Location: Three cuns inferior to ST 35 are located on the lateral tibia in the depression between the anterior tibial muscle and the toe extensor.
Needling Technique: Insert 2–3 cun deep.
Indications: Asthma, toothache, palpitations, epigastric pain, and gastrointestinal diseases.

77.09

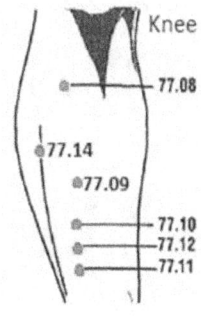

Knee
77.08
77.14
77.09
77.10
77.12
77.11

Fig. 8.77.4

Location: Located 4.5 cun inferior to 77.08.
Needling Technique: Insert 2–3 cun deep or perform bloodletting for acute conditions.
Indications: Shoulder, elbow, and index finger pain, epigastric pain, asthma, suffocation, emphysema, and eye disorders.

77.10
Location: Located 2.5 cun inferior to 77.09.

Needling Technique: Bleed with an injection needle.
Indications: Asthma, eye disorders, acute epigastric pain. Used with 77.09.

77.11

Location: Located 2.5 cun distal to 77.10.
Needling Technique: Insert 1–2 cun deep.
Indications: Gastroenteritis, abdominal distension, oedema, and teeth grinding. Used with 77.12.

77.12

Location: Located 1.5 cun superior to 77.11.
Needling Technique: Insert 0.5–1 cun deep.
Indications: Gastroenteritis, abdominal distension, epigastric pain, oedema, and teeth grinding.

77.13

Location: Located 1.2 cun medial to 77.09 on the medial border of the tibia.
Needling Technique: Insert 1.5–2 cun deep.
Indications: Knee pain and gastroenteritis.

77.14

Location: Located 1.5 cun lateral to 77.09.
Needling Technique: Insert 1–1.5 cun deep or bleed with an injection needle.

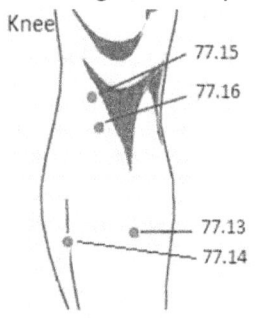

Fig. 8.77.5

Indications: Sciatica, shoulder and arm pain, earache, toothache, headache, migraine, intercostal neuralgia, facial paralysis, acute gastroenteritis, chest pain, asthma, rhinitis, and hypertension.

77.15

Location: Located on the lower lateral ridge of the patella.
Needling Technique: Bleed the point for quick effect.
Indications: Mouth disorders and knee pain.

77.16

Location: One cun inferior to the lower lateral ridge of the patella is located.
Needling Technique: Bleed the point for effect.
Indications: Lip pain and leukoderma around oral or genital areas.

77.17

Location: Located in the depression of the medial condyle of the tibia, 2.5 cun inferior to the knee joint.
Needling Technique: Insert 0.5–1 cun deep.
Indications: Acidity, GERD, diabetes, nephritis, hypertension, dizziness, and headache.

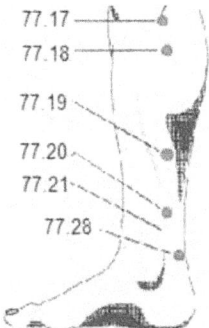

Fig. 8.77.6

77.18

Location: Located 1.5 cun inferior to 77.17 on the medial tibia.
Needling Technique: Insert 1–2 cun deep.
Indications: Shoulder periarthritis, frontal and orbital headache, nasal pain, neuropathy, GERD, epilepsy, dizziness, and diabetes. Use with 77.17.

77.19

Location: Located on the medial tibia, seven cun superior to the medial malleolus.
Needling Technique: Insert 1–1.8 cun at a 45° angle.
Indications: Nephritis, oedema, diabetes, impotence, premature and nocturnal ejaculation, difficult urination, fibroids, irregular menstruation, and lower back pain. Use with 77.18.

77.21

Location: Located on the posterior border of the medial tibia, three cun superior to the medial malleolus.
Needling Technique: Insert 0.5–1 cun deep.
Indications: Painful urination, impotence, premature ejaculation, lumbar and neck pain, dizziness, hand numbness, diabetes, nephritis, and neurasthenia.

77.22

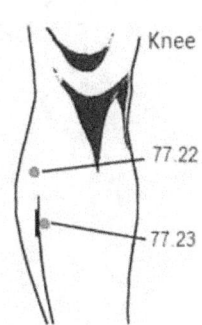

Fig. 8.77.7

Location: Located 1.5 cun lateral to 77.08.
Needling Technique: Insert 0.5–1 cun deep.
Indications: Toothache, facial paralysis, migraine, and trigeminal neuralgia. Use with 77.23.

77.23

Location: Located two cun inferior to 77.22.
Needling Technique: Insert 0.5–1 cun deep.

Indications: Toothache, facial paralysis, migraine, and trigeminal neuralgia. Use with 77.22.

77.24

Location: Located 0.5 cun lateral and two cun inferior to 77.27.
Needling Technique: Insert 1–2 cun deep.
Indications: Acute enteritis, shoulder and back pain, pharyngitis, tonsillitis, and thyroid enlargement.

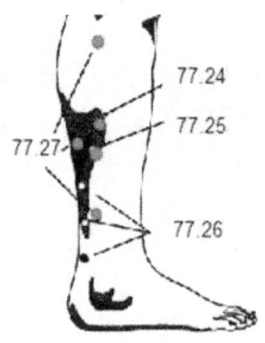

Fig. 8.77.8

77.25

Location: Locate two cuns that are directly inferior to 77.24.
Needling Technique: Insert 1–2 cun deep.
Indications: Shoulder and back pain, acute enteritis, pharyngitis, and thyroid enlargement.

77.27

Location: A group of three points on the line connecting the head of the fibula and the lateral malleolus.
Needling Technique: Insert 1–1.5 cun deep.
Indications: Tonsillitis, pharyngitis, and pain in the shoulder and arm.

8.8 Tung Points on Thigh – 88.xx

Tung acupuncture points on the thigh are grouped under the 88.xx series. There are 32 points on the thigh. According to holographic principles, the thigh corresponds to the opposite thigh, the upper arms, the chest, and the abdomen. The thigh is vital for treating muscular and cutaneous disorders, including lipomas.

88.01

Location: Located on the anterior midline of the femur, five cun superior to the knee crease.
Needling Technique: Insert 0.3–0.5 cun deep.
Indications: Gastrointestinal diseases, limb pain, dizziness, vertigo, and palpitations. It is commonly used with 88.02 and 88.03.

88.02

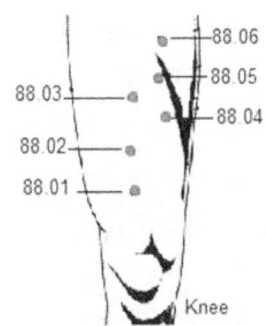

Fig. 8.88.1

Location: Located two cun superior to 88.01.
Needling Technique: Insert 0.5–0.8 cun deep.
Indications: Gastrointestinal disease, limb pain, dizziness, vertigo, and palpitations.

88.03

Location: Located four cun superior to 88.01.
Needling Technique: Insert 0.5–1 cun deep.
Indications: General body aches, limb pain, morning sickness, gastrointestinal diseases, dizziness, vertigo, and palpitations.

88.04

Location: Located one cun medial and superior to 88.02.
Needling Technique: Insert 1–2.5 cun deep.
Indications: Irregular menstruation, vaginal itching, endometritis, fibroids of the uterus, and abdominal pain.

88.05

Location: Located 2.5 cun above 88.04.
Needling Technique: Insert 1.5–2.5 cun deep.
Indications: Irregular menstruation, vaginal itching, endometritis, fibroids, intestinal pain, and gastric bleeding.

88.06

Location: Located 2.5 cun above 88.05.
Needling Technique: Insert 1.5–2.5 cun deep.
Indications: Irregular menstruation, vaginal itching, endometritis, fibroids, intestinal pain, and gastric bleeding. Commonly used with 88.04 and 88.05.

88.09

Location: Located on the superior and medial border of the patella.
Needling Technique: Insert 0.3–0.5 cun deep.
Indications: Impotence, premature ejaculation, nephritis, diabetes, dizziness, lower back pain, dysmenorrhoea, and leucorrhoea.

88.10

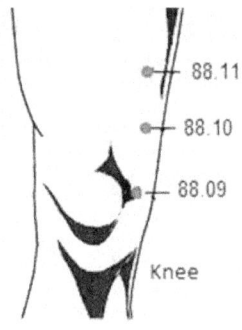

Fig. 8.88.2

Location: Located two cun superior to 88.09.
Needling Technique: Insert 0.5–1 cun deep.
Indications: Impotence, premature ejaculation, nephritis, diabetes, dizziness, lower back pain, dysmenorrhoea, and leucorrhoea.

88.11

Location: Locate four cuns superior to the medial-superior corner of the patella.
Needling Technique: Insert 0.5–1 cun deep.

Indications: Impotence, premature ejaculation, nephritis, diabetes, dizziness, lower back pain, dysmenorrhoea, and leucorrhoea.

88.12

Location: Located in the centre of the medial thigh.

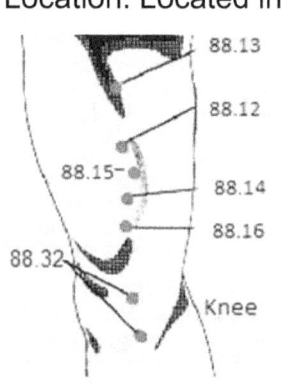

Fig. 8.88.3

Needling Technique: Insert 1.5–2.5 cun deep.
Indications: Cirrhosis, hepatitis, lower back soreness, eye pain, and indigestion.**88.13**
Location: Located three cun above 88.12.
Needling Technique: Insert 1.5–2.5 cun deep.
Indications: Cirrhosis, hepatitis, fatigue, lower back soreness, eye pain, indigestion, chorea, insomnia, vertigo, and Parkinson's disease.

88.14

Location: Located three cun inferior to 88.12.
Needling Technique: Insert 1.5–2 cun deep.
Indications: Jaundice and the same conditions as 88.12. Commonly used with 88.12 and 88.13.

88.15
Location: Located 1.5 cun superior to 88.14.
Needling Technique: Insert 1.5–2 cun deep.
Indications: Dizziness, back pain, and as an adjunct in jaundice and cholecystitis.

88.17

Location: Located three cun anterior to the point touched by the middle fingertips when standing erect with arms at the side.
Needling Technique: Insert 0.8–2.5 cun deep.
Indications: Pain of the hypochondrium, back, sciatica, chest, breast, sprains, rhinitis, pneumonia, asthma, deafness, tinnitus, facial paralysis, red eyes, hemiplegia, and psoriasis.

88.18

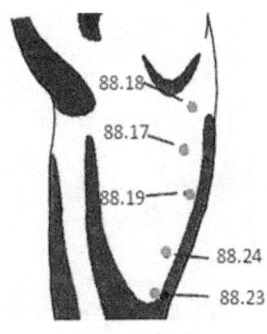

Fig. 8.88.4

Location: Located two cun superior to 88.17.
Needling Technique: Insert 0.8–2.5 cun deep.
Indications: Same as 88.17, with additional application for dermatoses.

88.19

Location: Located two cun inferior to 88.17.
Needling Technique: Insert 0.8–2.5 cun deep.
Indications: The same as 88.17. Points 88.17, 88.18, and 88.19 are collectively known as the "Four Horses" and are especially effective for systemic conditions and lipoma.

88.20

Location: Located 2.5 cun superior to the knee joint along the median line of the lateral thigh.
Needling Technique: Insert 0.3–0.5 cun deep.
Indications: Facial paralysis, facial tics, mouth and eye deviation, and Bell's palsy.

88.21

Location: Located two cun superior to 88.20.
Needling Technique: Insert 0.3–0.8 cun deep.
Indications: Facial paralysis, facial tics, and mouth-eye deviation.

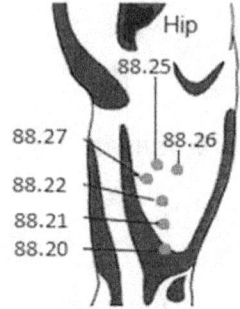

Fig. 8.88.5

88.22

Location: Located two cun superior to 88.21.
Needling Technique: Insert 0.5–1 cun deep.
Indications: Facial paralysis, tics, mouth-eye deviation, tinnitus, and hearing loss. Used in conjunction with 88.20 and 88.21, these are referred to as "Three Quan Points."

88.23

Location: Located one cun superior to the outer edge of the patella.
Needling Technique: Insert 0.3–0.5 cun deep.
Indications: Same as 88.22.

88.24

Location: Located 1.5 cun superior to 88.23.
Needling Technique: Insert 0.5–1 cun deep.
Indications: Epilepsy, headache, and sensitive skin.

88.25

Location: Located in the centre of the lateral thigh.
Needling Technique: Insert 1–2 cun deep.
Indications: Pain in the back, neck, and temples, migraine, limb numbness, hemiplegia, facial paralysis, dizziness, tinnitus, and eye distension.

88.26

Location: Located 1.5 cun anterior to 88.25.
Needling Technique: Insert 0.8–1.5 cun deep.
Indications: Anal pain, eye pain, and abdominal distension.

8.10 Tung Points on Head and Face – 1010.xx

The Tung acupuncture points on the head and face are grouped under the 1010.xx series. There are **25 points** in this region. These points correspond to the spine, lower abdomen, foot, and hand. Being closest to the brain, eyes, ears, and nose, the 1010. The xx series is particularly effective in treating nervous system disorders, as well as conditions affecting the head, spine, and lower abdomen.

Needling of Scalp Points

Some points in this series are located on the scalp. Chapter 9 covers detailed needling procedures. You should review those techniques before needling the scalp points of the 1010.xx series.

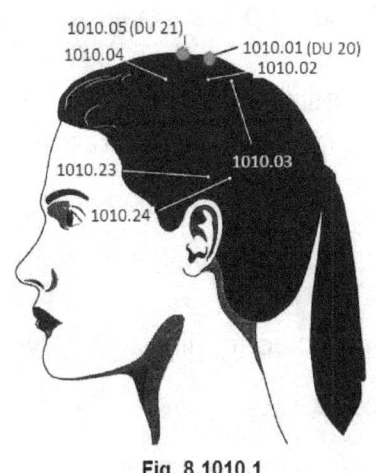

Fig. 8.1010.1

1010.01

Location: Located at the top centre of the head at the intersection of the midline and the line connecting the apices of both ears.
Indications: Tremors of limbs, deviation of mouth and eye, hemiplegia (when used with 22.05 and 22.04), nervous system disorders, and aphasia. Strong sedative effect.

1010.05

Location: Located 1.5 cun anterior to 1010.01.
Indications: Dizziness, distension in the head, and neurasthenia.

1010.06

Location: Located 1.5 cun posterior to 1010.01.
Indications: Spinal pain, particularly in the T12–L2 and coccygeal regions. Effective in aphasia due to paralysis. Commonly used with 1010.01.

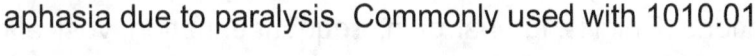

1010.07

Location: Located 0.8 cun above the posterior hairline.
Needling Technique: Bleeding with an 18-gauge injection needle is most effective, especially in children.
Indications: Neck pain, nausea, and vomiting. Strong sedative effect.

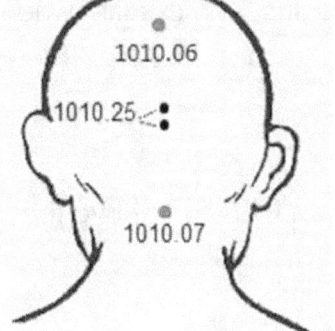

Fig. 8.1010.2

1010.08

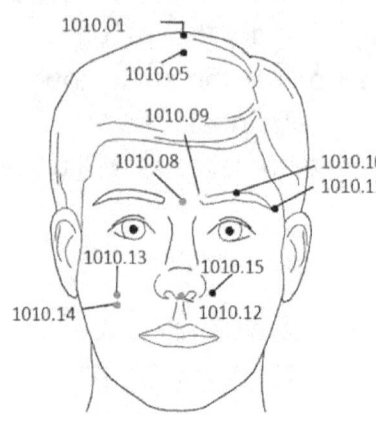

Fig. 8.1010.3

Location: Located 0.3 cun above the midpoint between the eyebrows.

Needling Technique: Insert the needle one cun above this point, subcutaneously toward the nose. This technique is most effective when combined with 1010.01.

Indications: Mental disorders, limb tremors, leg weakness, paralysis, insomnia, frontal headache, and trigeminal neuralgia.

1010.12

Location: Located at the tip of the nose, in the depression between the two small cartilages.

Needling Technique: Insert 0.1–0.2 cun deep without injuring cartilage.

Indications: Allergic rhinitis, nasal hypertrophy, nasal obstruction, psychosis, decreased mental function. Has a strong effect on resuscitation and mental clarity.

1010.13

Location: Located 1.5 cun below the lower border of the zygomatic bone, directly below the outer canthus.

Needling Technique: Insert 0.1–0.3 cun deep.

Indications: Rhinitis, chest pain on respiration, nephritis, lumbar sprain, and kidney stones.

1010.14

Location: Located 0.5 cun below the 1010.13 point.

Needling Technique: Insert 0.1–0.3 cun deep.

Indications: Rhinitis, lumbar pain, frequent urination, vesical calculus, and cystitis (when combined with 1010.13).

1010.16

Location: Located 1.5 cun lateral to the midpoint of the philtrum and 1.5 cun above the corner of the mouth.

Needling Technique: Insert 0.1–0.3 cun deep.

Indications: Urethritis (when combined with 1010.14).

1010.17

Location: Located 0.5 cun lateral to the corner of the mouth.
Indications: Facial paralysis and other related functions.

1010.18

Location: Located one cun superior and lateral to 1010.13.
Needling Technique: Insert 0.1–0.3 cun deep.
Indications: Gallbladder disorders.

1010.19

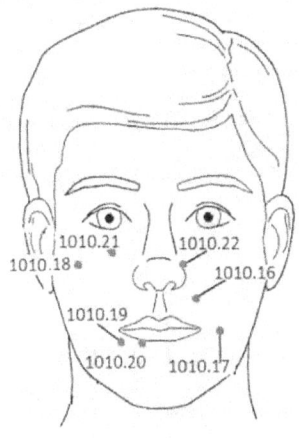

Fig. 8.1010.4

Location: Located 0.5 cun below the corner of the mouth.
Needling Technique: Insert obliquely towards the lateral side to a depth of 0.1–0.5 cun.
Indications: Rheumatism, lower back pain, acute lumbar sprain, and chest pain on breathing.

1010.20

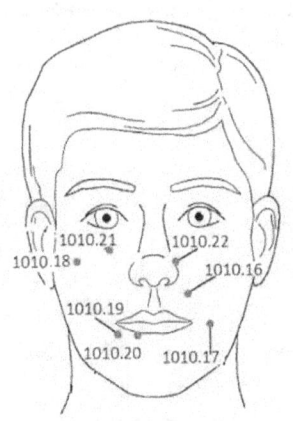

Fig. 8.1010.4

Location: Located 0.5 cun medial to 1010.19.
Needling Technique: Insert obliquely towards the lateral side to a depth of 0.1–0.5 cun.
Indications: Cold, cough, respiratory infections, asthma, nausea, vomiting, rheumatism, lumbar pain, and chest discomfort.

1010.21

Location: Located in the depression below the zygomatic bone, along a vertical line from the eye centre.
Needling Technique: Insert 0.1–0.3 cun deep.
Indications: Sciatica, pain in the shoulder, arm, limbs, knees, cheek, and maxillary region.

8.11 Tung Points on Dorsal Trunk – DT.xx

Tung acupuncture points located on the dorsal aspect of the neck and trunk are categorised under the **DT.xx** series. Over 160 Tung points are on the trunk's dorsal and ventral surfaces. Each dorsal point typically comprises a group of points arranged bilaterally on the neck or trunk, often corresponding to specific spinal vertebral levels and the functions of particular internal organs.

DT.03

Location: This group consists of seven points situated on and around the posterior neck:

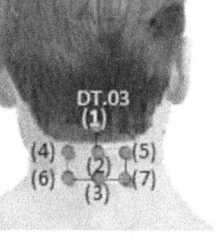

Fig. 8.DT.03

DT.03-1: 0.8 cun above the posterior hairline (same as 1010.07).

DT.03-2: 1 cun below DT.03-1.

DT.03-3: 2 cun below DT.03-1.

DT.03-4 & DT.03-5: 0.8 cun lateral to DT.03-2 on the left and right sides.

DT.03-6 & DT.03-7: 1 cun below DT.03-4 and DT.03-5, respectively.

Needling Technique: These points are primarily treated by **bloodletting using an injection needle**. To perform bleeding, gently pinch the skin between the thumb and index finger and puncture the site accurately with the needle. DT.03-1 to DT.03-3 are the primary points, while DT.03-4 to DT.03-7 are **auxiliary points**.

Indications: Nausea and vomiting, common cold with headache, high fever.

DT.04

Location:
Points of DT.04 are arranged in **five vertical lines** along the back:

- **1st Line**: Midline – 10 points extending from the level of the 2nd thoracic **vertebra (T2)** to the 12th thoracic vertebra (T12), each point positioned just below the spinous process.
- **2nd Line**: Four finger-breadths are lateral to the midline on each side, beginning at the level of T2 and descending vertically.

235

- **3rd Line**: Situated four finger-breadths lateral to the 2nd line on each side, starting at the level of T3 and extending downward.
  Each point along these lines is spaced one cun apart.

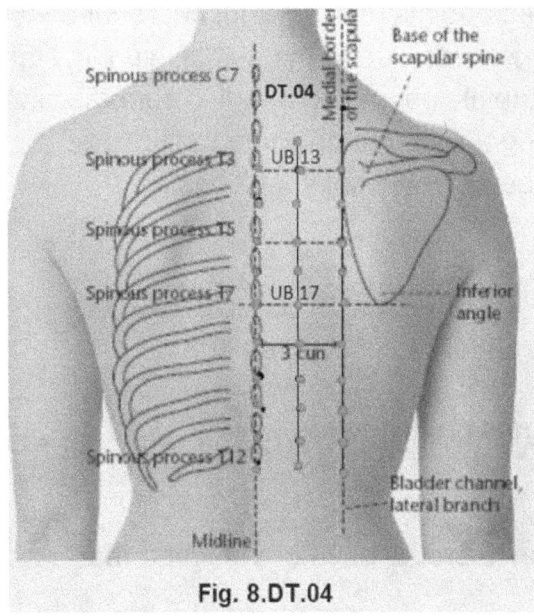

Fig. 8.DT.04

Needling Technique: Bleed with an injection needle. It is not necessary to treat all points simultaneously for a given condition; point selection should be symptom-specific.

Indications: Hypertension, acute low back pain, abdominal colic, severe cold and fever, chills, headache, sudden dizziness, numbness in hands or feet, hemiplegia, and vomiting.

DT.07

Location:

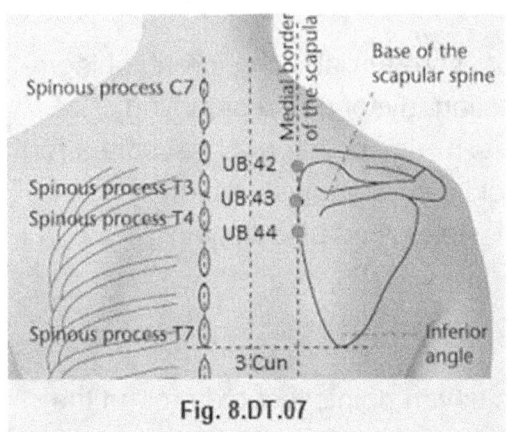

Fig. 8.DT.07

Three pairs of points are lateral to the spinous processes of the 3rd, 4th, and 5th thoracic vertebrae (T3, T4, T5). These points correspond to UB 42, UB 43, and UB 44 and lie within the 3rd, 4th, and 5th intercostal spaces of the shoulder line.

Needling Technique: Bloodletting with an injection needle. Pinch the skin and accurately puncture to let out a few drops of blood.

Indications: **Knee joint pain** – bleeding at these points often provides **instant relief** from knee pain.

8.12 Tung Points on Ventral Trunk – VT.xx

Tung acupuncture points located on the anterior aspect of the neck, chest, and abdomen are grouped under the VT.xx series. These points are powerful but require extreme caution, especially when needling over the chest, due to the risk of injuring vital structures such as the pleura and lungs. All chest points should be needled superficially and horizontally to ensure safety, ideally while lifting a skin fold between the fingers. These points are particularly effective for treating acute and local conditions.

VT.01

Location: This group consists of nine points in the anterior cervical region:

- The 1st point is at the Adam's apple (laryngeal prominence).
- The 2nd point is one cun below the first.
- The 3rd point is two cun below the 2nd.
- The remaining six points are located 1.5 cun lateral to each of the first three (three on each side).
  (Refer to Fig. 8.VT.01, 02, and 04 for visual orientation.)

Needling Technique: These points are pricked superficially using an injection needle for bloodletting. While puncturing, gently lift the skin fold between the fingers to avoid injury to deeper structures.

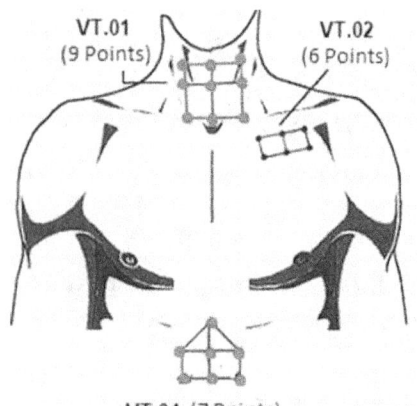

VT.01 (9 Points) VT.02 (6 Points)

VT.04 (7 Points)

Fig. 8.VT.01

Indications: Tonsillitis, sore throat, itchy throat, phlegm-induced throat congestion, dyspnoea resembling asthma, and thyroiditis. These points are best suited for acute throat and thyroid disorders, with rapid symptomatic relief possible using bloodletting.

VT.04

Location: Comprises seven points located around the xiphoid process:

- The 1st point is one cun below the lower border of the xiphoid process.
- The 2nd and 3rd points follow in a straight vertical line, each spaced one cun apart.
- The remaining four points are placed 1.5 cun lateral to each vertical point (two on each side).

- These correspond roughly to standard points: REN 15, REN 14, REN 13 (midline group) and ST 19, ST 20 (lateral group, 0.5 cun medial to the REN line). (Refer to Fig. 8.VT.01 for visual details.)

Needling Technique: Use an injection needle for shallow bloodletting. These points are used locally for acute symptoms, with a careful and superficial approach.

Indications: Local skin furuncles, acute abdominal disorders, palpitations, and gastric-related symptoms due to proximity to the stomach.

VT.05

Location: VT.05 includes twenty-three points distributed around the umbilicus:

The central vertical line includes:

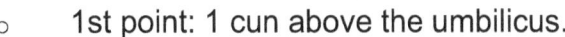

o   1st point: 1 cun above the umbilicus.
o   2nd point: 1 cun above the 1st.
o   Five points below the umbilicus, each spaced by one cun downwards.
- Two parallel vertical lines flank the central line, each containing four points, arranged symmetrically.

Fig. 8.VT.05

Needling Technique: Bloodletting with an injection needle is performed carefully, especially over the abdominal region.

Indications: Gastrointestinal disorders include gastroenteritis, as well as gynaecological conditions such as endometritis, nephritis, renal pain, and pain in the umbilical region.

8.13 Tung Extra Points – A.xx

The A.xx series of Tung acupuncture comprises extra points that do not fall within traditional meridian frameworks but have demonstrated powerful therapeutic effects in clinical practice. These points are primarily located on the hands and limbs, often at phalangeal junctions, and are especially effective for pain management, neurological disorders, and organ-related syndromes. Many are used in combinations with core Tung points for enhanced efficacy.

A.01 (Seven Miles)

Location: A.01 is two cun below point 88.25 on the thigh.

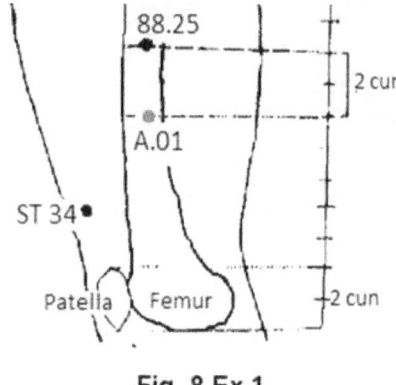

Fig. 8.Ex.1

Needling Technique: Insert the needle 1 to 2 cun (approximately 0.4 to 0.8 inches) deep.

Indications:
Back pain, cervical spondylosis, vertebral disc prolapse, neck stiffness, dizziness, vertigo, arm numbness, leg pain and weakness, cholecystitis, hypochondriac pain. It is particularly effective for pain involving the lateral body. The best results are obtained when combined with 88.25, especially in cases of hemiplegia.

A.02

Location: Located at the junction of the 2nd and 3rd phalanges on the dorsum of the hand when a fist is made.

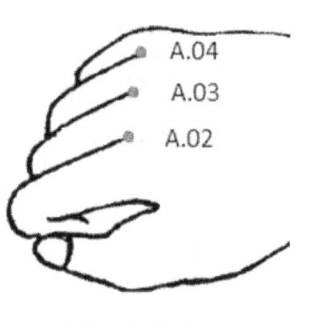

Fig. 8.Ex.2

Needling Technique: Insert 1 to 1.5 cun (approximately 0.4 to 0.6 inches) deep.

Indications:
Shoulder pain, upper and lower back pain, neck stiffness, hypochondriac pain, stomach pain, irregular menstruation, and metrorrhagia.

A.03

Location: Situated at the junction of the 3rd and 4th phalanges on the dorsum of the hand while making a fist. (See Fig. 8.Ex.2)

Needling Technique: Insert 1 to 1.5 cun (approximately 0.4 to 0.6 inches) deep.

Indications:
Knee joint pain, acute lumbar strain, and disorders of the five sense organs.

A.04

Location: Found at the junction of the 4th and 5th phalanges on the dorsum of the hand when a fist is made. (See Fig. 8.Ex.2)

Needling Technique: Insert 1 to 1.5 cun (approximately 0.4 to 0.6 inches) deep.

Indications:
Common cold, headache, shoulder pain, eye disorders (redness, swelling, pain), sore throat, tinnitus, palpitations, urticaria, leg pain, eyelid drooping or heaviness, fatigue, and myasthenia gravis.

A.05 (Small Joint)

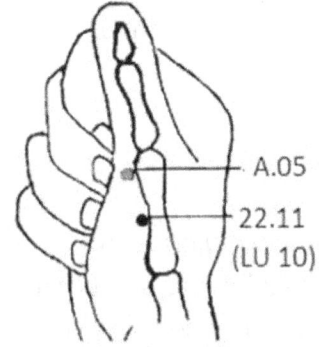

A.05
22.11
(LU 10)

Fig. 8.Ex.3

Location: On the Lung channel, at the radial side of the 1st metacarpal, at the junction of red and white skin, visible when the thumb is flexed into a fist.

Needling Technique: Insert 1 to 1.5 cun (approximately 0.4 to 0.6 inches) deep.

Indications:
It is most effective for ankle sprain (via holographic correspondence). It is also helpful for neck, shoulder, backache, sciatica, chest discomfort, stomach pain, chronic diarrhoea, and wrist and elbow pain.

A.06

Location: On the dorsum of the hand, 0.5 cun proximal to the junction of the 3rd and 4th phalanges, at the level of SJ 3, while making a fist.

Needling Technique: Insert 0.5 cun deep.

Indications:
Leg soreness, pain or distension, headache, and pain in the back and limbs.

9. Scalp Acupuncture

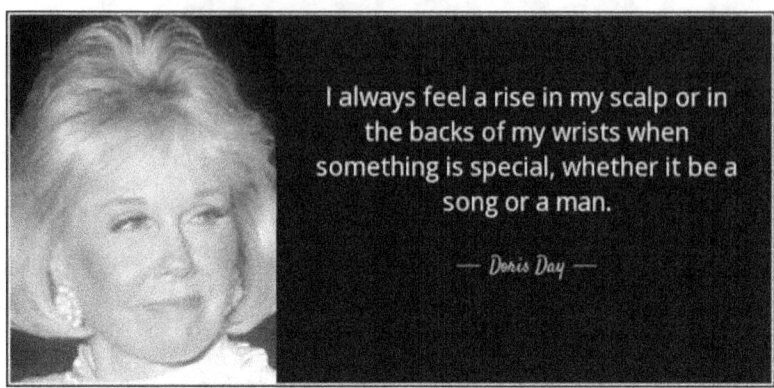

I always feel a rise in my scalp or in the backs of my wrists when something is special, whether it be a song or a man.

— Doris Day —

Scalp acupuncture is a relatively modern therapeutic modality that targets the functional areas of the brain by stimulating corresponding regions on the scalp. This technique is especially effective because the scalp lies near the brain's cortical surface, which governs various bodily functions. Scalp acupuncture does not follow traditional Chinese meridian systems; instead, it aligns with neuroanatomical principles, targeting brain areas underlying specific scalp regions.

Clinical Relevance to Acupuncture

The most practical use of scalp acupuncture is in treating paralysis following a stroke caused by ischemia, haemorrhage, or traumatic injury. It is also effective in spinal cord injuries, chronic pain syndromes, and various neurological and functional conditions. The treatment is based on stimulating brain areas that correlate to the motor, sensory, or functional impairment, thus bypassing TCM theories and classical meridians.

Mechanism of Action in Paralysis

Scalp acupuncture stimulates vasodilatation, enhances local blood flow, and increases glucose metabolism in affected cerebral areas. Neurophysiological research indicates that stimulating the cerebral cortex can activate hypoxic but salvageable neurons, reactivate dormant synapses, and reverse neural inhibition following a stroke. These effects mimic the principles of deep brain stimulation (DBS), a treatment used for Parkinson's disease and other neurological disorders.

Functional Areas of the Brain

Brain Region   **Function**

Brain Region	Function
Frontal Lobe	Executive functions – decision-making, planning, reasoning
Parietal Lobe	Sensory processing – touch, pressure, temperature
Temporal Lobe	Auditory processing, language comprehension, and memory
Occipital Lobe	Visual information processing
Basal Ganglia	Motor control and learning
Cerebellum	Coordination of movements, balance, and posture
Hippocampus	Memory formation and retrieval

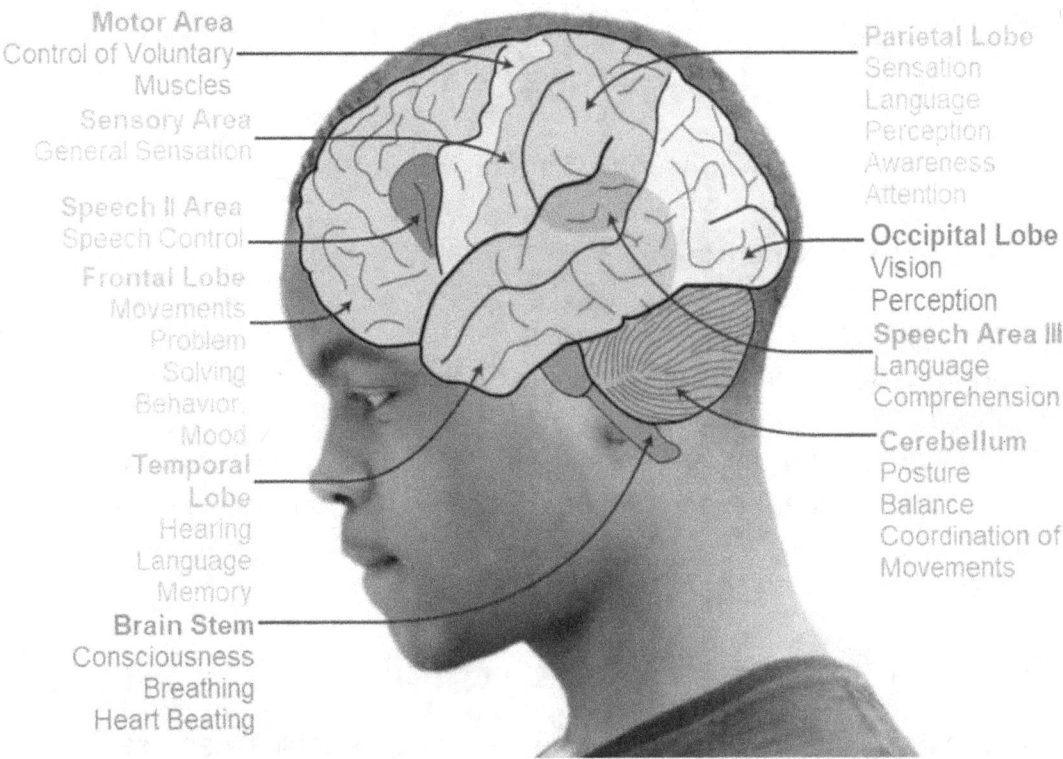

Source: Center for Biomolecular modeling

Fig. 9.1 Functions of Areas of Brain

These regions operate interdependently to regulate complex behaviours and physiological processes.

Structure of the Scalp

The scalp comprises multiple anatomical layers:
Skin → Hypodermis → Galea aponeurotica → Occipitofrontalis muscle → Sub-aponeurotic space → Pericranium

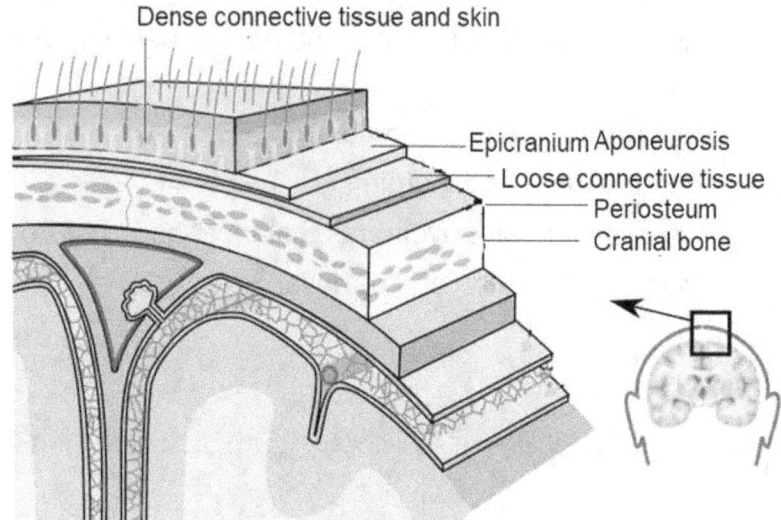

Fig. 9.2 Microscopic Structure of Scalp

Indications for Scalp Acupuncture

- **Paralysis** (post-stroke, spinal cord injury)
- **Cerebral disorders**: cerebral palsy, multiple sclerosis, dementia, aphasia, neurasthenia
- **Psychological conditions**: anxiety, neurosis, psychosomatic disorders
- **Pain conditions**: periarthritis, back and heel pain, chronic musculoskeletal pain

Scalp Needling Technique

Positioning:

- Patient should preferably be seated; lying down is acceptable if necessary.
- The acupuncturist must be positioned comfortably for precise access and control.

Insertion Protocol:

- Needles should pass through the sub-aponeurotic space, a loose connective layer between the galea and the pericranium.

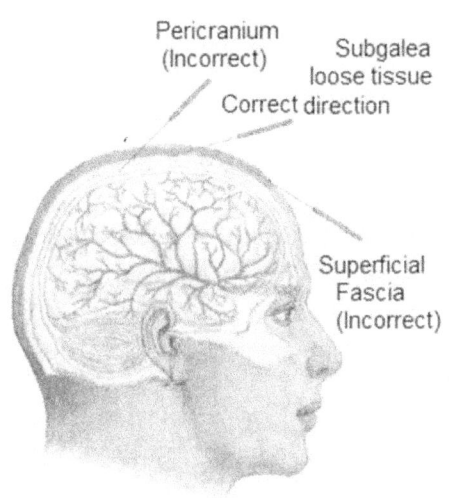

Pericranium (Incorrect)
Subgalea loose tissue
Correct direction
Superficial Fascia (Incorrect)

Fig. 9.3 Scalp Needling Technique

- Use 0.25 mm × 25 mm needles, avoiding hair follicles and underlying bone.
- Insertion angle: 15° to 30° to prevent painful contact with the skull or superficial misplacement.
- Insert needles horizontally for 1 to 1.5 cun, pointing toward the affected body region.
- During insertion, press the scalp, pull skin in the opposite direction, and ensure minimal pain.

Focus & Breathing:

- Encourage the patient to mentally direct breath toward the affected area during treatment.

Stimulation and Movement

- After insertion, stimulate the needle manually for 1 minute every 5 minutes over a 40-minute retention period.
- Electroacupuncture may be applied for continuous stimulation.
- Active or passive movement of the affected part is essential to reconnect peripheral signals to central pathways.
- Gradually add resistance or weights as strength improves.

Needle Removal Protocol

- Stimulate while the patient performs **breathing exercises**.
- **Pinch skin**, rotate the needle, withdraw slowly to the subcutaneous level, then **remove rapidly**.
- Apply **dry cotton pressure** and massage the site to avoid soreness.

Treatment Frequency

- Initially: daily for 5 days
- Then: every 2–3 days for 1–2 weeks
- Maintenance: twice weekly as needed
- Severe cases: twice daily

Methods of Scalp Acupuncture

The author endorses the clinically efficient and simplified methods developed by:

- **Dr. Shunfa Jiao**

- **Dr. Ming Qing Zhu**

Dr. Shunfa Jiao's Scalp Acupuncture

Standard Reference Lines

- **Antero-posterior line**: From the glabella to the external occipital protuberance
- **Eyebrow-occipital line**: From the midpoint of the eyebrow to the occipital protuberance

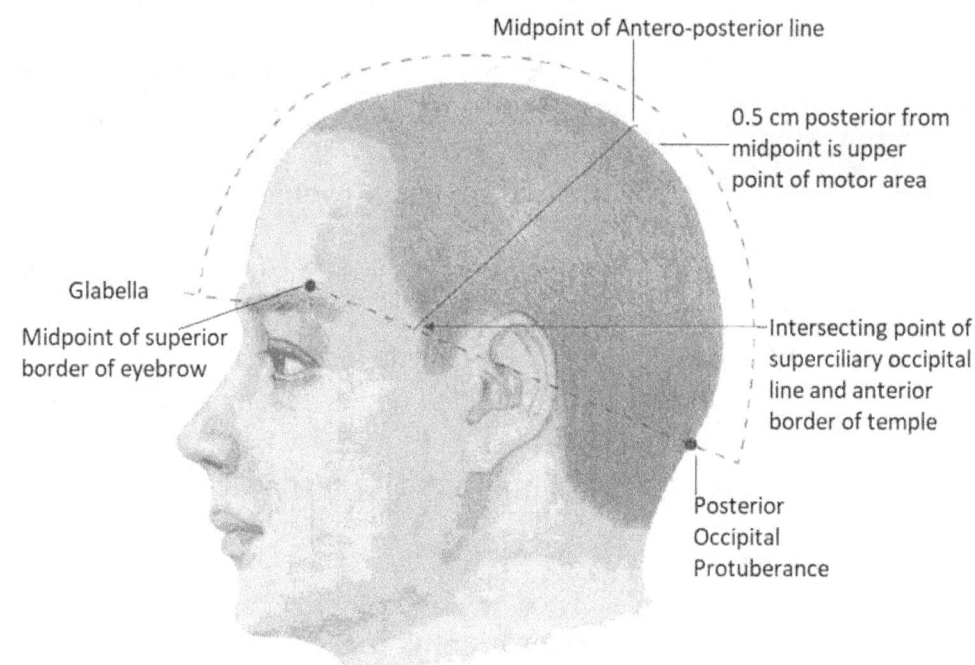

Fig. 9.4 Dr. Jiao Standard Lines

Motor Area

Located over the anterior central gyrus:

- Upper 1/5: Lower limb of the contralateral side
- Middle 2/5: Upper limb

Lower 2/5: Facial motor functions, aphasia

Sensory Area

Located 1.5 cm posterior to the motor line:

- Upper 1/5: Lumbar, leg, and neck pain
- Middle 2/5: Upper limb pain
- Lower 2/5: Facial pain, migraine, trigeminal neuralgia

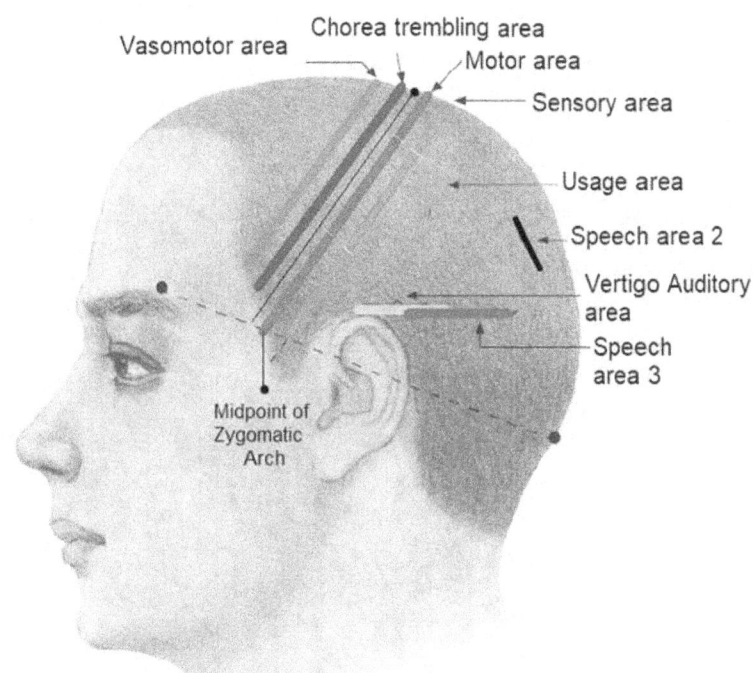

Fig. 9.5 Dr. Jiao Lateral Scalp Reaction Areas

Chorea-Tremor Control Area

1.5 cm anterior to the motor line – for Parkinsonism and chorea

Vertigo and Auditory Area

Horizontal line 1.5 cm above auricular apex, 4 cm long – for tinnitus, dizziness

Third Speech Area (Wernicke's)

Overlaps the posterior half of the auditory area – for sensory aphasia

Praxis Area

Three 3 cm lines meeting at the parietal tubercle – treat apraxia

Visual Area

Located 1 cm lateral to the midline, extending 4 cm upward, for cortical visual loss

Equilibrium Area

Located 3.5 cm lateral to the occipital protuberance, extending downward for balance issues

Second Speech Area

Vertical line 3 cm long, beginning 2 cm below parietal tubercle – for nominative aphasia

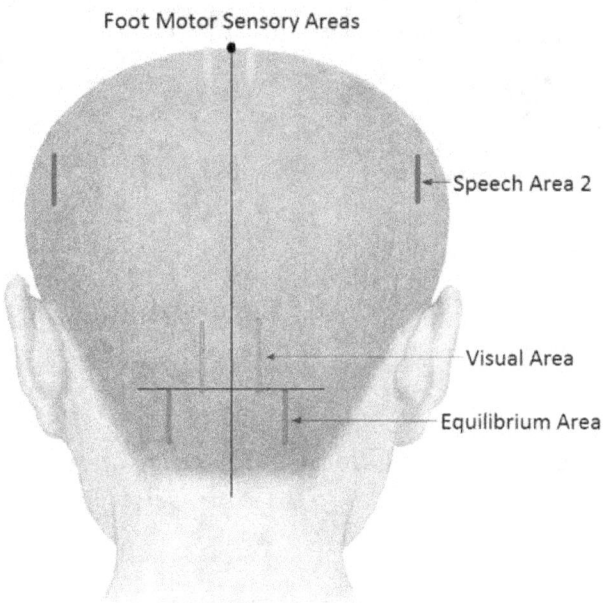

Fig. 9.6 Dr Jiao Areas on back of head

Foot Motor Sensory Area

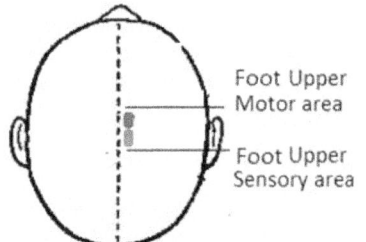

Fig. 9.7 Dr. Jiao's Foot Upper Motor & Sensory Areas

3 cm long, 1 cm lateral to midline – for lower limb motor disorders, lumbar pain, uterine prolapse

Stomach, Thoracic, Pelvic Areas

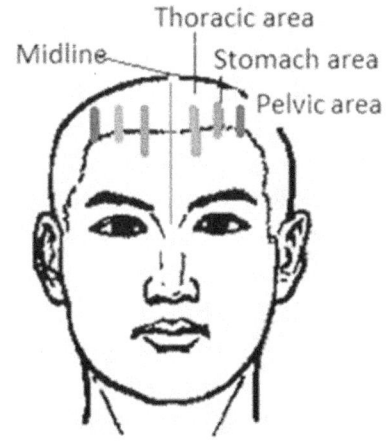

Fig. 9.8 Dr. Jiao's Thoracic, Stomach & Pelvic Areas

- **Stomach**: Above pupil, parallel to midline – for upper abdominal disorders
- **Thoracic**: Midway between the stomach area and the midline – for chest, cardiac, and pulmonary symptoms
- **Pelvic**: From head corner upward – for gynaecological and pelvic disorders

Dr. Ming Qing Zhu's Scalp Acupuncture

Eding Zone

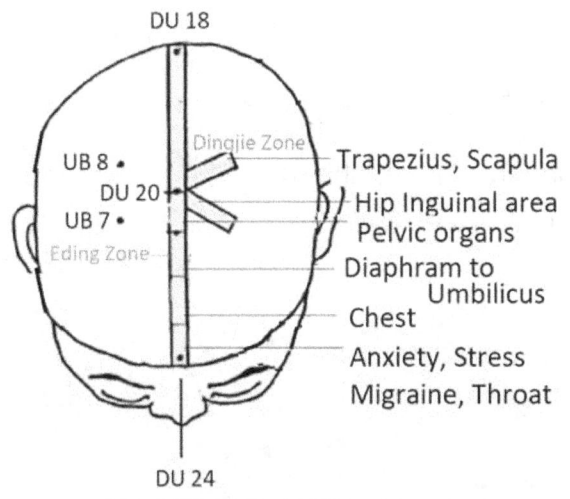

Fig. 9.9 Dr. Zhu's Eding Zone

1 cm wide strip from DU 24 to DU 20, divided into four zones:

1. **Head/Neck** (DU 24–23)
2. **Chest** (DU 23–22)
3. **Upper abdomen** (DU 22–21)
4. **Pelvis and lower limbs** (DU 21–20)

Dingjie Zone

Radiates from DU 20 to UB 7 (front) and UB 8 (back)

- Front: Hip and groin

- Back: Upper back, trapezius

Dingzhen Zone

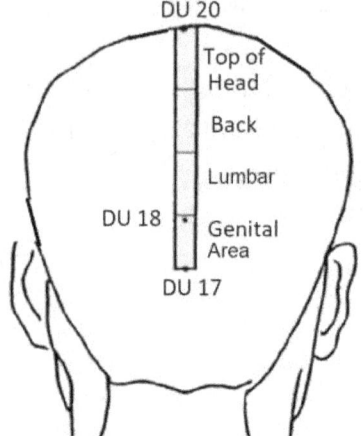

Fig. 9.10 Dr. Zhu's Dingzhen Area

Strip from DU 20 to DU 17, 1 cun wide

Treats pain from head to coccyx

Epang Zone

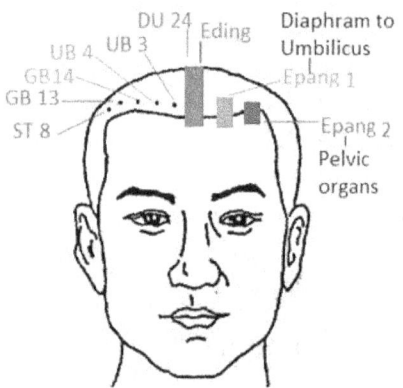

Fig. 9.11 Dr. Zhu's Epang Zones

Parallel short strips:

- **Epang 1**: Diaphragm to umbilicus
- **Epang 2**: Umbilicus to pelvis

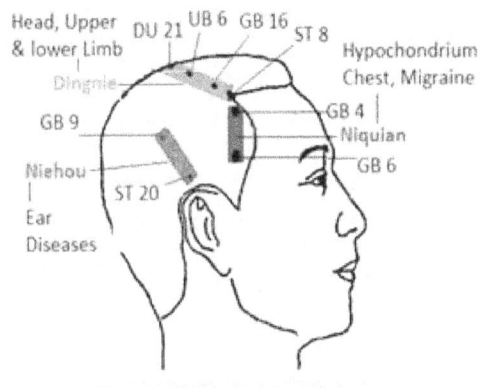

Fig. 9.12 Dr. Zhu's Niehou, Dingnie, Niquian Areas

Dingnie Zone

Temple region – treats motor and sensory issues of limbs and head

Nieqian Zone

From GB 4 to GB 6 – for hypochondriac pain, menstrual migraines

Niehou Zone

From GB 9 to SJ 20 – treats ear disorders

Summary Table of

Scalp Functional Zones and Clinical Use

Scalp Zone	Location	Clinical Indications
Motor Area	0.5 cm behind midline (anterior central gyrus)	Stroke paralysis, motor aphasia, and facial weakness
Sensory Area	1.5 cm posterior to Motor Area	Pain, numbness, and facial neuralgia
Chorea Tremor Control Area	1.5 cm anterior to Motor Area	Parkinsonism, tremors, spasms
Third Speech Area	Posterior half of Auditory Area (Wernicke's)	Sensory aphasia
Visual Area	1 cm lateral to midline, occipital region	Cortical vision loss
Praxis Area	3 lines from the parietal tubercle	Apraxia, loss of purposeful movement
Equilibrium Area	3.5 cm lateral to EOP, 4 cm vertical	Cerebellar ataxia, balance loss

Scalp Zone	Location	Clinical Indications
Eding Zones 1–4	DU 24 to DU 20 (frontal strip)	From migraine to pelvic dysfunction
Dingzhen Zone	DU 20 to DU 17 (midline posterior)	Back pain, spinal disorders
Dingjie (Ant/Post)	DU 20 to UB 7/UB 8	Inguinal or shoulder region disorders
Dingnie Zone	DU 21 to ST 8 (temple)	Limb and head motor/sensory disorders
Nieqian Zone	GB 4 to GB 6	Side head pain, gallbladder/liver syndromes, migraine
Niehou Zone	GB 9 to SJ 20	Ear diseases
Foot Motor Sensory Area	3 cm long, 1 cm lateral to midline	Lower limb paralysis, uterine prolapse
Thoracic Area	Between the stomach area and the midline	Chest pain, asthma, palpitations
Pelvic Area	Corner of head upward 2 cm	Gynaecological, bladder, and rectal disorders

10. Abdominal Acupuncture

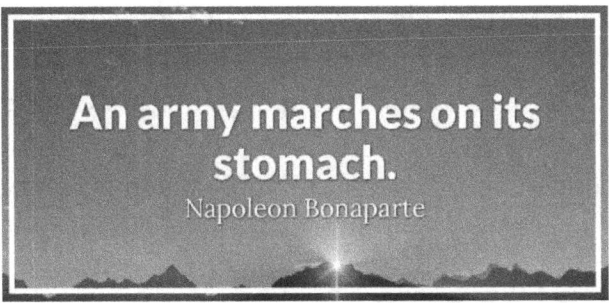

An army marches on its stomach.
Napoleon Bonaparte

The abdomen and pelvis are home to the digestive, excretory, and reproductive systems and contain the highest concentration of neurons outside the brain and spinal cord, earning the designation "second brain." This enteric nervous system is connected to yet capable of independent function from the autonomic nervous system, which comprises the sympathetic, parasympathetic, and enteric systems. The autonomic nervous system governs involuntary functions and maintains homeostasis through mutual antagonistic regulation of various organs.

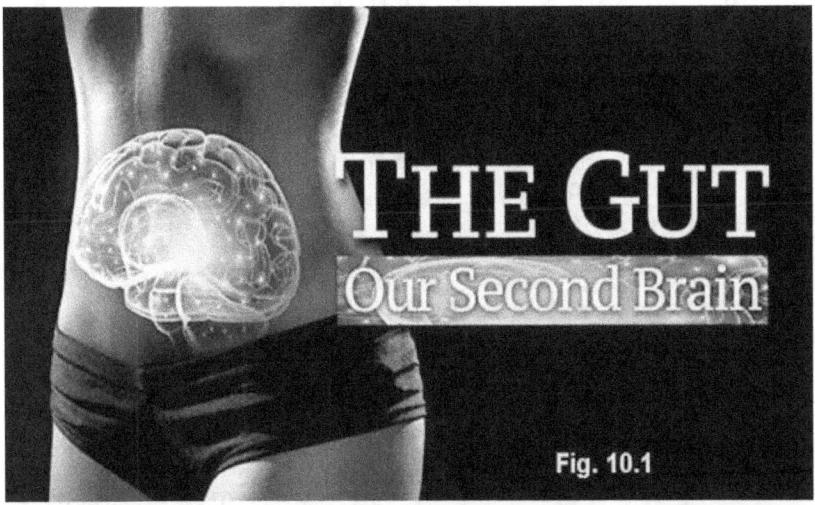

THE GUT
Our Second Brain
Fig. 10.1

The abdomen also produces many critical neurotransmitters and hormones. Notably, it synthesises approximately 95% of the body's serotonin, significantly influencing mood and emotional well-being. The spleen contributes by regulating serotonin levels via platelet function. Disruptions in serotonin metabolism, particularly in the intestines, are linked to conditions such as irritable bowel syndrome and obsessive-compulsive disorder. By correcting imbalances through acupuncture, emotional and physical health can be improved. Abdominal acupuncture leverages the dense neural network of the abdomen to influence a wide range of physiological functions, making it a powerful therapeutic modality.

Advantages of Abdominal Acupuncture

Abdominal acupuncture is particularly suitable for frail or elderly patients. It uses distal needling away from pathological sites, thereby reducing risk. This technique is less painful, has fewer complications, and may offer rapid therapeutic effects with minor needle depth or site adjustments. It is effective in stroke rehabilitation, fibromyalgia, and multiple simultaneous conditions. Practitioners find it unique, and patients often experience benefits quickly. Self-treatment is also feasible in some cases.

Cautions and Contraindications

Abdominal acupuncture should be avoided during pregnancy, in cases of venous dilation around the umbilicus, undiagnosed abdominal pain, peritonitis, hepatosplenomegaly, or abdominal malignancy.

Abdominal Acupuncture Points

The layout of abdominal acupuncture points is based on the image of a turtle. These include eight main Ab points and selected TCM points:

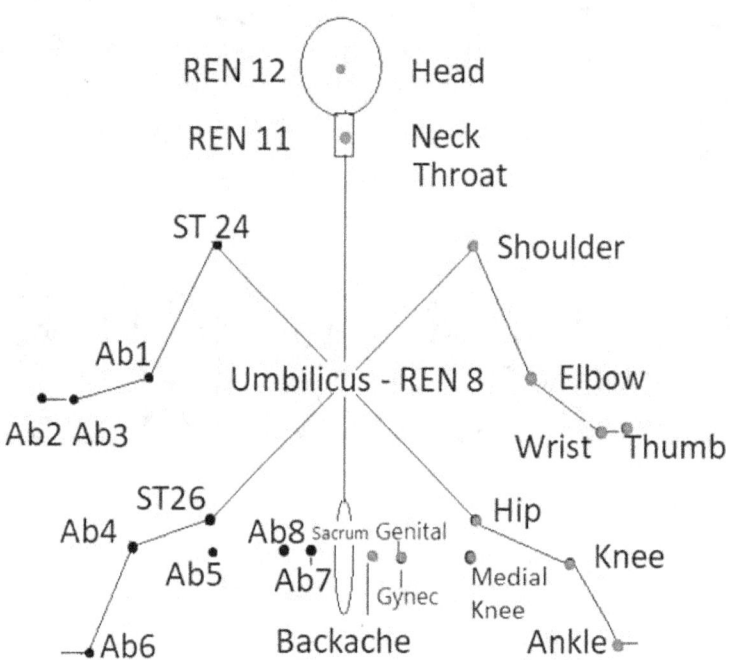

Fig. 10.3 Abdominal Points - Schematic Diagram

- **Ab1 (Elbow Point)**: ½ cun superior and ½ cun lateral to ST 24; used for elbow pain and dermatologic issues.

- **Ab2 (Wrist Point)**: ½ cun inferior and lateral to Ab1; treats wrist pain.
- **Ab3 (Thumb Point)**: 1 cun directly superior to Ab2; for thumb pain.
- **Ab4 (Knee Point)**: ½ cun inferior and lateral to ST 26; for knee pain.
- **Ab5 (Medial Knee Point)**: 1 cun medial to Ab4; targets medial knee pain.
- **Ab6 (Ankle Point)**: ½ cun inferior and lateral to Ab4; for ankle pain.
- **Ab7 (Sacrum)**: ½ cun lateral to REN 6; for lower back pain (L1-L2).
- **Ab8 (Coccyx)**: 1 cun lateral to REN 6; treats menstrual, abdominal, and digestive disorders.

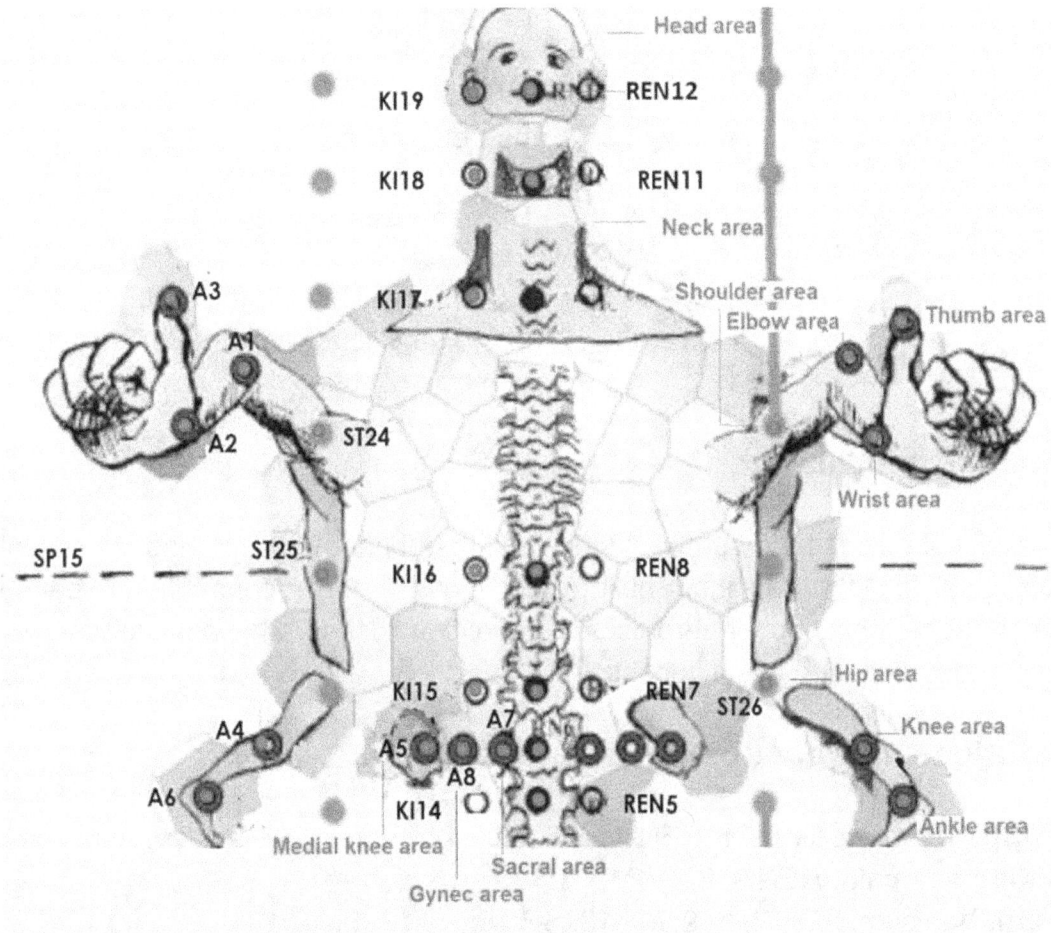

Fig. 10.2 Turtle Map of Abdominal Points

Key TCM Abdominal Points and Their Applications

REN Points:

- **REN 12**: Midway between the sternum and umbilicus; for headaches and sensory disorders.
- **REN 11 to REN 3**: Sequentially address issues from cervical spine disorders to genitourinary problems and lumbar pain.

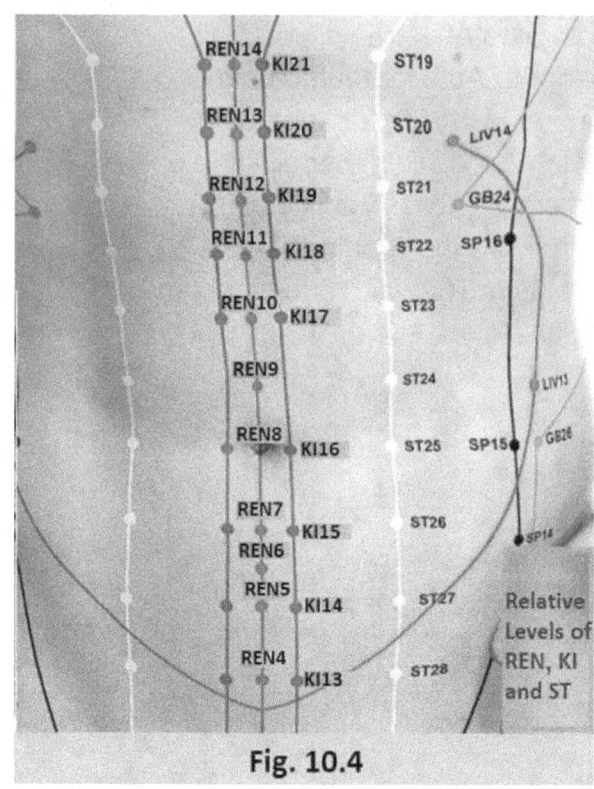

Fig. 10.4

Kidney Points:

- **KI 13, 17, 18, 19**: Support spinal, cervical, gastrointestinal, and reproductive issues.

Stomach Points:

- **ST 24, 25, 26, 27**: Useful for treating musculoskeletal, respiratory, digestive, and neurological conditions.

Spleen Point:

- **SP 15**: Lateral to the rectus abdominis at the umbilicus level; treats intestinal and muscular issues.

Treatment Protocols

The therapist should face the umbilicus directly. Insert needles from medial to lateral and from lower to higher regions. Shallow needling is preferred for acute and peripheral problems; deeper needling for chronic or visceral conditions. Ashi points around indicated zones enhance effectiveness.

Prescriptions for Pain Conditions

- **Upper back/Neck pain**: REN 12, 10, ST 24 bilaterally, KI 17, with Ashi points.
- **Mid back pain**: REN 9, 8, 7.
- **Lumbar pain**: REN 4, 6, 9, 10, 12, SP 15.
- **Shoulder pain**: ST 24, KI 17, REN 12, 10, 6, 4; Ab1, Ab2.
- **Arm, wrist, thumb pain**: Ab1–Ab3, REN 12, 4; KI 17; Ashi points.
- **Hip and Sciatica**: ST 26, REN 4–12, UB 25, KI 13, Ab7.
- **Knee pain**: Ab4.
- **Ankle pain**: Ab6, REN 9, SP 15, KI 13.

11. Ear Acupuncture

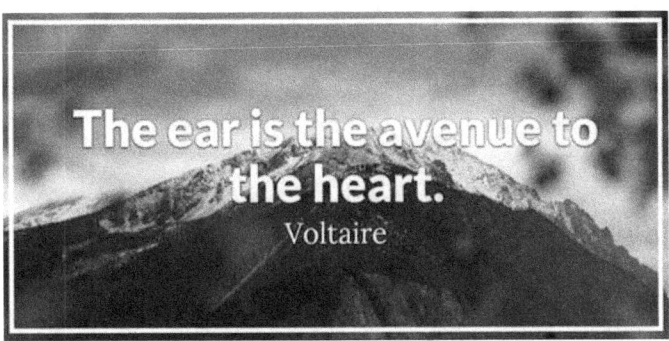

The ear is the avenue to the heart.
Voltaire

Ear acupuncture, or auriculotherapy, is a micro-acupuncture system based on the premise that the entire body is represented on the auricle in an inverted foetal pattern (Fig. 10.1). The head is located at the lower lobule, and the buttocks at the top of the helix. Stimulation of specific auricular points relieves corresponding body conditions, with clinical evidence showing immediate pain relief in many cases. Auricular points become reactive in pathological states, often confirming the diagnosis.

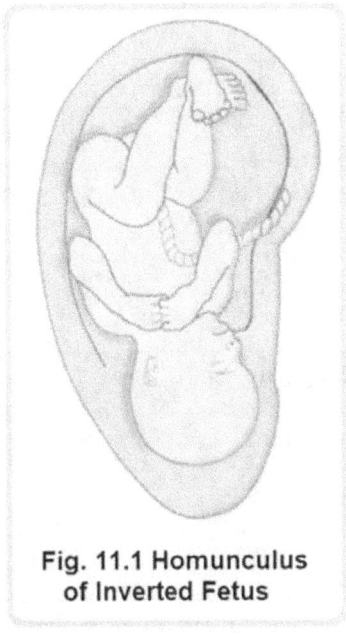

Fig. 11.1 Homunculus of Inverted Fetus

Condition	Percentage
Smoking cessation	68
Substance abuse	53
Weight control	53
Anxiety	43
Nausea	38
Insomnia	38
Depression	35
Allergies	35
Musculoskeletal pain	28
Attention deficit disorder	25
Neck and shoulder tension	25

Conditions Better Treated by Ear Than Body Acupuncture

Advantages of Ear Acupuncture

Auriculotherapy is widely used for:

- Chronic pain management
- Detoxification from addictive substances
- Nausea and vomiting relief
- Hypertension reduction
- Postoperative pain and inflammation
- Spasmodic conditions (e.g., gallstone colic)
- Fever, itching, and allergic responses

Usage of Ear Acupuncture

Ear acupuncture is commonly used to treat these conditions. It provides better relief than body acupuncture.

Anatomy of the Ear

The auricle consists of raised ridges, depressions, notches, and a lobule:

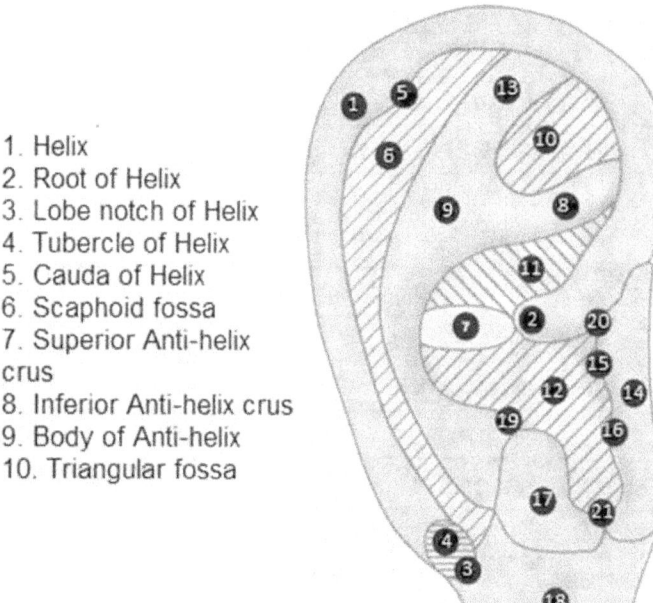

1. Helix
2. Root of Helix
3. Lobe notch of Helix
4. Tubercle of Helix
5. Cauda of Helix
6. Scaphoid fossa
7. Superior Anti-helix crus
8. Inferior Anti-helix crus
9. Body of Anti-helix
10. Triangular fossa
11. Superior Concha
12. Inferior Concha
13. Concha ridge
14. Tragus
15. Tragus - upper apex
16. Tragus - lower apex
17. Anti-tragus
18. Lobe
19. Anti-helix Anti-tragus
20. Supratragic notch
21. Intertragic notch

Fig. 11.2 Anatomy of Ear

- **Helix (1):** The outer rim; includes the root (2), tubercle (4), and cauda (5)
- **Antihelix (9):** Y-shaped ridge medial to the helix; divided into superior (7), inferior crus (8), and body

- **Scaphoid Fossa (6):** Groove between helix and antihelix
- **Tragus (14–16):** Anterior projection near the ear canal
- **Antitragus (17):** Small projection above the lobule, opposite the tragus
- **Lobule (18):** Soft lower part of the ear

Nerve Supply and Autonomic Influence

The auricle is innervated by the **Auricular Branch of the Vagus Nerve (ABVN)**, which projects to the Nucleus Tractus Solitarius (NTS) in the medulla. This forms the anatomical basis for the auriculo-vagal afferent pathway (AVAP), which potentially modulates autonomic and central nervous system functions, including cardiovascular, gastrointestinal, and respiratory regulation. Vagal stimulation may help prevent neurodegenerative diseases, although this remains under investigation.

Master Points:

These are the main points of auriculotherapy that support the actions of other auricular points. They bring the whole body towards homeostasis, producing a balance of energy, hormones, and brain activity. The following are ear masterpoints and their indications: Shen Men is used for stress, anxiety, and excessive sensitivity.

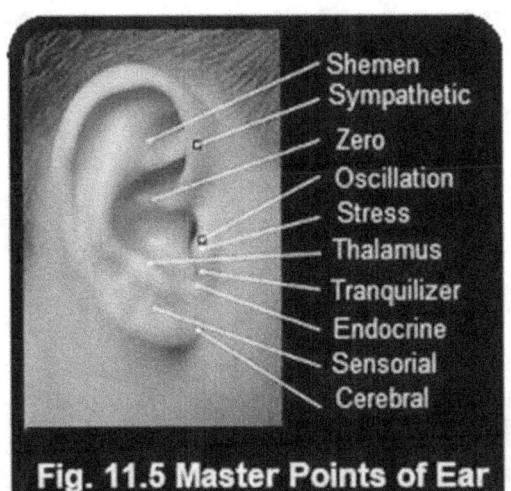

Fig. 11.5 Master Points of Ear

The autonomic point balances the sympathetic and parasympathetic nervous systems, helping to improve blood circulation.

Point Zero represents the level of the umbilicus. It represents the autonomic nervous system, which controls visceral organs through peripheral nerve ganglia.

The thalamus regulates treatment for shock and sweating.

The endocrine point manages balance, endocrine hormones, hypersensitivity, and rheumatism.

Master Oscillation point balances left and right hemispheres (proper for left-hand dominant clients).

Allergy points reduce allergic inflammation and eliminate toxicity.

The tranquilizer point is used for general sedation and anxiety.

The Master Sensorial (eye) point is indicated in tinnitus and blurred vision, and the Master Cerebral point is used in nervousness, anxiety, fear, and obsessive-compulsive disorder (OC.

Summary of Master Points, Indication, and Therapeutic Effects

Master Point	Primary Indication	Therapeutic Effect
Shen Men	Stress, anxiety, sensitivity	Neuro-emotional
Autonomic Point	Sympathetic-parasympathetic balance	Autonomic Regulation
Point Zero	Homeostasis, autonomic regulation	Homeostatic Control
Thalamus Point	Shock, excessive sweating	Neurological
Endocrine Point	Hormonal balance, hypersensitivity	Endocrine Balance
Master Oscillation	Brain hemisphere balance	Neurological Balance
Allergy Point	Allergic inflammation	Immune Modulation
Tranquilizer Point	General sedation	Sedative
Master Sensorial	Tinnitus, blurred vision	Sensory Support
Master Cerebral	Anxiety, OCD, fear	Psychological

Functional Ear Zones

Functional Ear Zones: Motor and Sensory Points

The auricle (external ear) is a microsystem that reflects the entire body, with specific motor and sensory zones corresponding to various anatomical regions. The image shows that auricular acupuncture utilizes this somatotopic arrangement to influence physiological and pathological functions.

- **Motor Points**: Located primarily along the antihelix and its branches, these points correspond to the musculoskeletal system. Key areas include joints (hip, knee, shoulder), limbs, and spine segments (sacral, lumbar, thoracic, and cervical). Stimulation of these zones aids in managing pain, paralysis, and motor dysfunction.
- **Sensory Points**: These are found mainly in the lobule and surrounding regions and correspond to cranial functions and sensory organs. They include points for olfactory, visual, auditory, and facial sensations. Additionally, zones related to the skull (frontal, temporal, occipital) modulate head-related symptoms such as headaches, sinus issues, and neuralgias.

This functional mapping of the ear enables targeted treatment for systemic conditions through a non-invasive, accessible approach in auriculotherapy.

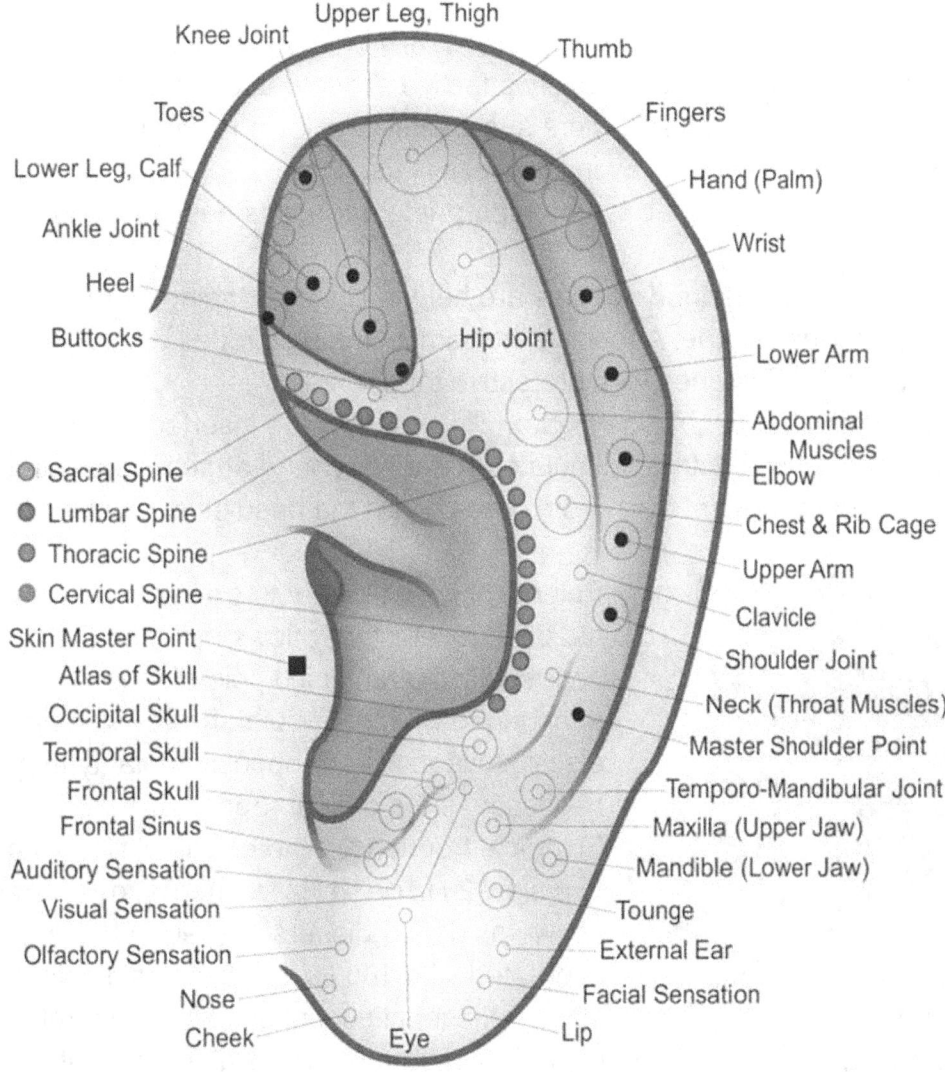

Fig. 11.4 Motor and Sensory Ear Points

Technique of Ear Acupuncture

- Use short (13 mm) sterilized needles
- Stabilise the ear with the non-dominant hand
- Insert manually at a 30°– 45° angle from the inferior aspect
- Avoid cartilage penetration
- Rapid insertion reduces pain
- Rotate needle gently to elicit De Qi (sensation of warmth, heaviness, energy)

- Stimulate every 5 minutes for 30 minutes
- Minor bleeding is beneficial and should not be suppressed

Electroacupuncture of the Ear

Electroacupuncture is an exceptionally effective accentuated mode of auricular therapy. It is typically more powerful and more successful in relieving pain and alleviating the problems of addiction. The following process is used.

Needling: Needles are applied to the appropriate ear points described in the previous section.

Secure needles: The inserted needles are held in place by taping them across the ear with medical adhesive tape. Attaching the stimulating electrodes will pull out the needles unless they are first fastened with protective tape.

Application of electrodes: Micro Alligator clips connect the inserted needles to the electrode leads of an electrical stimulator. It is also wise to attach the electrode wires to a secure anchor to prevent them from dragging on the needles and pulling them out.

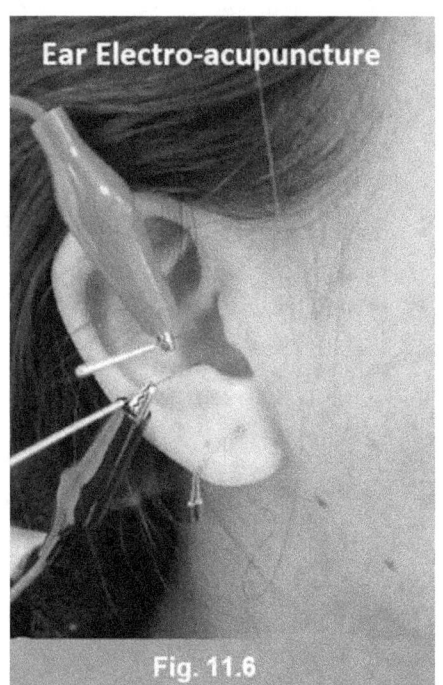

Ear Electro-acupuncture

Fig. 11.6

Polarity: It is necessary to stimulate between two needles, as electricity flows between the poles. It does not usually matter which pole of the stimulator is attached to which ear point; however, switching the electrode leads to the opposite polarity may be necessary if the patient reports any increase in pain.

Electrical frequency: The electrical frequency rate is set to a slow 2 Hz or 10 Hz frequency, or a parameter known as dense-disperse, where 2 Hz frequencies are alternated with 100 Hz frequencies. Lower frequencies, 10 Hz or less, affect enkephalins, endorphins, and disorders of both the visceral and somatic systems, whereas higher frequencies, 100 Hz or higher, affect dynorphins and neurological dysfunctions.

Current titration: The more straightforward method is to keep intensity to zero and slowly increase until the patient 'feels' the current. It should not be painful or uncomfortable; the patient should be aware of their current state.

Frequency of treatment: As with auricular acupuncture without electrical stimulation, leave the needles in place and maintain the stimulation current for 30 minutes. Treat the patient daily for three days, assess the response, and reduce the frequency to alternate days, twice a week, and once a week until optimal results are achieved.

Press-Needles/ Tacks/ Pellets/ Seeds

Ear acupressure treatments include pellets, seeds, or tacks on specific ear points to prevent or treat disease or pain. They may be used as an adjunct to regular acupuncture treatments to enhance and prolong their effects, or can be used alone as the primary form of therapy. Press needles are another modality of ear tacks, somewhat similar to seeds and pellets.

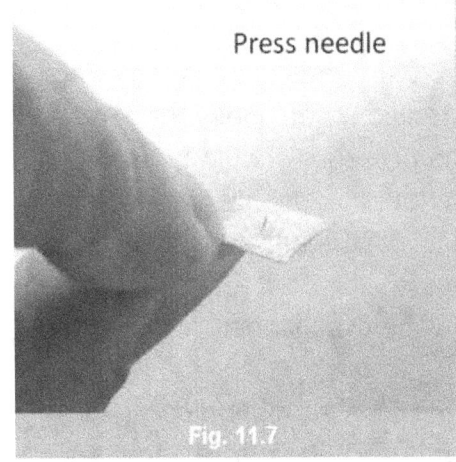

Press needle

Fig. 11.7

They resemble small thumbtacks and are available in several sizes: extra small, small, medium, and large. The bigger the tack, the stronger the stimulus obtained in the ear. Extra small or small-sized tacks seem the most comfortable for patients, yet still offer a suitable stimulus. The tacks come affixed to skin-colored tape and can be applied to the ear with tweezers or forceps. The typical retention time is theoretically 3 to 5 days. Because their stimulus is so strong, a patient may only be able to tolerate a few hours of stimulation a day. Exposure to water through swimming, bathing, or high humidity levels can increase the risk of infection.

Bloodletting:

Ear bleeding is effective when applied to specific ear points. The patient should be in a reclining position to bleed. The practitioner should wear gloves to protect themselves from touching the patient's blood. Clean the ear and apply an antiseptic solution.

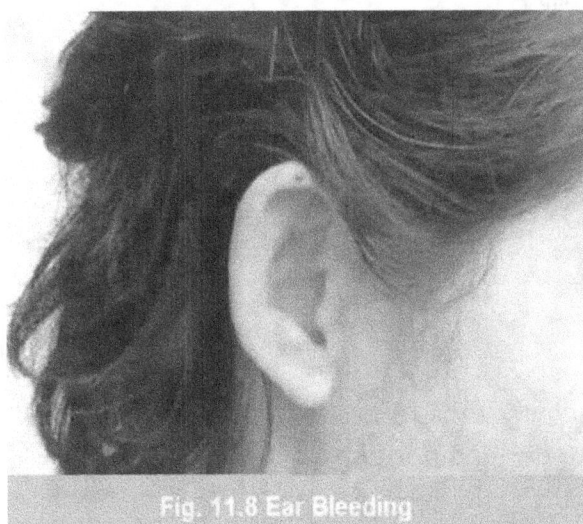

Fig. 11.8 Ear Bleeding

Massage the ear to promote capillary congestion, which increases bleeding by enhancing blood flow to the ear. Use 20 or 18-gauge injection needles. Injection needles have the advantage of a two-edge point, creating a minute cut as desired by an acupuncturist. The ear cannot be bled quickly with a regular acupuncture needle, and lancet penetration can be uncontrolled, causing cartilage injury. Areas such as petechiae or red spots may be bled. Direct the needle at 30 - 45 degrees to the skin's surface with the bevel facing up to cause bleeding in the limited depth available on the ear. Puncture quickly and to the same depth as recommended.

Absorb the blood droplets by placing a cotton ball over the point and applying gentle pressure. This small amount of blood-tinged cotton may be disposed of in the garbage basket. Do not bleed more than three points at a time; bleeding at one end is the norm and is often sufficient. High blood pressure responds instantly to bleeding the ear's hypertension point. The ears of patients with high blood pressure may bleed more quickly than those with normal blood pressure. Specific points, such as Shen Men and Occiput, are more likely to bleed than others.

Stimulation:

The ear tack should be pressed gently and rhythmically 3 to 5 times daily for several seconds. It should produce a mild sensation of heat, distension, heaviness, or soreness. The sensation is a sign that the treatment is working. The pressure should not be 3 to 5 seconds each time, as irritation may develop. Pressure should be sufficient to feel the discomfort of a needle. When bathing, it is essential not to get the ear wet. All such ear attachments should be replaced every 3 to 5 days. It ensures the best results and protects the ear against infection. The patient must follow the practitioner's advice on when to return to the office to change the ear therapy.

Important Note: If the ear therapy becomes too painful, the tape should be carefully peeled off. The tape will come off with the seed, pellet, or tack. If the ear tape comes off accidentally, the patient should not attempt to replace it herself (unless she is sure where it goes), as she may place it on the incorrect point. Some bleeding may occur when removing the ear tape, although this should not happen unless the patient has been pressing too hard on the end of the tape. The point should be pressed lightly to absorb the blood, and the blood-tinged cotton ball should be disposed of in the garbage. If someone else removes the patient's ear tape, they should wear disposable gloves to guard against infection transmitted through the blood.

Side Effects, Precautions, and Contraindications

Possible Side Effects:
Fainting, convulsions, local pain, infection (rare)

Precautions:

- Do not puncture cartilage
- Avoid treatment with alcohol or sexual activity within 6 hours before/after
- Aviation/diving personnel should be grounded temporarily
- Only sterile equipment should be used

Contraindications:

- Unwilling patient

- Local ear infection or malignancy
- Immunocompromised state
- Severe bleeding disorders

Expected Outcomes

- Acute disorders resolve quickly; chronic ones need multiple sessions
- Initial aggravation may indicate a healing crisis
- Endocrine disorders require multi-point prescriptions
- Patients may feel tired—rest is advised after treatment

Clinical Prescriptions

Prescriptions of Ear Acupuncture

Addictions

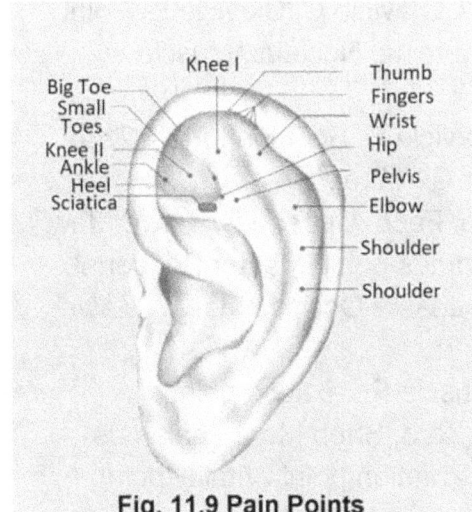

Fig. 11.9 Pain Points

Smoking Cessation: Nicotine is far more addictive than other drugs and, therefore, more challenging to treat. Ear acupuncture point reduces cravings and enhances mental well-being to relieve smoking addiction. It is more effective than other methods of treating smoking addiction. Nicotine, Lung 1, Lung 2, Mouth, Point Zero, Shen Men, Sympathetic Autonomic point, Brain (Electroacupuncture on Lung points at 80 Hz for 2 minutes or needle for 20 minutes), Adrenal Gland, Aggressiveness, Limbic System.

Alcoholism: Stimulation of the Alcohol points on the conchae of the ear's pinna is likely to reduce relapse after detoxification treatment by many folds. The alcoholic points are the liver, Lung, Brain, Occiput, Forehead, Kidney, Point Zero, Shen Men, Lesser Occipital nerve, Thirst point, Sympathetic Autonomic point, Endocrine Tranquilizer point, Master Cerebral, Master Oscillation, Limb System, Aggressiveness, and Antidepressant point.

Drug Addiction: Lung 1, 2, Shen Men, Sympathetic, Autonomic Point, Liver, Kidney, Brain. Occiput, Adrenal Gland C, Limbic System.

Pain Conditions

Musculoskeletal pain: Thoracic Spine, Lumbosacral Spine, Buttocks, Sciatic Nerve, Lumbago, Lumbar Spine on the conchae ridge, Lumbar Spine Phase III on the Tragus, Point Zero, Shen Men, Thalamus point, Darwin's point, Muscle Relaxation point, Liver, Urinary Bladder, Adrenal Glands.

Shoulder pain, frozen shoulder, bursitis: Shoulder, Shoulder phase, Master Shoulder, Clavicle, Cervical Spine.

Tennis elbow: Elbow Phase, Forearm, Arm, Thoracic Spine, Point Zero, Shen Men, Thalamus point, Muscle Relaxation point, Adrenal Gland, Kidney, Occiput. Oscillation point, Kidney, Spleen, Occiput, San Jiao, Apex of Ear, Helix.

Migraine headaches: Temples, Lesser Occipital nerve, Vagus nerve, Shen Men, Kidney, Thalamus point, Cervical Spine, Sympathetic, Autonomic point, Point Zero, Tranquilizer point, Master Oscillation, Master Sensorial, Master Cerebral, Muscle Relaxation Point.

Temporo-mandibular joint dysfunction: TMJ, Upper Jaw, Lower Jaw, Cervical Spine, Trigeminal nerve, Occiput, Master Cerebral, Point Zero, Shen Men, Thalamus point, Master Sensorial, San Jiao, Muscle Relaxation, Psychosomatic Reactions.

Torticollis, neck strain: Cervical Spine, Neck, Occiput, Clavicle C, Clavicle E, Point Zero, Shen Men, Thalamus point, Endocrine point, Trigeminal Nucleus, Muscle Relaxation.

Whiplash injury: Neck, Cervical Spine, Clavicle C, Clavicle E, Shoulder, Point Zero, Shen Men, Muscle Relaxation, Thalamus point, Master Cerebral.

Trigeminal neuralgia, facial neuralgia: Trigeminal nerve, Face, Upper Jaw, Lower Jaw, Mouth, Occiput, Shen Men, San Jiao, Point Zero, Thalamus point, Master Sensorial, Master Cerebral, Temples, Shoulder, Brainstem, Liver, Lesser Occipital nerve, Master Oscillation, Wind Stream.

Fibromyalgia: Thoracic Spine, Lumbosacral Spine, Muscle Relaxation point, Antidepressant point, Psychosomatic Reactions, Point Zero, Shen Men, Thalamus point, Abdomen, Kidney, Sympathetic chain, Master Oscillation point, Vitality point, Tranquilizer point.

-Modern Acupuncture-

12. Periosteal Acupuncture

The periosteum is a specialised membrane that envelops the outer surface of bones, except at joint surfaces. It is distinct from the endosteum, which lines the inner medullary cavity of long bones. The periosteum comprises dense, irregular connective tissue and is anatomically divided into two functional layers: an outer fibrous layer and an inner cambium (osteogenic) layer. The fibrous layer contains fibroblasts that maintain structural integrity, while the cambium layer houses progenitor cells capable of differentiating into osteoblasts, which are essential for bone formation and repair.

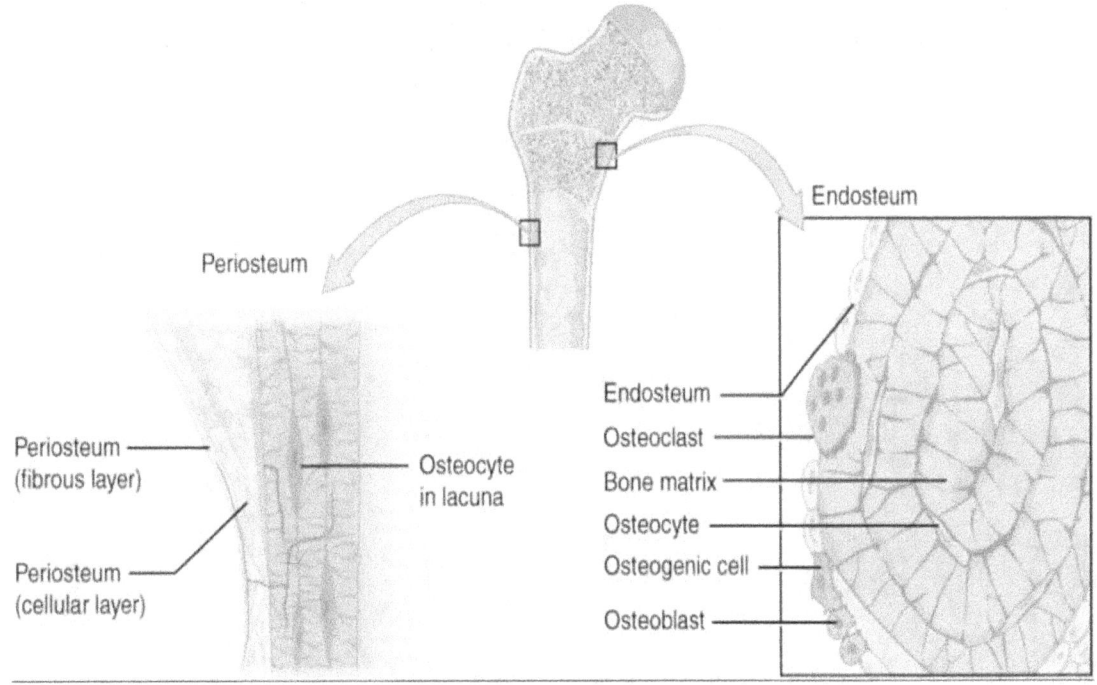

Fig. 12.1 Structure of Periosteum

These osteoblasts contribute to bone growth and thickness during development and play a critical role in bone regeneration after injury or fracture. Upon fracture, the progenitor cells of the cambium layer proliferate and differentiate into osteoblasts and chondroblasts, initiating the healing process. Furthermore, the periosteum facilitates vascular nourishment of the cortical bone and marrow, owing to its extensive vascular supply.

Structurally, the periosteum is anchored to the underlying bone matrix by strong collagen fibres called Sharpey's fibres, which penetrate the outer lamellae. It is also a firm anchorage point for muscles, ligaments, and tendons. Unlike the relatively insensate skeletal tissue, the periosteum is abundantly supplied with nociceptive (pain-sensing) nerve endings, making it highly sensitive to mechanical stimuli and an ideal target for therapeutic periosteal acupuncture to achieve profound analgesic effects.

Technique of Periosteal Acupuncture

Periosteal acupuncture is a therapeutic method popularised by Dr. Felix Mann. It involves stimulating the periosteum's rich nerve supply via acupuncture needling. The rationale lies in the periosteum's dense innervation, which makes it exceptionally responsive to micro-traumatic mechanical signals. The technique elicits potent analgesia by engaging local and segmental neurophysiological pathways.

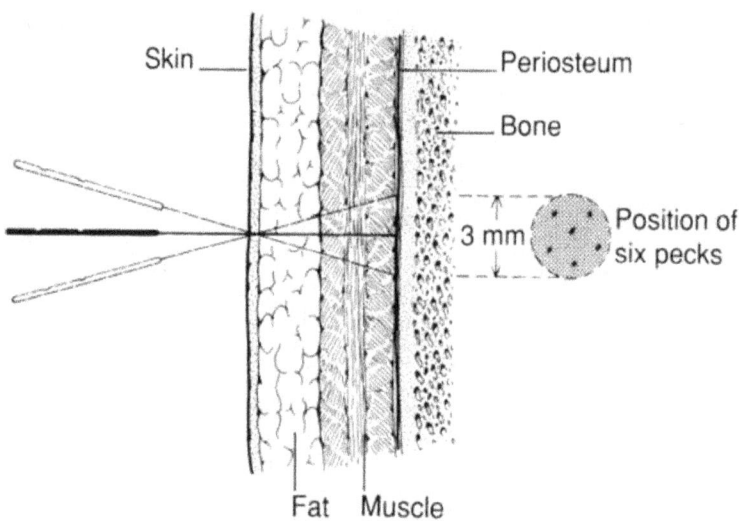

Fig. 12.2 Technique of Periosteal Needling

Source Reinventing Acupuncture, Dr Felix Mann

To perform periosteal acupuncture, the practitioner first identifies a tender or reactive bony area, often correlating with the patient's complaint site. The acupuncture needle is inserted in the standard perpendicular manner until it reaches the bony surface, ensuring it gently contacts the periosteum. This direct contact should be firm but gentle enough to activate the periosteal receptors without damaging the bone. Alternatively, the needle may be inserted adjacent to the bone so that it glides or brushes along its surface, as is practiced at specific points such as 22.04 and 22.05, particularly in Tung acupuncture.

Crucially, twisting or rotating the needle is avoided to prevent excessive trauma. Instead, the needle may be repeatedly re-angled or 'pecked' through the same dermal puncture to stimulate multiple adjacent periosteal sites. Although the needling site is local, the perceived analgesic effect is often distal or proximal, reflecting broader segmental and systemic modulation of nociception.

Care must be taken during cranial applications, as intense stimulation, especially when contacting the skull's periosteum, may exacerbate discomfort or lead to delayed pain that persists for several days. Therefore, the precise technique, depth control, and patient feedback of this modality are essential.

Indications of Periosteal Acupuncture

Periosteal acupuncture is highly effective in managing various types of pain, particularly those of musculoskeletal origin. Its use is most prominent in chronic and degenerative pain conditions that involve deep structures near the bone. Some of the standard clinical applications include:

- Osteoarthritis of the knee
- Chronic and acute sciatica
- Back and neck pain with bony tenderness
- Refractory musculoskeletal pain syndromes
- Subcutaneous nodules such as lipomas
- Dermatological conditions (where segmental dermatomal connections exist with skeletal structures)

This technique influences pain perception, inflammation, and local tissue healing by stimulating periosteal nerve fibres and initiating local cytokine release and reflex arcs. It represents a unique blend of mechanical stimulation and neurohormonal modulation, setting it apart from conventional acupuncture techniques focusing solely on muscular or meridian-based stimulation.

-Modern Acupuncture-

13. Myofascial Trigger Points

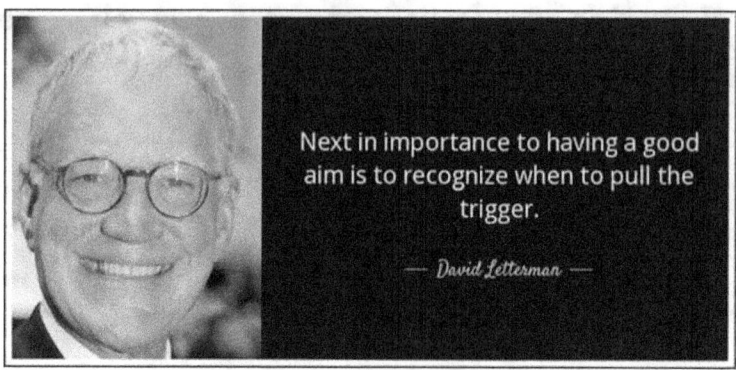

Next in importance to having a good aim is to recognize when to pull the trigger.

— David Letterman —

A myofascial trigger point (MTrP) is a hypersensitive, palpable nodule within a taut skeletal muscle band (Simons, Travell, and Simons). Typically, 2–10 mm in size, these nodules are tender upon palpation and may cause characteristic referred pain, motor dysfunction, and autonomic responses.

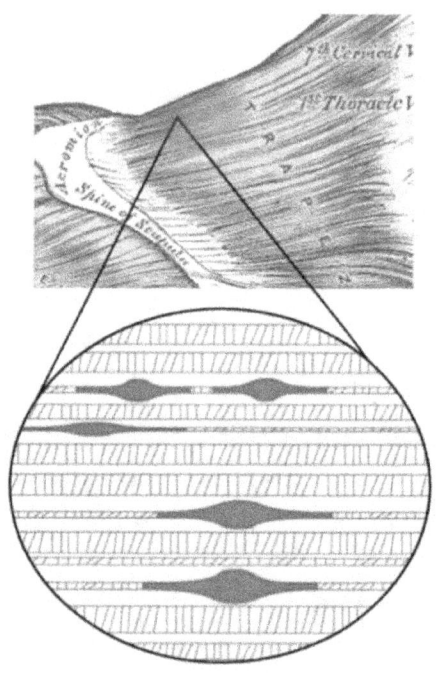

Fig. 13.1
Myofascial Trigger Point Structure

MTrPs commonly arise in the myofascia, particularly in the muscle belly where the motor endplate enters (primary or central MTrP). When these trigger points cause regional pain originating from soft tissue, the condition is referred to as Myofascial Pain Syndrome (MPS). MPS often presents with somatic dysfunction, psychological distress, and impaired daily functioning. Patients may exhibit muscle and fascial tenderness at multiple focal points, each just a few millimeters in diameter. Additionally, MTrPs may occur in ligamentous structures such as the anterior longitudinal spinal ligament, ligamentum patellae, fibular collateral ligament, and tendon-to-bone junctions. If left untreated, MTrPs can cause degenerative changes in adjacent joints due to sustained dysfunction.

Types of Trigger Points

- **Active vs Inactive (Latent):**
  - *Active MTrPs* are painful upon palpation and produce referred pain patterns. Typically, central MTrPs are active, and some satellite MTrPs may also be active.

- o *Inactive MTrPs* are not painful but can present as palpable lumps. These may contribute to muscle stiffness and may become active if provoked by trauma or strain.
- **Primary vs Secondary:**
  - o *Primary (central) MTrPs* are found in the muscle belly, producing local and referred pain.
  - o *Secondary (satellite) MTrPs* emerge in muscles surrounding a primary MTrP, usually resolving when the primary MTrP is treated. In severe postural abnormalities, multiple primary and secondary MTrPs may coexist, forming a diffuse pattern known as *diffuse MTrP*.

Causes of Trigger Points

Multiple factors contribute to the formation of MTrPs:

- Prolonged low-level muscle contractions
- Uneven intramuscular pressure
- Direct trauma

Additional associated factors include:

- Sedentary lifestyle (especially in adults aged 25–55, with 45% being men)
- Poor posture (e.g., swayback, crossed postures, telephone posture)
- Muscle overuse and microtrauma (e.g., weightlifting)
- Chronic psychological stress, anxiety, and depression
- Vitamin deficiencies
- Sleep disturbances
- Joint hypermobility
- Age-related muscular changes

Symptoms of Trigger Points

Pain is the hallmark symptom. Other associated symptoms may include:

- Headaches
- Generalised muscle aches
- Morning stiffness
- Temporomandibular joint (TMJ) dysfunction
- Tinnitus
- Movement-induced pain
- Muscle weakness or imbalance

- Restricted range of motion
- Postural abnormalities

Diagnostic Features of Trigger Points

Palpable taut band with a discrete, tender nodule

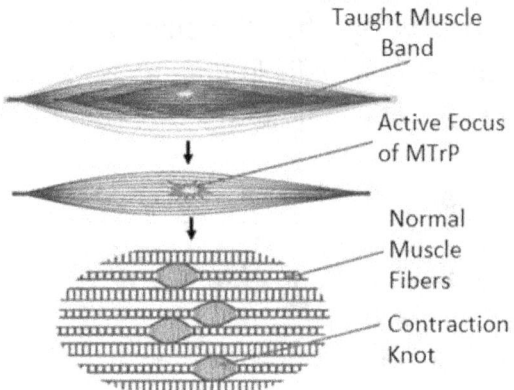

Fig 13.2 Myofascial Trigger Complex

Reproducible referred pain patterns that do not follow dermatomes, myotomes, or nerve root distributions

Absence of joint swelling or neurological deficits

Jump sign: An exaggerated pain reaction, often with involuntary movement or vocal response upon palpation

Local twitch response (LTR): A transient visible or palpable muscle contraction on snapping palpation or needling

These features are pathognomonic for MTrP and crucial for clinical diagnosis.

Locating Trigger Points

Identifying MTrPs is essential for effective pain management. No imaging or laboratory test confirms MTrPs; diagnosis relies on:

- Detailed clinical history
- Observation of movement patterns
- Pattern recognition of muscle-related pain

Two palpation techniques are employed:

- **Flat palpation**: Firm pressure applied with fingers/thumbs perpendicular to muscle fibres
- **Pincer palpation**: The muscle is grasped between the examiner's fingers

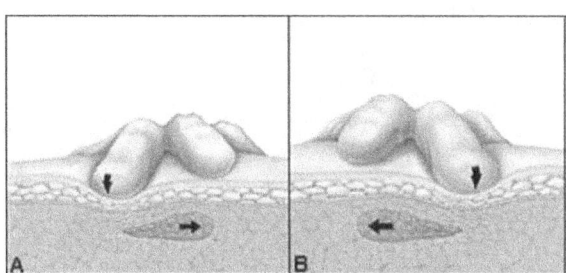

Fig. 13.3a Locating MTrP

Once a taut band is identified, the clinician searches its length for a discrete, hardened, tender nodule. Pressing this point should reproduce deep, dull, or aching pain, occasionally burning or tingling in superficial muscles. Patient recognition of this pain strengthens diagnostic certainty. The elicited *local twitch response* confirms the presence of an MTrP.

Management of Trigger Points

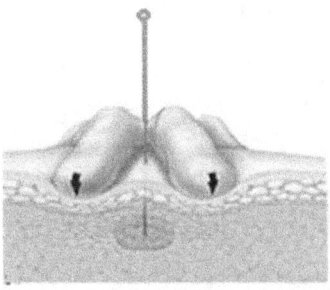

After accurate identification, treatment is straightforward. **Precise needling of the MTrP**—either dry needling or acupuncture—provides rapid and significant pain relief in over 97% of cases. Though other modalities exist (e.g., massage, ultrasound, stretching), none match the effectiveness of needling.

Fig. 13.4 Treating MTrP

MTrP Pain Maps

Referred pain from MTrPs follows predictable patterns, as mapped by Adrian White, Mike Cummings, and Jacqueline Filshie. Readers are encouraged to consult their comprehensive work, **An Introduction to Western Medical Acupuncture,** for further study.

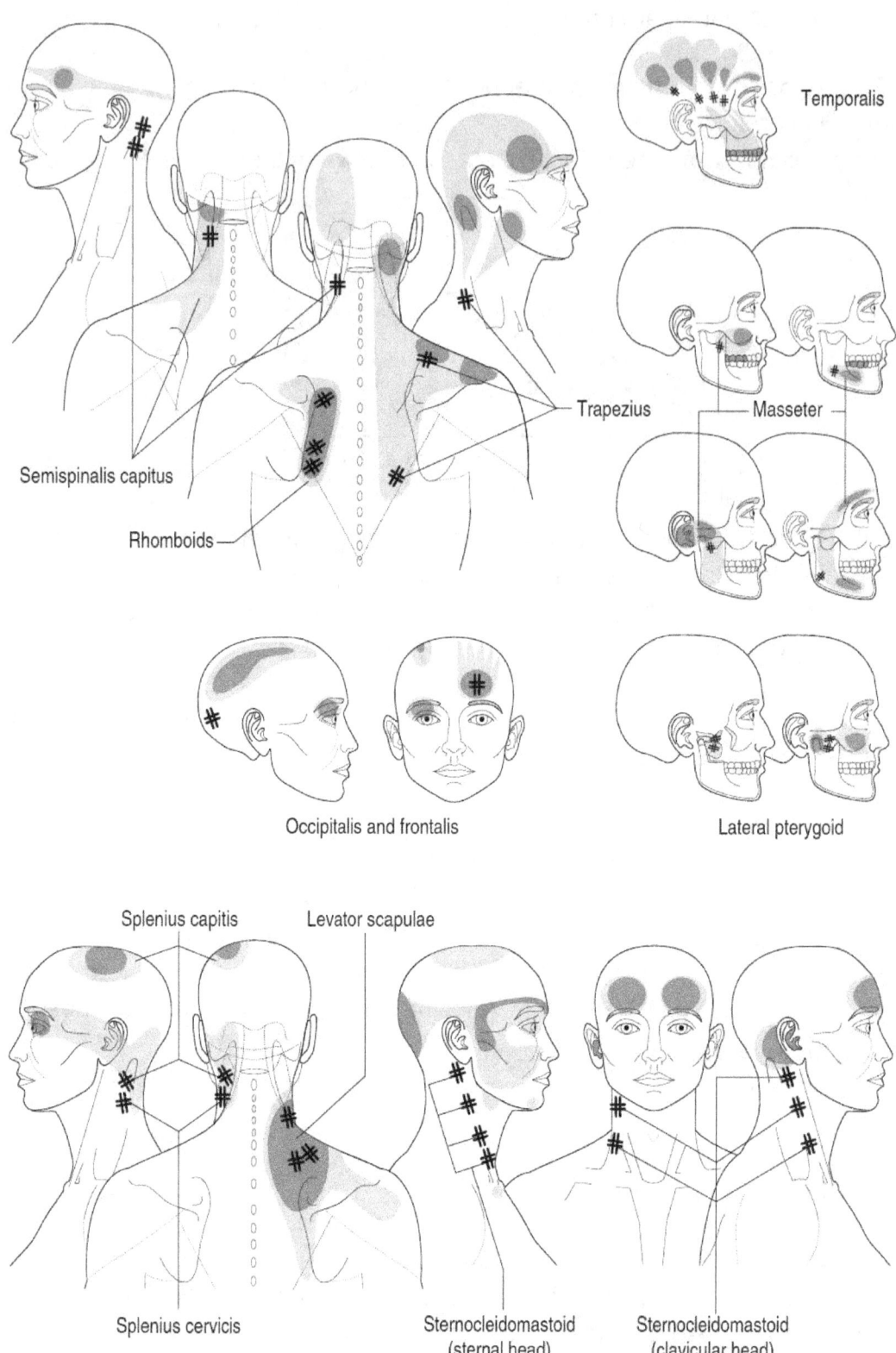

Fig. 13.5 MTrP on Head, Face and Neck and Reference Zones

Source Introduction to Western Medical Acupuncture
Adrian White, Mike Cumming and Jacquiline Filshie

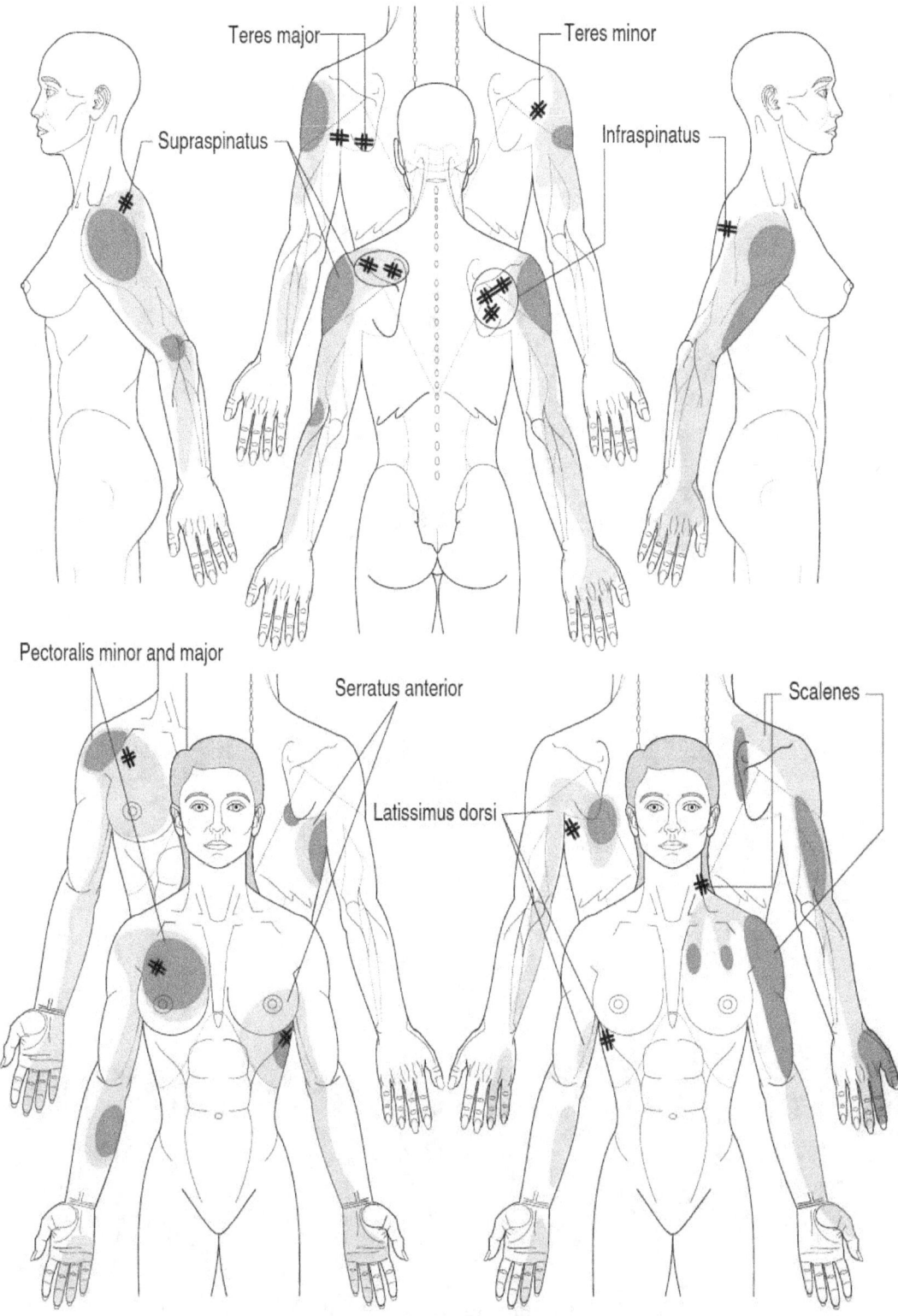

Fig. 13.6 MTrP on Shoulder and Arm and Reference Zones

Source Introduction to Western Medical Acupuncture
Adrian White, Mike Cumming and Jacquiline Filshie

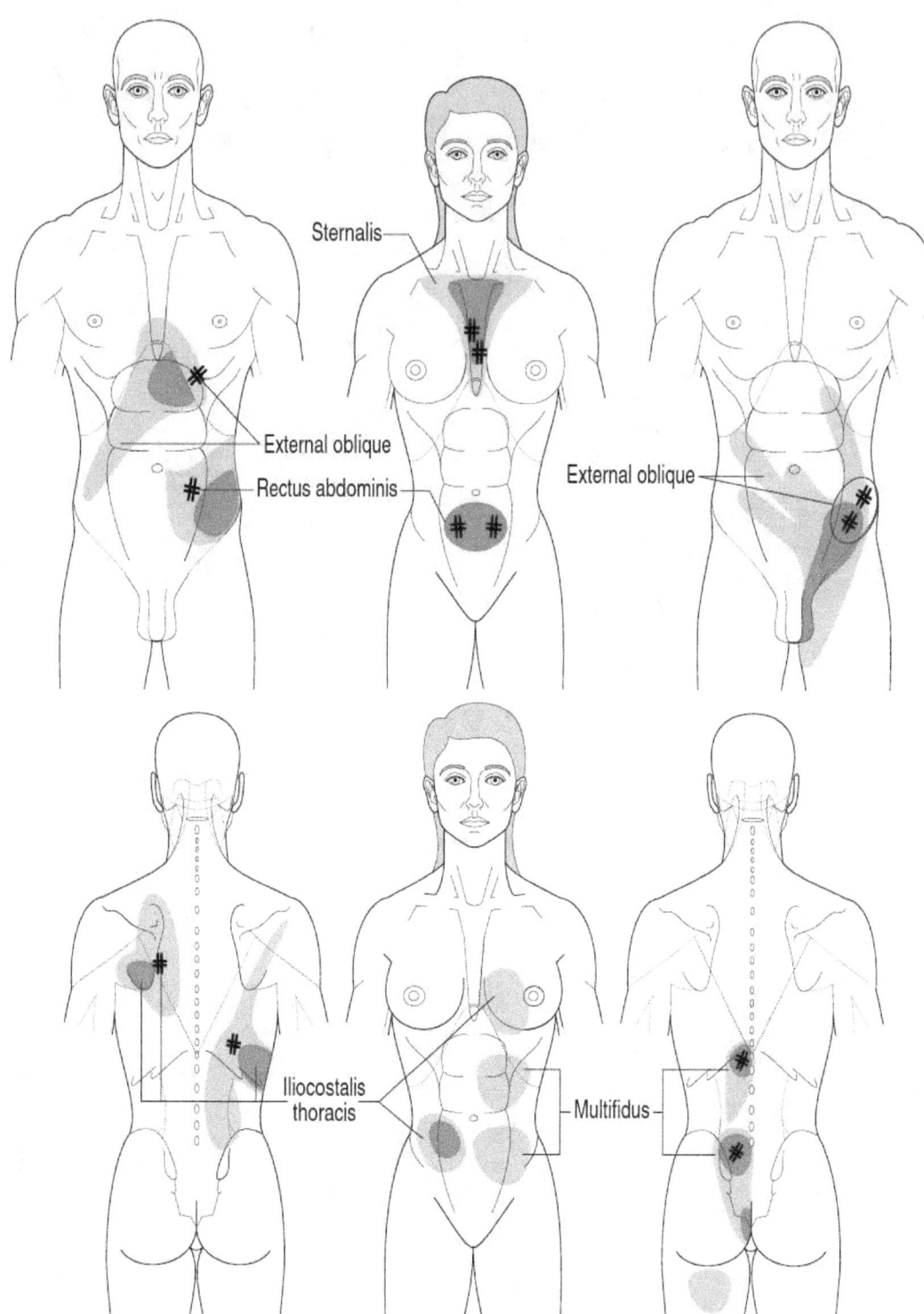

Fig. 13.7 MTrP on Thorax and Abdomen and Reference Zones

Source Introduction to Western Medical Acupuncture
Adrian White, Mike Cumming and Jacquiline Filshie

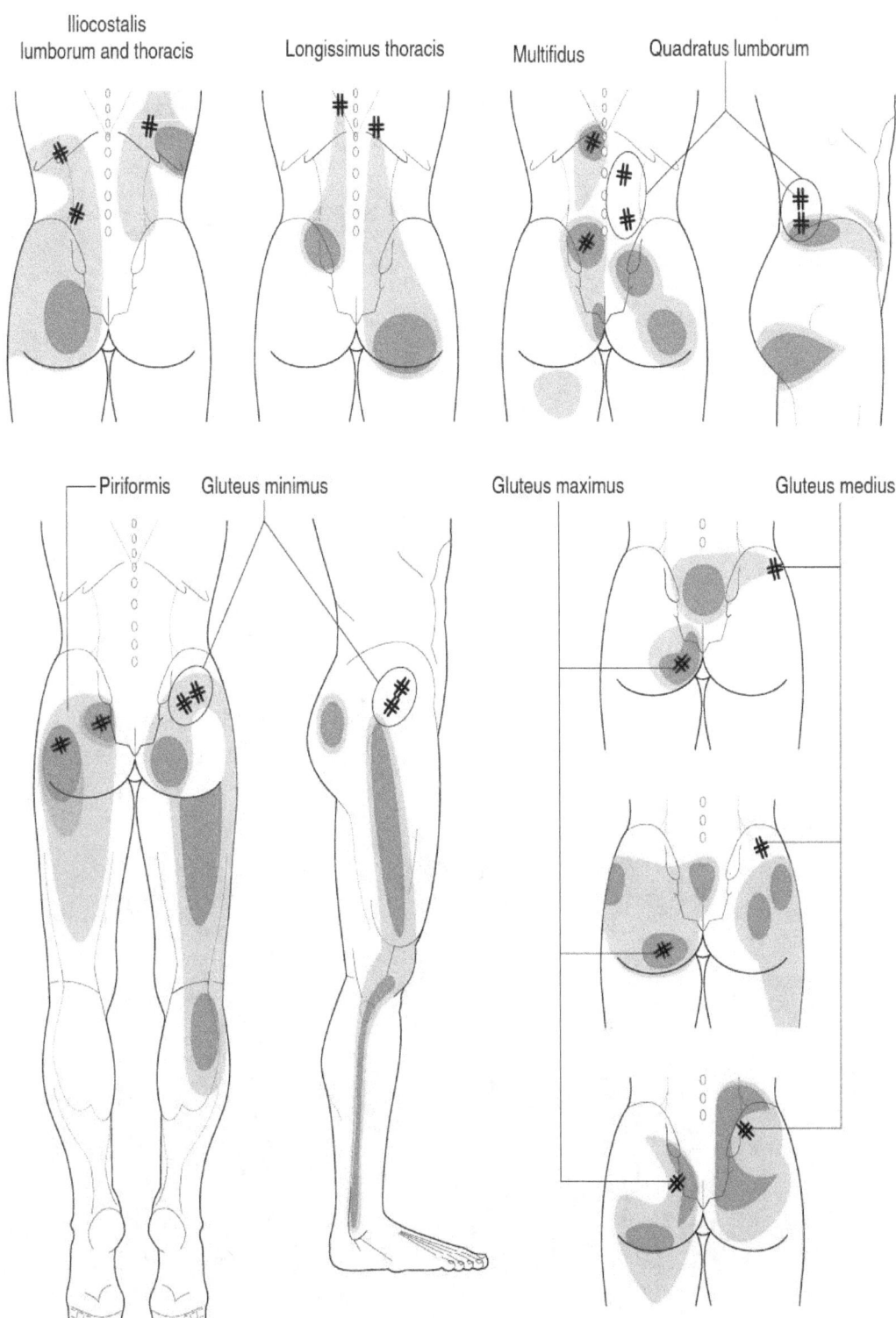

Fig. 13.8 MTrP on Low Back Hip Girdle and Reference Zones

Source Introduction to Western Medical Acupuncture
Adrian White, Mike Cumming and Jacquiline Filshie

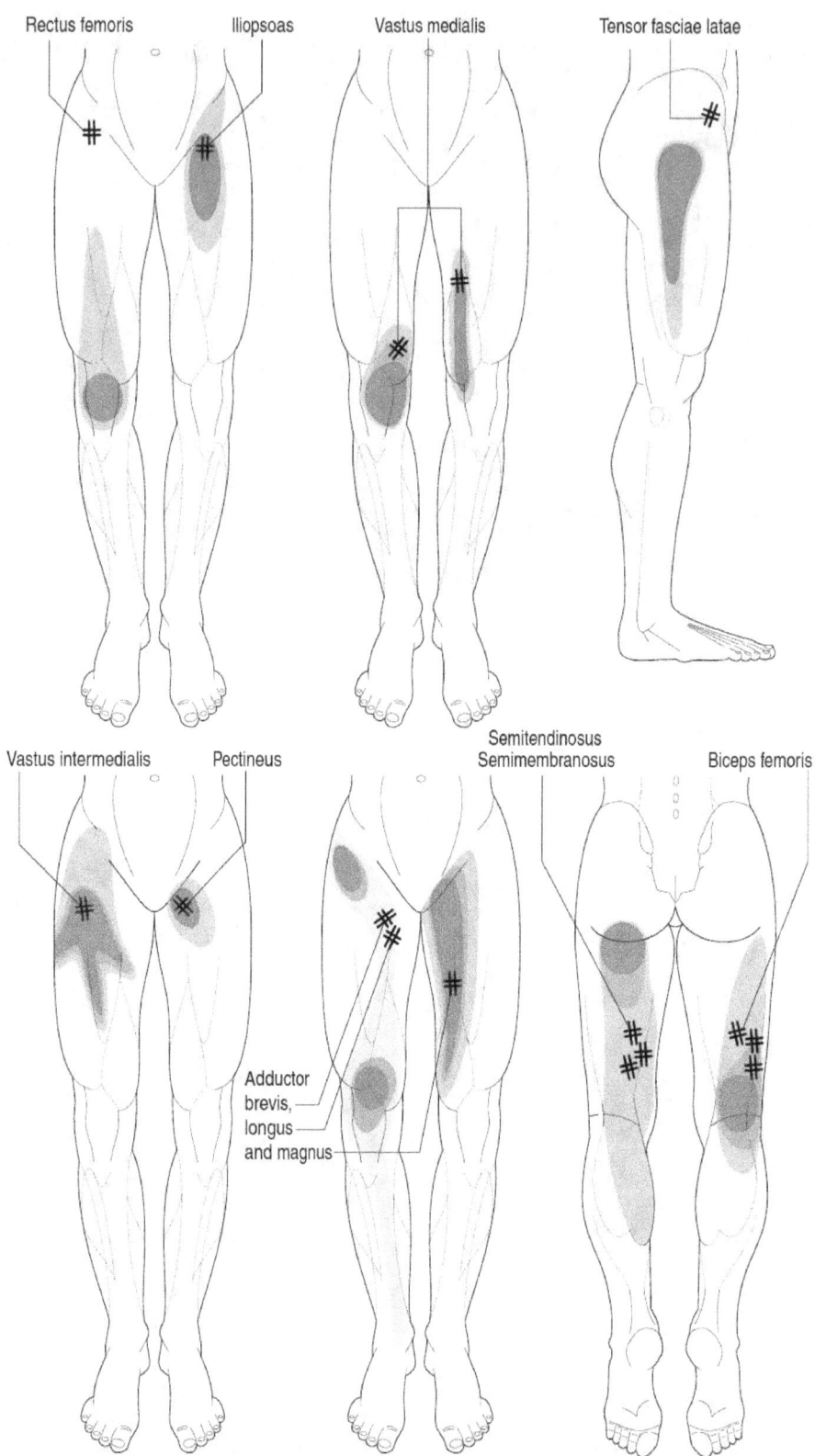

Fig. 13.9 MTrP on Lower Limb and Reference Zones

Source Introduction to Western Medical Acupuncture
Adrian White, Mike Cumming and Jacquiline Filshie

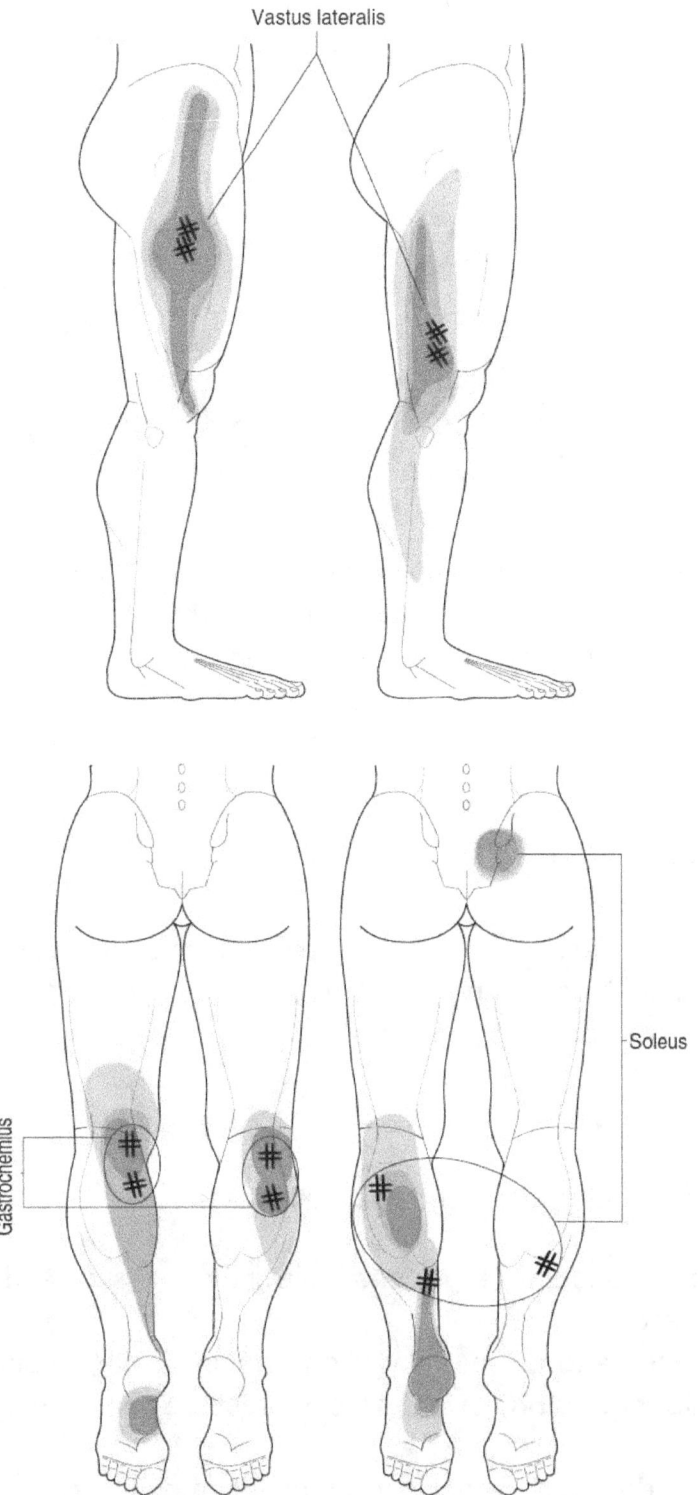

Fig. 13.10 MTrP on Vastus Lateralis, Gastrocnemius
& Soleus and Reference Zones

Source Introduction to Western Medical Acupuncture
Adrian White, Mike Cumming and Jacquiline Filshie

-Modern Acupuncture-

14. Bloodletting Therapy

"Let the blood flow, and the disease go." – Ancient Medical Adage.

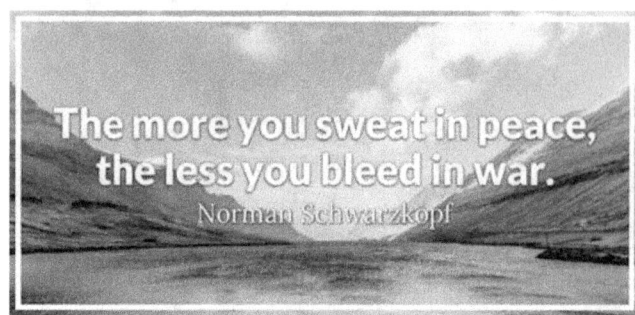

Bloodletting therapy is the deliberate withdrawal of a small quantity of blood from the body surface at specific anatomical sites for therapeutic purposes. This technique, one of the oldest in medical history, has been documented in ancient Chinese, Greek, and Ayurvedic medical systems. It is advantageous in resistant conditions where conventional acupuncture or drug therapies fail to relieve pain, congestion, or systemic imbalance.

Historical Background

In Ayurveda, *Raktamokshana*—bloodletting by leeches or surgical methods—has been used to expel "impure blood." It persisted for over 2,000 years in Europe and was once considered a panacea for most ailments.

Mechanism of Action

Modern research suggests that bloodletting stimulates:

- **Reflex neurovascular responses**, relieving congestion and restoring microcirculation.
- **Local detoxification**, especially when combined with cupping.
- **Autonomic regulation**, lowering blood pressure and calming excitatory neural activity.
- **Immune modulation**, reducing inflammatory mediators in chronic disorders.

Techniques of Bloodletting

A. Collateral Pricking Technique

- Ideal for visible venules (e.g., UB 40, LI 11).
- Apply a rubber band proximally to distend the vein.
- Hold a disposable needle at 15–30° and puncture the vein bevel up.
- Let 0.5–2 ml of blood drip naturally.
- Clean and compress with sterile cotton after bleeding.

B. Pinching and Pricking Technique

- Used at distal points on fingers, toes, or auricle.
- Pinch the area firmly to induce hyperaemia.
- Prick superficially (1–2 mm) and squeeze 1–3 drops.
- Applied in micro-acupuncture and auriculotherapy.

C. Clumpy Pricking Technique

- Multiple shallow pricks are made over red, swollen, or inflamed skin.
- Often combined with **fire cupping** for suction-enhanced drainage.
- Effective for furuncles, carbuncles, or herpes outbreaks.

Some Clinical Indications

Condition	Suggested Site	Rationale
Resistant sciatica	UB 40 (Weizhong)	Unlocks stagnation and clears meridian obstruction
Osteoarthritis with joint swelling	Periarticular veins	Reduces local pressure and inflammation
Hypertension	Ear apex, Taiyang region	Balances sympathetic tone
Acute tonsillitis	Shaoshang (LU 11)	Clears heat from the throat and lung meridian
Herpes zoster	Local dermatomal veins	Reduces neural congestion and relieves burning pain
Acne and skin boils.	Back shu points with cupping	Clears internal heat and toxins

Some Examples of Bloodletting

Bloodletting at Point 77.18

Title: Venous Bloodletting on the Lower Limb and Back
Description: Controlled venous bloodletting performed at point 77.18 using a sterile gauze pad to collect blood after puncture. This site is effective for sciatica, leg pain, and venous congestion.

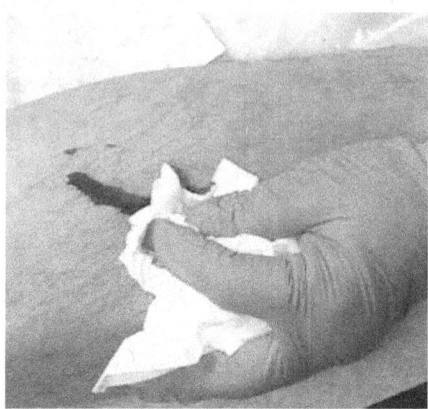

Blood Letting

Headache Relief Points (Tung 1010.xx Series) Fig. 14.1

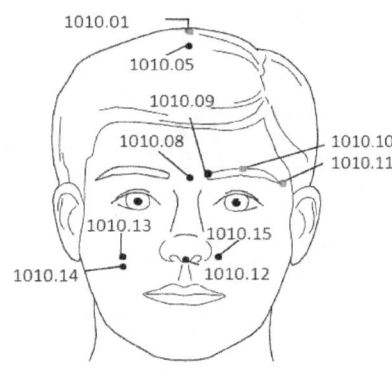

Fig. 14.1

Title: Tung Head and Face Points for Neurological Conditions
Description: The 1010.xx Tung acupuncture points on the face and scalp, including 1010.01 (vertex), 1010.10–11 (temples), and 1010.15 (infraorbital), are highly effective in treating trigeminal neuralgia, facial palsy, and migraine when combined with bloodletting.

Jinjin and Yuye (Ex HN 12, 13) Fig. 14.2

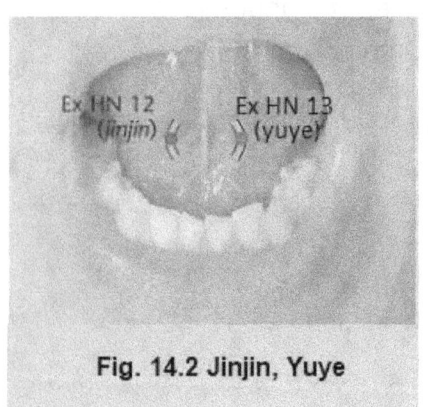

Fig. 14.2 Jinjin, Yuye

Title: Emergency Bloodletting Points under the Tongue
Description: Jinjin (Ex HN 12) and Yuye (Ex HN 13) are under the tongue and used in emergencies such as aphasia, coma, and stroke. Bloodletting at these points may restore consciousness rapidly.

GB 41–43 on the Foot Fig. 14.3

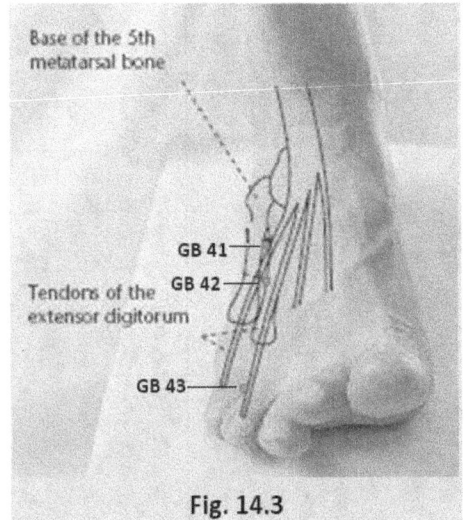

Fig. 14.3

Title: Bloodletting Points for Gall Bladder Channel Disorders
Description: GB 41 to GB 43 are distal points used for migraine, eye disorders, and lateral body pain. These sites are prone to resistant lateral leg and hip pain syndromes.

LI 15 and SJ 14 for Frozen Shoulder Fig. 14.4

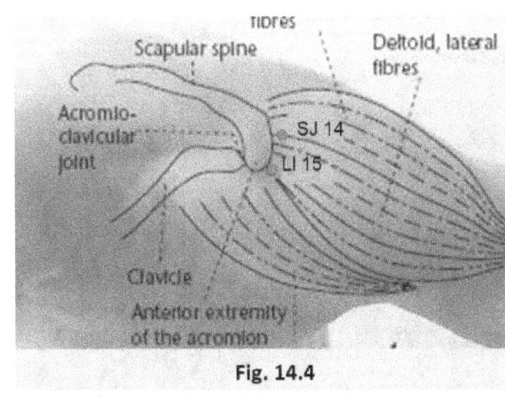

Fig. 14.4

Title: Bloodletting in the Shoulder Region for Adhesive Capsulitis
Description: LI 15 and SJ 14 are commonly used for shoulder stiffness and pain. Bloodletting here reduces inflammation and improves joint mobility, especially in frozen shoulder.

UB 40, UB 56, and UB 57 for Lower Limb Pain Fig. 14.5

Title: Key Bloodletting Points on the Posterior Leg
Description: UB 40 is crucial for low back pain and sciatica, while UB 56 and UB 57 target calf spasms and plantar fasciitis. Bloodletting facilitates decompression and pain relief.

UB 57 for Haemorrhoids Fig. 14.6

Title: Bloodletting at UB 57 for Anorectal Disorders
Description: UB 57, located midway between the popliteal crease and heel, is

specifically indicated for internal and external haemorrhoids. Bloodletting here improves venous drainage and reduces anal swelling.

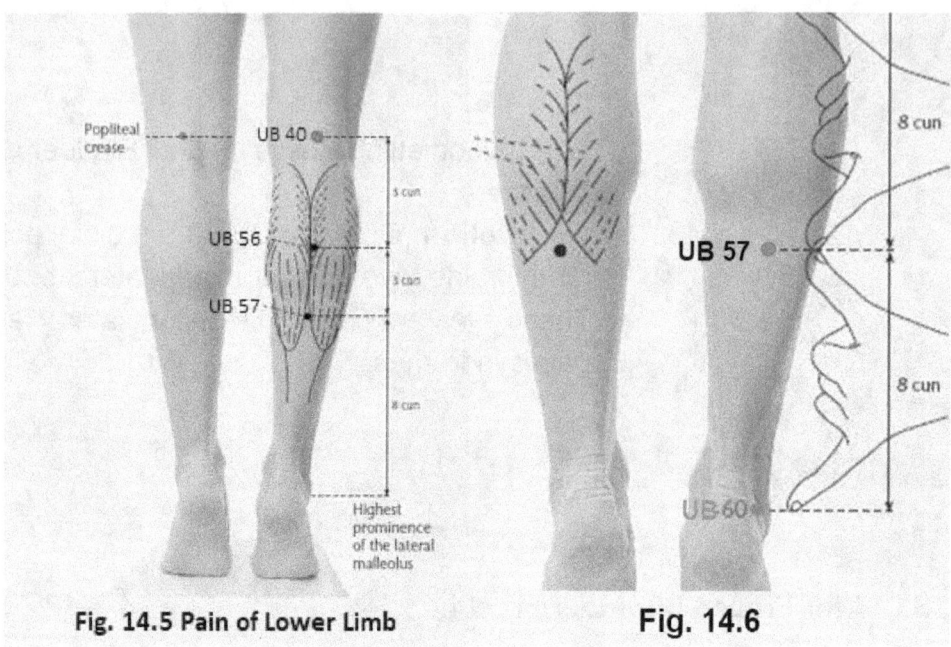

Fig. 14.5 Pain of Lower Limb   Fig. 14.6

Ex B 8 and UB 31–34 for Gynaecological Conditions 14.7

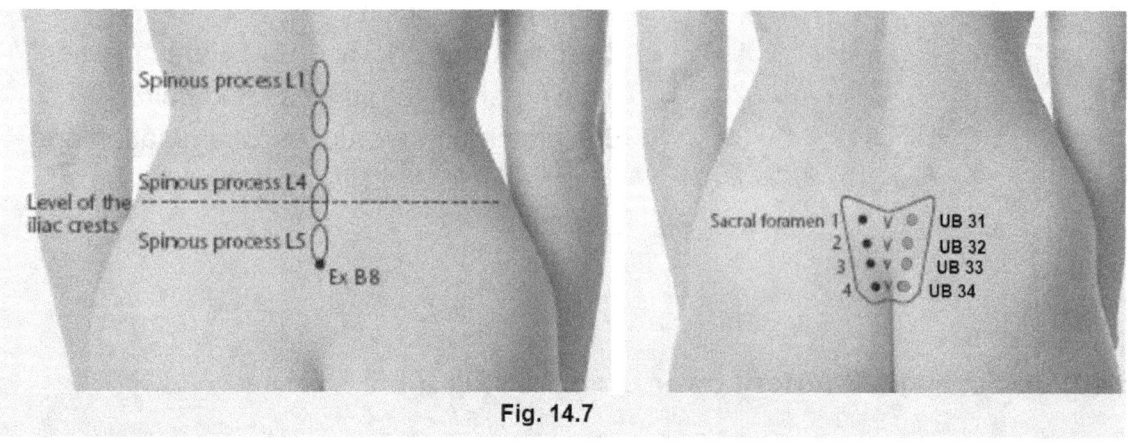

Fig. 14.7

Title: Sacral Bloodletting Points for Pelvic Pain and Dysmenorrhoea
Description: Points over the sacral foramina (UB 31–34) and Ex B8 treat menstrual disorders, pelvic inflammatory disease, and lumbar pain. Bloodletting here modulates autonomic pelvic innervation and improves uterine blood flow.

Jing-Well Points of the Hands and Feet
Title: *Fig. 14.8 – Jing-Well Points on Hands and Feet*
Description:

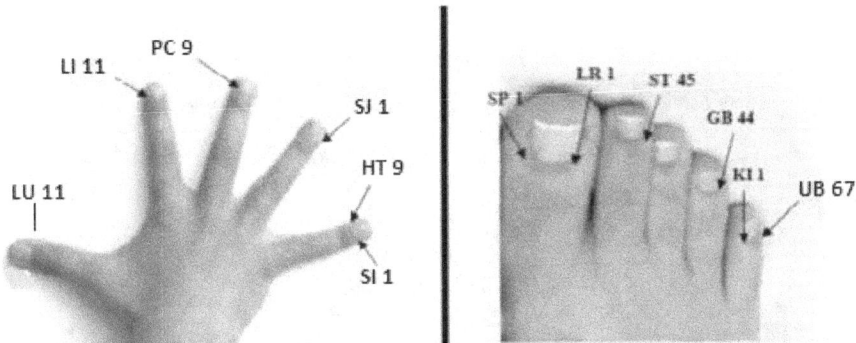

Fig. 14.8 Jing well Points

This diagram shows the Jing-Well points located at the tips of the fingers and toes, each representing the starting (or ending) point of the twelve primary acupuncture meridians. These points are highly sensitive and are commonly used in emergency acupuncture for revival, mental disorders, and acute conditions. Notable points include LU 11 (Lung), LI 1 (large intestine), PC 9 (Pericardium), and ST 45 (Stomach), among others.

Precautions and Contraindications

- Avoid in patients with coagulopathies, severe anaemia, or hypotension.
- Do not exceed 5 ml in frail patients.
- Always use sterile, disposable instruments.
- Monitor for dizziness, especially during the first session.

Post-Procedural Care

- Apply gentle pressure for 30–60 seconds.
- Cleanse the area with antiseptic.
- Observe for signs of persistent bleeding or secondary infection.
- Advise adequate hydration.

Conclusion

Bloodletting is a powerful adjunctive therapy for chronic and resistant conditions. When applied rationally, it offers immediate symptom relief, improved circulation, and homeostatic balance, without the side effects associated with pharmacotherapy. In the hands of trained practitioners, bloodletting is a safe, cost-effective, and potent acupuncture modality.

15. Electroacupuncture

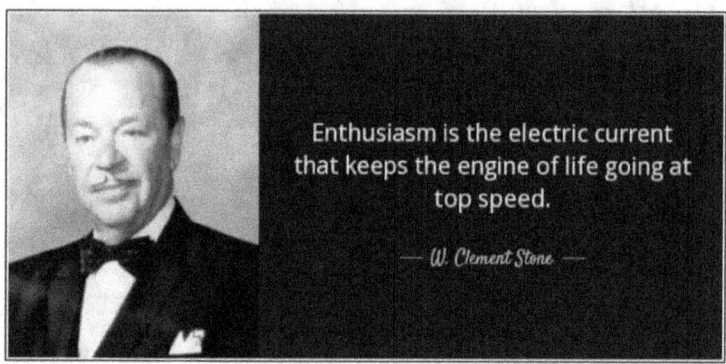

Enthusiasm is the electric current that keeps the engine of life going at top speed.

— W. Clement Stone —

Electroacupuncture involves stimulating acupuncture points using a low-intensity electrical current. Two acupuncture needles serve as electrodes—one positive and one negative—through which impulses are passed across tissues. These needles are connected via small clips to an electroacupuncture device capable of generating various pulse types. The frequency and intensity of stimulation can be customised according to the therapeutic requirement. As the current disperses through a larger tissue area than manual needling alone, precise point location sometimes becomes less critical.

Actions of Electroacupuncture

Electroacupuncture provides more substantial and sustained analgesia than traditional acupuncture, especially in musculoskeletal disorders. The electrical stimulus induces cell membrane depolarisation, leading to faster nerve conduction to the central nervous system. Three neuroanatomical centres—the spinal cord, mesencephalon, and pituitary gland are activated and release endogenous neurochemicals that modulate pain perception.

In addition to analgesia, electroacupuncture exerts:

- Muscle relaxation
- Sedative and hypnotic effects
- Antidepressant and anti-inflammatory actions

Different frequencies elicit specific neurohormonal responses:

- Low-frequency (1–10 Hz) stimulation promotes the release of enkephalins and β-endorphins from the brain and spinal cord.
- High-frequency (50–200 Hz) stimulation enhances dynorphin release in the spinal cord.

- These opioids, along with serotonin and oxytocin, mediate profound pain relief and emotional balance.

Thus, the distal stimulation of acupuncture points influences central neural pathways, validating the efficacy of the neurohumoral mechanism behind electroacupuncture.

Applications of Electroacupuncture

Electroacupuncture is particularly useful when:

- Stronger and more consistent stimulation is desired.
- Manual stimulation needs to be substituted.
- Pain relief, muscle relaxation, or anti-inflammatory effects are required.
- Treating neurological disorders, muscle spasms, or acute nausea (e.g., from chemotherapy).
- Manage skin conditions such as acne or internal colic like renal colic.

Modulating systemic responses, such as lowering blood pressure or improving cardiac health via endorphin release.

Electroacupuncture Machine Specifications

Modern electroacupuncture devices should ensure **maximum safety** and **precise control**. Minimum features include:

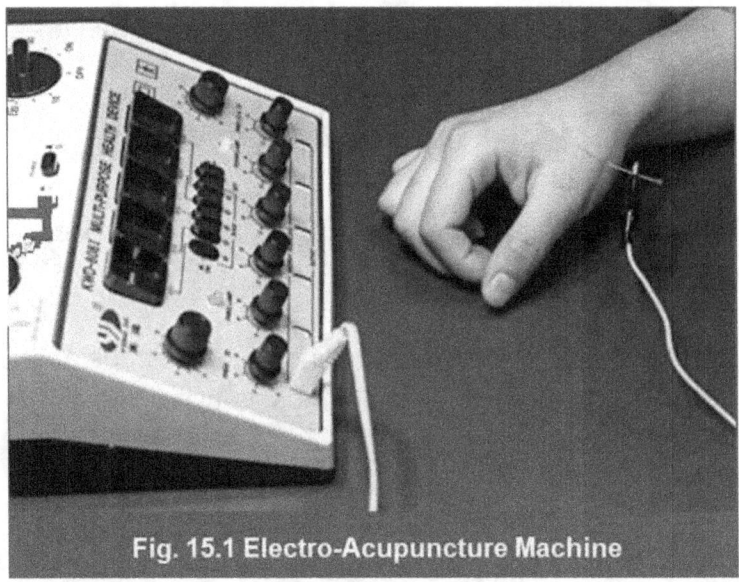

Fig. 15.1 Electro-Acupuncture Machine

- Two or more independent channels with polarity control.
- Adjustable settings for:

- o Modulation type: continuous, burst, dense-disperse.
- o Polarity: positive, negative, or biphasic.
- o Frequency: shown in Hz (typically 2–200 Hz).
- o Intensity: displayed in mA (usually 0.5–2 mA).
- o Timer: pre-settable treatment duration in minutes.

Care and Contraindications

Electroacupuncture must be used with caution. It is contraindicated in:

- Patients with pacemakers, deep brain stimulators, or other electronic implants.
- Individuals with a history of seizures or epilepsy.
- Placement directly over the heart.
- Cross-body stimulation, where the current path crosses the midline.

Electrode options:

- Alligator clips (for needle connection)
- Probes with metal tips
- TENS pad terminals

Technique of Electroacupuncture

- The patient should lie down comfortably, free from distraction.
- Acupuncture points are selected as per classical manual needling protocols.
- Whenever possible, distal points are preferred. The painful area should lie between the two electrodes.

Connect LI 4 (right hand) and LV 3 or 77.07 (left leg) for right shoulder pain.

- The patient should be encouraged to focus mentally and occasionally move the affected area.
- Sensations expected:
  - o High-frequency (15–200 Hz): tingling or paraesthesia.
  - o Low-frequency (1–10 Hz): visible muscle twitches.

Frequency guidelines:

- High-frequency (segmental): fast-acting, used in acute or subacute pain.
- Low-frequency (extra-segmental): generalised, longer-lasting effect.
- Mixed-frequency (e.g., 2 Hz alternating with 80 Hz): combines both benefits for chronic conditions.

Session duration: Typically, 30–45 minutes. Patients should rest for 5 minutes post-treatment.

Best Practice Settings (Author's Recommendation)

- 10 Hz for chronic pain
- 50 Hz for acute pain
- Burst modulation
- Unipolar stimulation
- Rectangular wave shape

While evidence remains inconclusive, these settings have yielded reliable clinical results. Practitioners are advised to explore and refine parameters through safe experimentation.

Transcutaneous Electrical Nerve Stimulation (TENS)

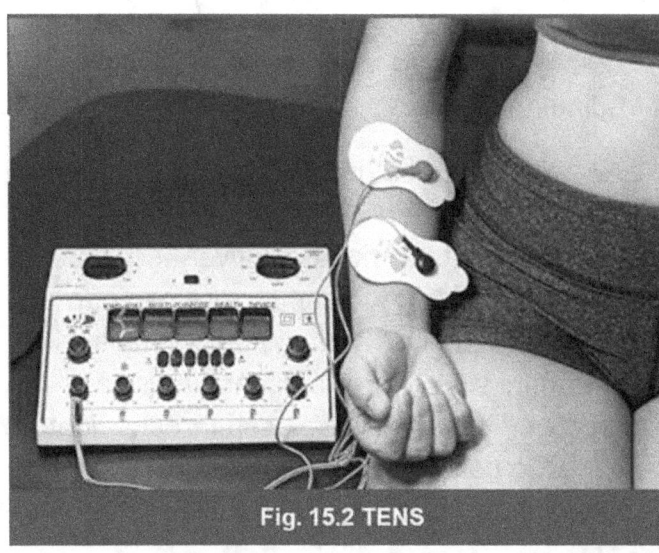
Fig. 15.2 TENS

TENS is a non-invasive, needle-free method using surface electrodes to relieve pain. Though less effective than electroacupuncture in depth penetration, TENS is useful for:

- Short-term pain management
- Wound healing and tendon repair
- Skin flap survival post-surgery

It likely works via neurochemical release, improved blood flow, and tissue repair stimulation.

Acupuncture Pen

A miniaturised, portable version of TENS, the **acupuncture pen** delivers low-frequency (1–2 Hz) impulses directly to pain points. It is helpful for:

- Back and joint pain
- Sports injuries
- Migraine and headache
- Fatigue, toothache, and even hangovers

It is safe, cumulative, and overdose-free. It is also usable through light clothing. Some devices claim effectiveness for non-invasive acupuncture applications.

Acupuncture Pen:

A smaller version of Transcutaneous Electrical Nerve Stimulation (TENS) is an easy but equally effective alternative for relief and pain management.

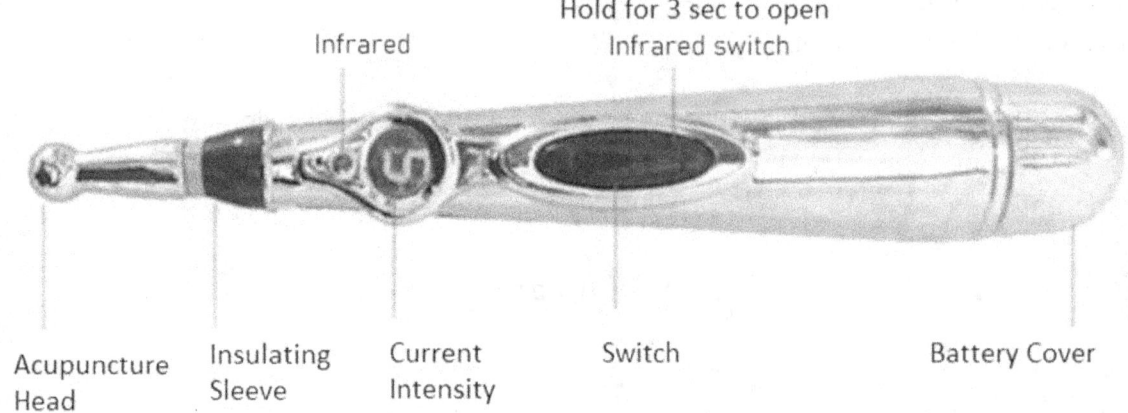

Fig. 15.3 Electrical Stimulation Pen

This device uses a low-frequency (1 - 2 Hz) stimulator fed by quartz crystals. The pen is held against the pain point, and a button is pressed; the patient receives a small electrical impulse that acts similarly. Repeated treatments work cumulatively, so more severe conditions may be treated over an extended period. An acupuncture pen can relieve backache, shoulder pain, arm and leg pain, headache and migraine, tennis elbow, sports injuries, and sciatica. It has no harmful side effects and can be used as often as required. It is impossible to "overdose," and it can even be used through light clothing. It is claimed that stimulation pens can also be used for non-invasive acupuncture to relieve many everyday conditions, such as tired eyes, toothache, fatigue, and even a hangover.

-Modern Acupuncture-

16. Acupressure and Other

Allied Traditional Chinese Therapies

Acupressure is a non-invasive therapeutic technique that involves applying manual pressure to specific points on the body surface to achieve desired physiological effects. These points are usually located on meridians recognised in acupuncture theory. Acupressure is rooted in the same principles as acupuncture but uses fingers, palms, elbows, or blunt tools instead of needles.

It is especially beneficial for:

- Needle-sensitive individuals
- Geriatric or paediatric patients
- Self-treatment or remote care protocols

Acupressure is widely used worldwide, particularly in home remedies, physiotherapy, and integrative medicine. It is now supported by growing scientific evidence validating its effects on pain modulation, emotional balance, and autonomic regulation.

Mechanism of Action

Both traditional meridian theory and modern neurophysiology can explain the action of acupressure:

- **Local Mechanical Stimulation:** Pressure on acupoints stimulates cutaneous mechanoreceptors and underlying muscle spindles, which send afferent signals via A-delta and C-fibres to the spinal cord and brainstem.
- **Neurohormonal Release:** Mechanical stimulation releases endogenous opioids such as endorphins, enkephalins, and serotonin. These chemicals help reduce pain, induce relaxation, and modulate mood.
- **Gate Control Theory:** Acupressure may close the "gate" to pain perception in the spinal cord by activating non-nociceptive fibres, thereby inhibiting pain signals to the brain.
- **Autonomic Nervous System Balance:** Regular stimulation of specific acupoints may reduce sympathetic overactivity and enhance parasympathetic tone, helping regulate heart rate, respiration, and digestive function.

Techniques of Acupressure

Different techniques are used based on condition severity, patient age, and therapeutic intent:

Technique	Method
Finger Pressure	Use the tip or pad of the thumb or index finger to apply steady, circular, or pulsatile pressure.
Palm Pressure	Broader surface contact; used for abdominal, lumbar, or thoracic areas.
Knuckle Pressure	Focused deep pressure on larger muscular areas or stubborn points.
Elbow Pressure	Used by therapists to target deep trigger points in the back or gluteal.
Tool-assisted Pressure	Blunt tools (e.g., acupressure probes, spoons, or rollers) for precision or self-treatment.

Duration: Each point is typically pressed for 30 seconds to 2 minutes.
Frequency: Once or twice daily for chronic conditions; more frequently in acute issues.

Clinical Indications

Acupressure has shown benefits in the following conditions:

Condition	Effective Points	Remarks
Headache & Migraine	LI 4, GB 20, Taiyang	Relieves pain, tension, and vascular spasm
Insomnia	HT 7, Anmian, Yintang	Calms Shen and promotes sleep
Dysmenorrhoea	SP 6, Ren 4, LI 4	Regulates blood flow, relieves cramping
Constipation	ST 36, LI 11, SP 15	Stimulates bowel motility
Anxiety & Palpitations	PC 6, HT 7, REN 17	Harmonises heart and mind
Shoulder Pain	LI 15, SJ 14, SI 11	Releases muscular tension
Knee Pain	ST 35, GB 34, UB 40	Enhances local circulation

Special Applications

1. Auricular Acupressure:
Small seeds (e.g., Vaccaria seeds) or metal beads are taped on auricular points.

Continuous mild stimulation improves conditions like hypertension, insomnia, addiction, and weight control.

2. Acupressure Bands and Mats:

Commercially available wristbands (for nausea) and foot mats stimulate reflex zones and are helpful for travel or home care.

3. Emotional First Aid:

A technique called "Emotional Freedom Technique (EFT)" combines acupressure with affirmations to help manage emotional trauma, PTSD, and stress.

Safety and Precautions

- Avoid pressing over open wounds, varicose veins, fractures, or inflamed skin.
- Excessive pressure may cause bruising, especially in elderly or bleeding-prone individuals.
- Pregnant women should avoid stimulating forbidden points such as LI 4, SP 6, and BL 60 unless under expert supervision.
- Always ensure hand hygiene and use blunt tools to avoid accidental skin injury.

Advantages of Acupressure

- Painless and non-invasive
- Self-administered with minimal training
- Safe for all age groups
- Cost-effective and portable
- A valuable adjunct to acupuncture and physiotherapy

Conclusion

Acupressure is an invaluable modality in integrative medical practice. While its principles are derived from traditional Chinese medicine, its effectiveness can now be understood through modern neurophysiology. It empowers patients with a self-care tool, offers therapists a non-invasive intervention, and bridges conventional and holistic care. When used judiciously, acupressure relieves symptoms and enhances the body's natural healing mechanisms.

Moxibustion

Moxibustion is a traditional warmth-based therapy that involves burning dried herbal substances—primarily **moxa**, made from the leaves of *Artemisia vulgaris* (Chinese

Mugwort)—near or directly on the skin at specific acupuncture points. The principal therapeutic goals are to warm meridians, invigorate the flow of Qi and blood, expel cold and dampness, and restore balance within the organ systems.

There are two primary forms of moxibustion:

- **Direct Moxibustion:** Small moxa cones are placed directly on the skin and lit. They may be removed before burning the skin or allowed to burn down for scarring effects.
- **Indirect Moxibustion:** The moxa is burned above the skin, typically held over an acupuncture point or attached to the end of an inserted needle.

Moxibustion is widely used for:

- Warming the uterus in cases of infertility
- Treating cold-damp arthralgia
- Correcting breech presentation in pregnancy (notably at **UB 67**)
- Boosting immunity and preventing diseases through general tonification

Cupping Therapy

Cupping therapy involves creating a sub-atmospheric pressure (vacuum) inside glass, plastic, or bamboo cups and applying them to the skin to stimulate the underlying tissues. The suction mobilises blood flow, clears stagnation, and promotes healing.

There are two primary types:

- **Dry Cupping:** Only suction is applied; the skin remains intact.
- **Wet Cupping (Hijama):** A small skin incision is made before cupping to extract a small amount of blood.

Vacuum Generation Methods:

- Flame method: A flame is briefly introduced into a glass cup to consume oxygen, creating suction upon skin contact.
- Mechanical suction: A hand pump or valve system removes air after placing the cup.

Common Application Sites: The back, shoulders, chest, thighs, and occasionally the face. Cups may remain static or be moved after oil is applied to facilitate gliding.

Mode of Action of Cupping

Cupping therapy appears to exert its effects through a combination of mechanical, circulatory, neurological, and immunological mechanisms:

- Increases peripheral blood circulation
- Enhances local anaerobic metabolism
- Modulates inflammatory mediators
- Raises pain thresholds through cutaneous stimulation
- Stimulates immune function by influencing cytokine activity
- Relieves stagnation of Qi and Blood by drawing them to the surface

Clinical Indications for Cupping

Cupping is used for both therapeutic and preventive purposes. Reported benefits include:

- Musculoskeletal conditions: Lower back pain, neck stiffness, shoulder pain, knee arthritis, sciatica
- Neurological disorders: Headache, migraine, facial paralysis
- Systemic conditions: Hypertension, diabetes mellitus, asthma
- Peripheral neuropathies: Carpal tunnel syndrome
- Emotional and autonomic disorders

Side Effects of Cupping

Though generally safe, potential side effects include:

- **Mild:** Bruising, local pain, erythema, itching, fatigue
- **Moderate:** Small hematomas, headaches, vasovagal responses
- **Severe (rare):** Skin burns, abscesses, hyperpigmentation, or infections from poor technique

Recovery: Most bruising and marks resolve spontaneously within 7–10 days.

To avoid complications:

- Monitor suction strength and duration
- Avoid repeated cupping in the exact location within short intervals
- Use sterile technique in wet cupping

Contraindications for Cupping

Cupping should not be performed in the following conditions:

- Bleeding disorders (e.g., haemophilia) or use of anticoagulants
- Over large arteries, varicose veins, or deep vein thrombosis
- Over fractures, inflamed skin, or open wounds
- Severe dermatological conditions
- On or near orifices, the eyes, or mucosal surfaces
- In unwilling patients or those unable to communicate discomfort

Laser Acupuncture

Laser acupuncture involves stimulating acupuncture points using low-intensity, non-thermal laser light. This modality offers a painless, sterile, and minimally invasive alternative to traditional needle acupuncture.

Advantages:

- **No skin penetration**—ideal for paediatric, geriatric, and needle-phobic patients
- **Short treatment time**—10 to 60 seconds per point
- **Reduced risk** of infection or trauma
- **Portable**—suitable for remote or mobile healthcare settings

Clinical indications include:

- Musculoskeletal pain
- Neuropathies
- Wound healing
- Rehabilitation after stroke

While promising, the efficacy of laser acupuncture depends heavily on appropriate **wavelength, intensity, pulse frequency**, and **dosing protocols**. More high-quality research is needed for universal standardisation.

Embedding Therapy

Embedding therapy involves inserting absorbable material, such as sterile catgut, into acupuncture points for prolonged stimulation. The material is typically inserted via hypodermic needles into the subcutaneous layer.

Purpose: To provide continuous stimulation of points over several days or weeks.

Clinical applications: Chronic pain syndromes, obesity, and digestive disorders:

Contents of Volume 2

'Modern Acupuncture - *Learn from The Master'*

Sections III - Treatment of Diseases

References

I am indebted to the following books and their authors for their valuable contributions, without which this book would not have been possible.

A Manual of Acupuncture – Peter Deadman & Mazin Al-Khafaji with Kevin Baker

A Study on Acupuncture, Therapeutics, and Points – Yong

Acupuncture – Anatomical Approach – Houchi Dung, Curtis P Clogston

Acupuncture 1, 2, 3 – Richard Tan

Acupuncture for Dysphagia in Acute Stroke - Xie Y, Wang L, He J, Wu T

Acupuncture for Gastrointestinal and Hepato-biliary Disorders – David L. Diehl

Acupuncture in Musculoskeletal Medicine – Grant Cooper, Stuart Kahn, Paul Zucker

Acupuncture for Pain Management – Yuan Chin Lin, Eric Shen Zen Hsu

Acupuncture for Palliative Care – British Acupuncture Council

Acupuncture in Clinical Practice – Nadia Ellis

Acupuncture in Eye Disease – Eastland Press

Acupuncture in Modern Medicine – Lucy L. Chen, Tsung A. Chen

Acupuncture in Pain Management – Lucy Chen

Acupuncture in Practice – Anthony Campbell

Acupuncture Point Combination – Jeremy Ross

Acupuncture Textbook and Atlas – Gabriel Stux, Bruce Pomeranz

Acupuncture Theories and Evidence – Hong Hai

Acupuncture Therapy for Neurological Diseases – Ying Zia, Xiaoding Cao

Acupuncture Treatments for Head and Face Pain – David Legge

Acupuncture: Review and Analysis of Controlled Clinical Trials – World Health Organization

Advanced Electro-Medicine – Darren Starwynn

Advanced Tung Style Acupuncture, Anesthesiology, and Pain Management – James H Maher

Advanced Tung Style Acupuncture, Internal Medicine – James H. Maher

An Introduction to Western Medical Acupuncture – Adrian White, Mike Cummings, Jacqueline

Atlas of Acupuncture – www.AcupunctureProducts.com

Auricular Acupuncture Diagnosis – Marco Romoli

Biomedical Acupuncture for Sports and Trauma Rehabilitation – Yun-tao Ma Chen

Chinese Auricular Acupuncture – Skya Abbate

Clean Needle Technique – Council of Colleges of Acupuncture and Oriental Medicine

Clinical Practice Guideline of Acupuncture for Bell's Palsy – Xi Wu, Ying Li, Yi-Hui Zhu,

Clinical Acupuncture Scientific Basis – Gabriel Stux, Richard Hammerschlag

Contemporary Medical Acupuncture – Guan Yuan Jin, Jia X, Louis Jin

Cupping Therapy – Ilkay Zihni Chirali, David S. Rosenthal

Death – Point Striking – Erle Montaigue

Diagnosis in Chinese Medicine – Giovanni Maciocia

Diagnostic and Therapeutic System of Stroke, XNKQ – Shi Xuemin, Doherty-Gilman

Dr. Tan's Strategy of Twelve Magical Points – Richard Tan

Dr. Zhiyum Bo's Turtle Acupuncture – Zhiyum Bo

Effects of Electroacupuncture Vs. Manual Acupuncture on Human Brain – Vitaly Napadow

Efficacy of Acupuncture for Acute Migraine Attack – Lin-Peng Wang and Others

Electroacupuncture: An Introduction and its use for Peripheral facial Paralysis - David F Mayor

Lectures on Tung Acupuncture Points – Wei Chieh Young

Management of Postoperative Pain with Acupuncture – Sun Peilin

Master Tong's Acupuncture – Miriam Lee

Myofascial Pain Dysfunction – Acupuncture Point Manual – Janet Travel, David Simon

Obstetrics and Gynecology – Giovanni Maciocia

Pain Assessment Scales – National Institute of Pain Control

Reinventing Acupuncture – Felix Mann

Scalp Acupuncture Theory and Application – Yuzing Liu

Sports Injuries and Acupuncture – British Acupuncture Council

Surface Anatomy and Surface Markings – Henry Grey

Synopsis on Scalp Acupuncture – Shubhuti Dharmendra, Edythe Vickers

The Foundations of Chinese Medicine – Giovanni Maciocia

The Use of Acupuncture in Sports Medicine – Melanie Sfara

Tung's Acupuncture – Dechen Pladan, Ching Chan Tung

Twelve and Twelve in Acupuncture – Richard Tan

Twenty-four More in Acupuncture – Richard Tan

Western Medical Acupuncture – Adrian White, Mike Cummings, Jacqueline Filshie

What Experts Say About the Book

Dr. Chandra Sekhar Pardeshi is a renowned Gynaecologist as well as Acupuncture Physician. He has explained nicely the basics of Human Anatomy, Physiology and Philosophy of Acupuncture Therapy in his book. Diseases are discussed and guide line given for management by Acupuncture Therapy. This book will be helpful to Students of Acupuncture Therapy and Acupuncture Practitioners.

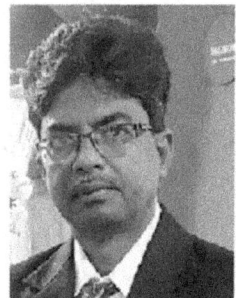

Hiralal Samanta

Director
Dr. B. K. Basu Memorial Research & Training
Institute of Acupuncture
Kolkata - 700045
Govt. of West Bengal

"Modern Acupuncture" may be the first all-inclusive book to make learning and practising 'Acupuncture' so easy by integrating T.C.M. into modern medicine. Section on 'How to start practice' is a bonus to every new and practising acupuncturist.

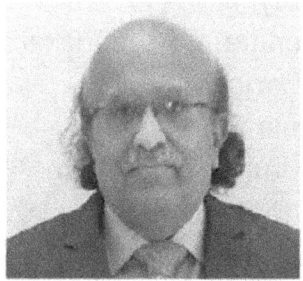

Dr. Mohan S. Sali
M.D., DGO.
'Get Well Hospital'
India

Anand Pain Relief & Rehabilitation Institute
Hubli School of Knee & Back Care

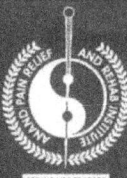

Dr. VINAY VARMA
MBBS, D. Ac. M.Ac.F. (Sri Lanka), M.I.Ac. S (Hong Kong)
MD (Med. Alt). P.G.C.R. (Mumbai) Ph.D.
SENIOR MEDICAL ACUPUNCTURIST
PHYSIATRIST & FAMILY PHYSCIAN

Dr. ANAND VARMA
MBBS, DNB-PMR, MNAMS
CONSULTANT PHYSIATRIST

"Modern Acupuncture" is a comprehensive acupuncture guide and reference book for new and senior acupuncturists.

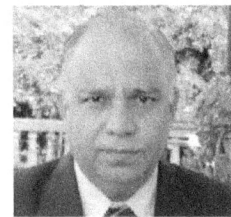

Medical Director &
Sr. Acupuncturist.

Dr. Pardeshi's comprehensive book on acupuncture will serve as a most useful practical guide for practitioners of this wonderful system of medicine
— Dr. Ravindra Shirde M.D. D.G.O.

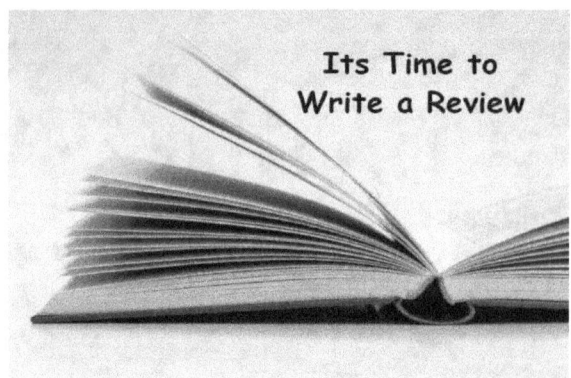

Thank You for Choosing Modern Acupuncture!

I am sincerely grateful that you chose Modern Acupuncture from the many available options. Your decision to learn more about acupuncture is inspiring, and I hope the book has enriched your understanding and practice.

Your Feedback Matters:
Whether you enjoyed the book or found it particularly helpful, I would greatly appreciate your feedback. Sharing your thoughts through an Amazon review will not only help others learn, but it will also provide valuable insights and encouragement for my future writing endeavours.

Scan to Review This Book

Dr. Chandrashekhar Pardeshi, MBBS, DGO, MD
Obstetrician, Gynecologist, and Acupuncturist
Ex-Vice President, Maharashtra Acupuncture Council

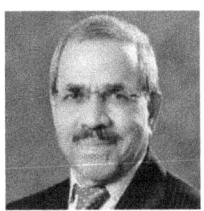

Dr. Chandrashekhar Pardeshi, MBBS, DGO, MD, is a distinguished Indian medical professional internationally recognized for his work in integrative medicine and acupuncture. A postgraduate in obstetrics and gynaecology with over 45 years of active clinical experience, he has spent the past two decades mastering and applying the science of acupuncture in both acute and chronic conditions, often where conventional medicine alone offers limited success.

Trained in modern medicine and certified in acupuncture, Dr. Pardeshi brings a unique dual perspective that blends scientific rigour with the therapeutic depth of traditional healing systems. He is known for his rational, evidence-based application of acupuncture, particularly for conditions involving neurogenic pain, functional disorders, and rehabilitation. His contributions to the field include novel insights into non-retentive needling, neurohormonal mechanisms of action, and simplified teaching approaches for allopathic practitioners.

Modern Acupuncture: Learn From The Master is the culmination of his decades-long journey as a clinician, educator, and reformer. Through this book, he aims to bridge the long-standing gap between traditional Chinese principles and modern anatomical logic, making acupuncture more accessible, acceptable, and clinically relevant for today's healthcare professionals.

Dr. Pardeshi currently lives in Nashik, India, where he practises medicine, teaches acupuncture, and continues to advocate for integrative care that is cost-effective, scientific, and patient-centric.

www.ingramcontent.com/pod-product-compliance
Lightning Source LLC
Chambersburg PA
CBHW080944290526
45795CB00009B/2915